DATE DUE

DEC 0 5 1994	
APR 2 4 1996	
MAY 1 7 1996	
DEC 2 0 1996	
MAY 2 0 1998	
JUN 0 9 1998	

DRUGS IN AMERICA:
Crisis or Hysteria?

DRUGS IN AMERICA: Crisis or Hysteria?

AN EDITORIALS ON FILE BOOK

Editor: Oliver Trager

Facts On File Publications
New York, New York • Oxford, England

DRUGS IN AMERICA:
Crisis or Hysteria?

Published by Facts On File, Inc.
460 Park Ave. South, New York, N.Y. 10016
© Copyright 1986 by Facts On File, Inc.

International Standard Book Number: 0-8160-1775-1

Library of Congress Cataloging-in-Publication Data
Main entry under title:

Drugs in America

(An Editorials On File book)

Includes index
Summary: A collection of editorials on the use and abuse of drugs and the treatement of that topic by law enforcement and the legal system.
1. Drug abuse--United States. [1. Drug abuse.
2. Drugs] I. Trager, Oliver. II Series.
HV5825.D84 1987 362.2'93'0973 87-6812
ISBN 0-8160-1775-1

PRINTED IN THE UNITED STATES OF AMERICA

9 8 7 6 5 4 3 2 1

Contents

Preface

The preoccupation with drugs has reached a fever pitch nationwide. Countless lives have been lost, careers wrecked, heroes toppled, homes broken, businesses crippled, policemen and politicians corrupted. Virtually every aspect of public and private life has been tainted, and billions bled from the economy. Since the late 1950s when drugs were found strictly in the domain of the underground, the scourge has escalated into a national scandal—an epidemic as pervasive and poisoning as the medieval plagues. Small-time drug runners have been replaced by ruthless, nontraditional modes of organized crime that continue to flourish. Crime in American cities is rising with drugs implicated in more than half of them, and governments have been compromised by drug traffickers and their millions.

In 1986, the President's Commission on Organized Crime reported that marijuana "was firmly entrenched" in American society, heroin had a steady half million customers and cocaine had as many as as five million regular users. The National Institute on Drug Abuse (NIDA) reported in July 1986 that as many as 80% of "today's young adults" had "tried an illicit drug" by their mid-20s. More than half had used a drug besides marijuana. America's "high school students and other young adults still show a level of involvement with illicit drugs which is greater than can be found in any other industrialized nation in the world," according to the report. Indeed, hardly a day passes where some mention of drugs does not appear in the media. The so-called 'crack' epidemic, the government's war on drugs and the growing prospect of employee drug testing have fueled the national controversy.

But while drug abuse has undoubtedly resulted in many personal tragedies throughout the country, its importance as a problem may be exaggerated by politicians all too eager to appease a concerned public. *Drugs in America* explores the U.S. government's and the American public's often contradictory attitude concerning this thorny issue through the words and images of America's leading editorial writers and cartoonists.

April, 1987 — Oliver Trager

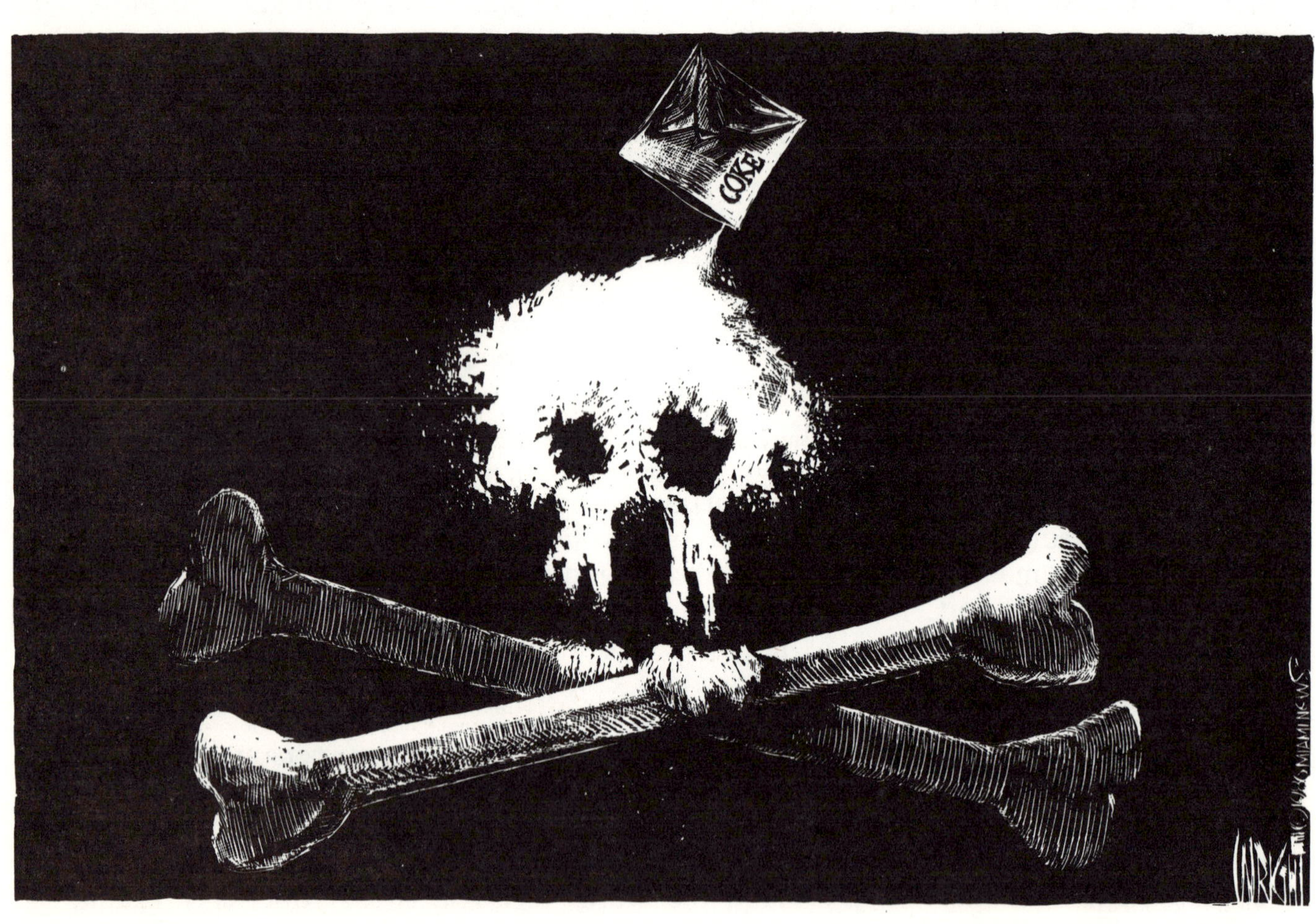
COKE
WRIGHT
THE MIAMI NEWS

Part I:
Schedule I Substances: Marijuana, Cocaine and Heroin

Drugs had been used in America long before the Europeans landed on eastern shores. The native peoples taught the explorers how to smoke and grow tobacco. Not long after, the settlers used their skills to distill grain into alcoholic beverages and the rum trade blossomed in New England early on. A century later, cocaine became popular as an ingredient not only in many elixers but in the original recipe for the popular soft drink Coca-Cola. Cannabis was widely grown by Virginia colonists as a source of hemp, and in the 19th century large hemp plantations were found throughout the South. Cultivation of marijuana actually continued into the late 1930s and it is estimated that at that time the commercial crop covered 10,000 acres. Marijuana was used medicinally and recreationally during the 18th and 19th centuries, but on a minute scale compared to today. The use of opium was rampant during the 19th century, as it was an ingredient in numerous patent medicines and sold at extremely low prices.

In modern times, the popularity of heroin developed in the early part of the 20th century, when it was discovered that heroin was a more potent drug. Heroin has remained a problem drug since the early 1900s but the number of heroin dependent people has stablized since the mid-1970s. During the 1940s and 1950s the abuse of other substances began to be a major concern. The use of newly developed drugs became widespread before their addictive qualities were acknowledged or made known. "Minor tranquilizers" were widely prescribed by doctors as a way of dealing with symptoms rather than treating them, and amphetamines were in widespread use as an "energizer." These patterns not only continue today; they are greatly magnified. Cocaine, previously not used to any great extent, is now a leading drug of abuse. When it gained popularity in the late 1960s and 1970s it was considered a drug of the affluent because of its high cost, but despite that fact its use has now spread to many segments of the population, especially with the emergence of the powerful new form known as "crack." Marijuana is the popular controlled substance. It has been estimated that 30 million people in the United States have used marijuana, though the actual number of users, whether regular or occassional, is impossible to pinpoint as sources of marijuana include not only imports from other countries but the vast amounts that are grown domestically. The U.S. government estimates that 7% of the marijuana used in America today is domestically cultivated; however, the number of people who grow plants in the backyard for personal use, with no thought of selling or trafficking, could increase this estimate substantially.

John Belushi, TV & Movie Comic, Dies of Cocaine, Heroin Overdose

John Belushi, comic actor on television and in movies, died March 5, 1982 of an overdose of cocaine and heroin. The 33-year-old actor had appeared on the television series "Saturday Night Live" and in several feature films, including *Animal House*, *The Blues Brothers*, and *Neighbors*. Initial reports attributed Belushi's death to natural causes, but after an autopsy was performed, the news was announced March 10 that death was caused by injections of heroin and cocaine. Both drugs were found in the actor's Hollywood bungalow. The coroner's report said Belushi had been drinking heavily as well as taking drugs. He was described as being in poor physical condition, suffering from, among other things, obesity, lung congestion and an enlarged heart. Belushi's satiric, manic style made him an instant audience favorite when he started with "Saturday Night Live" in 1975. He left the show in 1979 to act in films, often satirizing the drug culture.

A year later, Cathy Evelyn Smith surrendered to authorities in Toronto, Canada after she had been indicted for murder in connection with Belushi's death. She was also charged with 13 counts of supplying and administering dangerous drugs. According to the coroner's report, Smith had accompanied Belushi during his last week in Los Angeles. The report characterized that week as a binge of drinking and drug use.

The Detroit News

Detroit, MI, March 14, 1982

Headlines announced the other day that John Belushi died, not of natural causes as originally reported, but of cocaine and heroin.

We're sure the warning implicit in those news reports wasn't lost on Mr. Belushi's thousands of young fans, and we have no wish to belabor the obvious here.

One report that did catch our eye, however, quoted the actor's Beverly Hills doctor. Mr. Belushi knew better than to take cocaine, the unidentified doctor said. "On the other hand," he added, "let's say he got drunk, *which we all have a right to do*, and somebody gave it to him."

Well, a high tolerance of substance abuse — including alcohol abuse — is one of the hallmarks of Hollywood culture, where many important fads and fashions are said to originate.

God only knows what miscalculations or private torment drove Mr. Belushi to self-destruction. But one thing's certain: His social *milieu* had no behavioral brakes to offer.

The San Diego Union

San Diego, CA, March 17, 1982

There was nothing funny about the accident that nearly killed comedian Richard Pryor two years ago. He is now dead-serious when he talks about the menace of cocaine, which caused it. As for John Belushi, another comedian and cocaine-user, he is simply dead.

Most of the news about the rising popularity of cocaine comes from the entertainment world. But most of those getting hooked on this "in" drug are not celebrities. They are, to use a recent term from Hollywood, ordinary people.

If John Belushi's sad death from a combination of heroin and cocaine was startling to his fans, it was not as alarming as the statistics coming from the National Institute of Drug Abuse. The number of Americans severely dependent on cocaine is now estimated at between 100,000 and 200,000, and if the trend of the past few years continues, the number could surpass the 500,000 believed to be addicted to heroin.

Deaths associated with cocaine quadrupled between 1975 and 1980. Persons who have sniffed, injected, smoked, or swallowed cocaine now constitute a major category of drug-abusers showing up in hospital emergency rooms and entering treatment programs to break their habit. That cocaine is "safe" compared to other psychoactive drugs is a dangerous myth.

What does this mean? For one thing, it poses a major new problem for enforcement agencies already struggling to keep up with the traffic in heroin, marijuana, and other illegal drugs. Cocaine, which comes mainly from South America, now accounts for more illicit income than marijuana on the underworld market.

But the more pertinent meaning is for our society as a whole. We see yet another insidious drug working its way into our midst, even as we worry about the implications of the pot-smoking habit that took root among young people during the 1960s.

Officials of drug abuse agencies believe the use of cocaine would be even more widespread if it were not so expensive. That's the irony. Those who are "doing cocaine" are typically well-educated members of the upper middle class — people who ought to know better.

St. Louis Globe-Democrat

St. Louis, MO, March 18, 1982

It's obvious that John Belushi, who became a tv and movie star portraying a consummate slob, wasn't always play acting. Belushi lived like a slob and died like a slob.

According to the Los Angeles coroner's report, the 33-year-old actor's last days were spent in heavy drinking and drug ingestion, leading to his death from acute cocaine and heroin intoxication.

A rock singer who spent a week in a Sunset Strip hotel with the married actor before his nude body was found, told police that she and Belushi had stayed up all night drinking wine and inhaling cocaine. At one point he vomited. That was nothing new for Belushi.

Multiple fresh needle puncture marks were found on both of his arms, and quantities of cocaine, morphine and other drugs were found in Belushi's blood, bile and urine.

What has happened to America when a bum like Belushi can be considered a hero and role model for young people?

Belushi is not alone in setting a bad example for youngsters.

Elvis Presley, the original king of rock, made millions and died a junkie. Twelve drugs, including codeine, morphine and barbiturates, were found in blood and tissue samples taken from his body after his death at the age of 42 in 1977.

Janis Joplin, the "Judy Garland of rock," whose performances were described as "writhing, wailing and sometimes profane," died of a drug overdose in 1970 with fresh needle marks on her arms. She was 27.

Judy Garland herself, who went from pigtails to pigsty in her raucous roller coaster career, died of a drug overdose at age 47 in 1969.

There's a lesson to be learned from these human tragedies — drugs and debauchery are a one-way ticket to deadly disgrace. John Belushi may have left millions, but he left no memory worth admiring.

Rocky Mountain News

Denver, CO, March 18, 1982

A RECENT study which received prominent attention in the news media suggested that "recreational" sniffing of cocaine carries small threat to health.

The death of comedian John Belushi from a cocaine-heroin overdose ought to put that study into better perspective.

A major risk in "recreational" use of drugs is that it often leads to dependence and dangerous experimentation to achieve bigger kicks. John Belushi no doubt started out as a recreational sniffer.

THE COMMERCIAL APPEAL

Memphis, TN, March 23, 1982

THE DEATH OF comedian John Belushi due to an overdose of heroin and cocaine, has focused new attention on the use of illegal drugs. If something good comes of that attention, then perhaps his death will not come as a total loss to those people who admire his comic genius.

If it could happen to Belushi, someone at the zenith of success, could it not happen to anyone? The answer, of course, is yes.

What is so frightening about heroin use in this country is that it is spreading — from adults to the young, from the wealthy to the destitute, from those who fail life's lowest challenges to those who achieve its greatest rewards.

To those people who are unimpressed by Belushi's death (don't all movie stars do that? the skeptics ask), we offer the frightening observations of Dr. Forest Tennant, the director of the largest drug treatment center in Los Angeles, who says he has seen a 1,000 per cent increase in heroin addiction among young people.

Three months ago, he says, the center only saw one or two heroin addicts daily under the age of 20. Today more than 1,000 addicts in that age range pass through the center every day.

"To us it's a shocker because to be an addict at 16, it means they would have had to start smoking and drinking at eight, moved on to marijuana, then something like PCP (or 'angel dust') and then try heroin," he says.

Psychologist Richard Rawson, director of operations at the clinic, says there has been a "tremendous surge of first-time, new heroin users."

THE STATISTICS coming out of Los Angeles are alarming, particularly in view of that city's reputation as a trend-setter for the nation's drug culture. Authorities there report a 25 per cent rise in heroin seizures over last year, a 16 per cent jump in arrests for heroin possession and a 100 per cent increase in heroin overdose deaths.

"In the '60s and '70s there were drugs and then there was heroin, which rarely was used by people outside the real hardcore drug scene," says Rawson. "Now it's being used at parties . . . It's become more available and more acceptable as a recreational drug, and then one day the kids find out it's no longer recreational."

Belushi, like others before him, found out the hard way.

OKLAHOMA CITY TIMES

Oklahoma City, OK, March 22, 1982

IN the wake of the latest drug caused death of a popular personality, actor John Belushi, there has been much discussion of cocaine. The argument seems to be that cocaine is "safe" to use, since it is not really a narcotic but a stimulant.

Los Angeles coroner's office doctors who performed the autopsy disagree. Cocaine, they insist, was one of the substances that caused Belushi's death.

The law that put cocaine under the misnomer of a narcotic years ago has been used by defense lawyers to secure acquittals in drug cases, although in other cases it has been upheld. It is reported that this history led to the present nomenclature of the Bureau of Narcotics and Dangerous Drugs. The fact is that cocaine is a dangerous drug — as are a number of other stimulants.

In recent months, while highly publicized drives to educate American youth to the dangers of drug abuse were aimed at preventing the initial trial and addiction, there has been a trend toward another kind of education. Richard Pryor has taken a role in drug education since his brush with death. His message: Don't start.

John Phillips, founder of the Mamas and the Papas rock group, and his daughter, Mackenzie Phillips, John Lucas, the basketball star, guitarist Keith Richards of the Rolling Stones and several well-known professional football players have

been talking to those who have not only tried drugs but are using them now.

Michael Howard, who was fired as editor of The Rocky Mountain News by the newspaper chain his grandfather helped found, has submitted to interviews in which he talked frankly about what the cocaine habit did to his life. He is articulate and convincing, since those who have read his remarks often felt that they knew him as a prominent and highly visible Denver figure.

But, despite the testimony of its victims, cocaine's dangers are still not widely believed. Critics still have little credibility with those who have tried it without becoming addicted, or who see it used openly at parties. The courts and law enforcement officials do not treat its use or trafficking the way they do so-called hard drugs like heroin.

It has taken nearly 20 years for the medical professions to learn enough about marijuana to be able to say positively that it has long-term effects that can destroy a person's health. It will be years more before a majority of young people are convinced — and avoid it. Clearly, it is going to take the word of a lot of cocaine victims to make an effective case against it, too.

But the bottom line is that a drug is a drug, and while there are life-saving uses for most drugs, abuse of any drug is dangerous and can be fatal.

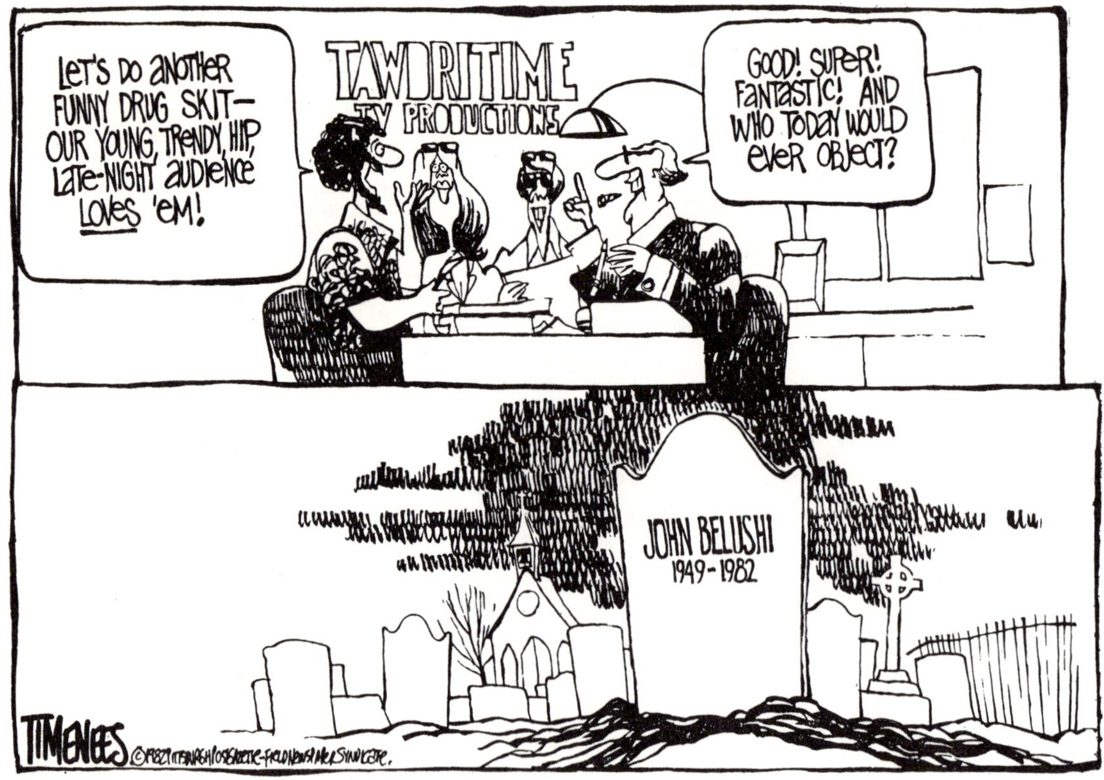

THE ARIZONA REPUBLIC

Phoenix, AZ, March 13, 1982

SOMETIMES it's useful to hold up celebrities from the fantasyland of show business as examples for young people *not* to emulate.

A case in point is John Belushi, who snuffed out his life by "speedballing" with injections of cocaine and heroin.

No matter how people viewed Belushi's manic, irreverent humor, the irrefutable fact is that he was one of America's established and most successful young film comedians.

He reached the pinnacle of his craft after humble beginnings on the low-budget TV series, "Saturday Night Live," a program that gave space in which the Belushi brand of comedy flourished.

So, having achieved that, what did Belushi do with his life?

He apparently did what an increasing number of the "beautiful people" of the arts and theater do, when success becomes heady and their fortunes flourish.

They turn to hard drugs and the almost irreversible slide into addiction and, therefore, flirtations with death.

Graveyards of the world are littered with tombstones of the meek and the mighty of the world, whose yen for the opaque twilight zone of drug stimulation and depression cut their lives short.

The National Clearinghouse For Drug Abuse has found, in a sampling of 26 major U.S. cities, that:

✔ More than 290,000 persons were rushed to hospital emergency rooms in 1979 for treatment of drug overdoses.

✔ In 1979, some 9,800 persons died from drug overdoses.

✔ At least 250 persons are known to have died from the use of cocaine alone, or in conjunction with heroin or alcohol.

Untold thousands of young people seeking excitement, and emulating the fast track habits of the glamorous, are at the bottom of the drug ladder and risking the fate of Belushi.

From marijuana, many inevitably must find higher highs in hard drugs.

Time magazine estimates that 10 million Americans are regular users of cocaine.

Drug traffickers are willing to please.

By current estimates cocaine fetches some $40 billion from users looking for new thrills.

For users, there are no thrills.

The big winners are drug peddlers who weep for their victims all the way to the banks.

the Charleston Gazette

Charleston, WV, March 25, 1982

THE death of John Belushi by OD, as drug overdose is known on morgue charts, angers Nickie McWhirter, columnist for Knight-Ridder News Service.

"Anger," says McWhirter, "is a strange response to the death of a stranger who, only incidentally, gave me some pleasure with his TV and movie slapstick. Anger is an odd emotion to feel because some stranger named John Belushi goofed up his morning fix."

The anger is justified. Funny as Belushi was, and at times he was very funny, he abused the one great gift given him: life.

Two of McWhirter's acquaintances have multiple sclerosis. They don't take drugs for cheap thrills. Think, McWhirter says, what they would give for good health. "How dare (then) John Belushi or anyone else shoot cocaine and heroin into healthy veins just for kicks?"

Neither does McWhirter want any shrine built memoralizing this fallen dolt. He sympathizes for family and close friends who loved him, did their utmost to assist him and finally lost because of Belushi's own foolishness.

But no tears or sorrow are reserved for Belushi. Just anger.

The Dispatch

Columbus, OH, March 15, 1982

THEY BURIED comedian John Belushi on Martha's Vineyard last Tuesday, four days after he was found dead in a Hollywood bungalow. As family and friends described him as a genius and a dear man, officials in California were describing the cause of death: a fatal overdose of heroin and cocaine.

Even as Belushi was being laid to rest, federal officials in Florida were wrapping up a hectic 48 hours in which they confiscated nearly $1.1 billion in cocaine, marijuana and methaqualone en route from South America to the United States. The two-day period was one of the most successful ever in the government's efforts to halt the flow of illegal substances to this country.

But the flow continues and the death toll mounts. Cases like Belushi's involving prominent people get the most attention, but thousands of other people die virtually unnoticed every year: shriveled human beings, their bodies wracked by months or years of drug abuse, lie strewn across the landscape of a society that struggles, most of the time impotently, against the drug menace.

The government estimates that drug abuse kills about 4,000 people each year, and that the loss in health costs, income and reduced productivity runs into billions of dollars annually.

Some progress has been made. Greater emphasis is being placed on closing the country's borders to the flow of illegal substances from other countries. Last week's Florida seizures capped a five-month period during which custom officials in the Miami office intercepted 5,500 pounds of uncut cocaine and 203,000 pounds of marijuana while confiscating 89 vehicles, 91 boats and 59 airplanes used in illegal drug traffic.

But there will be more graveside ceremonies, more wasted lives, more grief as long as people afflict their bodies with drugs. Government and society can do just so much. Each individual is responsible for his or her own body, and the problem will continue for as long as people fail to appreciate the human body as the precious creation that it is.

THE ATLANTA CONSTITUTION

Atlanta, GA, March 12, 1982

The family of comic John Belushi is complaining about the way the Los Angeles coroner's office made public the findings of the autopsy on the comic's body. Sympathy is due the survivors in their personal loss, but Coroner Thomas Noguchi acted in the public interest, as he did in the deaths of actors William Holden and Natalie Wood — two other celebrities whose deaths brought the coroner criticism for doing his job.

Whether they want it or like it, people who enter the public spotlight are seen as role models by many who think their behavior is to be copied. The public is given the impression, many times, that some very harmful forms of behavior are commonplace, ordinary and safe. It increases chances of experimenting, which can lead to tragic results.

Noguchi's report said Bulushi died of an overdose of heroin and cocaine, taken intravenously. One of Belushi's in-laws was critical of Noguchi for telling Belushi's brother the cause of death, then telling the news media. She felt there should have been delays, so that the whole family could be informed.

In the case of death, public officials usually ask the news media to withhold names until the next of kin have been told. However, autopsy reports are a different thing. It's not the same as the shock of finding out someone is dead.

Autopsies are public information. The public has a right to know about them and the coroner has a responsibility to issue his findings.

This particular event comes at a time when the National Institute on Drug Abuse reports that at least 15 million Americans have tried cocaine. So many are experimenting that it is creating a problem for federally funded drug treatment centers. By the way, a survey shows the average drug-clinic patient is male, white and aged 20-29.

Noguchi was correct to bring attention to the drugs linked to the death of Belushi, a talented man who could have had a long career ahead of him. Maybe it will make somebody on drugs or considering using them stop and think what can flow from such abuse.

The Boston Herald American

Boston, MA, March 23, 1982

There was nothing funny about the accident that nearly killed comedian Richard Pryor two years ago. He is now dead-serious when he talks about the menace of cocaine, which caused it. As for John Belushi, another comedian and cocaine-user, he is simply dead.

Most of the news about the rising popularity of cocaine comes from the entertainment world. But most of those getting hooked on this "in" drug are not celebrities. They are, to use a recent term from Hollywood, ordinary people.

If John Belushi's sad death from a combination of heroin and cocaine was startling to his fans, it was not as alarming as the statistics coming from the National Institute of Drug Abuse. The number of Americans severely dependent on cocaine is now estimated at between 100,000 and 200,000, and if the trend of the past few years continues, the number could surpass the 500,000 believed to be addicted to heroin.

Deaths associated with cocaine quadrupled between 1975 and 1980. Persons who have sniffed, injected, smoked, or swallowed cocaine now constitute a major category of drug-abusers showing up in hospital emergency rooms and entering treatment programs to break their habit. That cocaine is "safe" compared to other psychoactive drugs is a dangerous myth.

What does this mean? For one thing, it poses a major new problem for enforcement agencies already struggling to keep up with the traffic in heroin, marijuana, and other illegal drugs. Cocaine, which comes mainly from South America, now accounts for more illicit income than marijuana on the underworld market.

But the more pertinent meaning is for our society as a whole. We see yet another insidious drug working its way into our midst, even as we worry about the implications of the pot-smoking habit that took root among young people during the 1960s.

Officials of drug-abuse agencies believe the use of cocaine would be even more widespread if it were not so expensive. That's the irony. Those who are "doing cocaine" are typically well-educated members of the upper middle class — people who ought to know better.

Attitudes Regarding Drugs Vary Throughout Nation

The counterculture of the 1960s is usually blamed for the increased popularity of drug use and abuse in America. When the term was coined, it was used to describe those who were in favor of the use of such drugs as LSD and marijuana. Many of these individuals were also antigovernment, antipolice and antiwar. But America's diversity and complexity suggest that the situation is more serious and can't be justly pinned on a minority of dissidents. The various social and ethnic classes that comprise the fabric of American life hold many different views toward drug use and abuse. For example, upper-class groups generally have a more permissive attitude toward drinking and do not regard it as a moral problem. Lower socioeconomic groups take this attitude less often and generally contain a greater number of abstainers although, on the surface, their problem drinkers may seem more obvious. Until recently, the abuse of cocaine was originally found only among members of the upper-classes, a fact attributable to the high cost of the drug. But that trend is now changing as cocaine is thought of as a status symbol. The high incidence of heroin abuse among lower-class groups is centered in the ghettos of metropolitan areas and is attributed to to the easy availability of narcotics "on the street," and to feelings of helplessness in individuals living in these areas and to their need to belong to a group. These factors are also responsible for the relapse of rehabilitated addicts who return to their old neighborhoods. Whether because of its availability or its relatively cheap cost, marijuana is not restricted to a particular social class. Its use seems to be as widespread among the teenage children of blue-collar workers as it is among college-educated adults in their 30's. But aside from illegal drugs, America does seem to have an obsession with drugs of all kinds to alleviate the day-to-day angst of life. Alcohol, tobacco, caffeine and even aspirin are consumed in quantities that would certainly justify concern.

The Dispatch

Columbus, OH, December 12, 1983

The findings of a study that indicate a youth's tendency to take up cigarettes, alcohol or marijuana can be determined through early psychiatric testing may prove useful in fully utilizing society's resources to combat illegal drug and alcohol use. But the knowledge gleaned from this study should be used carefully so as not to paint too broad a stroke in predicting teen behavior.

The study is one facet of a 13-year look into the behavior of 15,-000 pupils in six middle-class Boston suburbs. One of the researchers, Dr. Gene Smith of Massachusetts General Hospital, said that he and his colleagues were able to conduct a series of interviews with selected pupils during the course of the study and correlate early test results with later behavior. They found that it is possible to identify certain types of personalities that lend themselves to alcohol and drug abuse. Their research was published recently in *Contemporary Drug Problems*.

This study could be useful in targeting anti-abuse resources toward those most likely to engage in such activity. Counselors would have to be careful in their use of the information, however, since a child knowing that he or she is likely to abuse substances might be encouraged to accelerate abusive activities. And it would be important for counselors to keep in mind that the students surveyed possessed certain demographic characteristics which could affect their behavior in unique ways. It would have to be determined to what extent behavior characteristics can be transferred to youngsters in other demographic groups.

Nevertheless, the research should help shed some additional light on why young people engage in abusive activity and this, in turn, will help adults prevent or limit those activities. The researchers should be congratulated.

The Pittsburgh PRESS

Pittsburgh, PA, March 26, 1983

How to help keep decent citizens of a neighborhood under the oppression of drug dealers who operate in the open on crowded street corners:

A suspected heroin dealer is being arrested by police.

He resists arrest and calls for help from a crowd of bystanders.

The crowd responds and pelts the arresting officers with rocks and bottles in an attempt to make them turn the suspect loose.

★ ★ ★

How to help rid a neigborhood of drug dealers who are trying to keep decent citizens under their oppression:

A man and his sister are suspected by neighborhood residents of dealing in marijuana.

Concerned about the drug possession and trafficking going on under their noses, the residents furnish information to the police, who arrest the man and woman, to the delight of those who live nearby.

★ ★ ★

Both scenarios are true.

The first occurred this week in the Hill District when a convicted drug dealer who was being apprehended by police called for help from a crowd of about 75 people on the corner of Wylie Avenue and Erin Street.

The crowd turned on the cops and didn't relent until police reinforcements arrived. Two detectives were struck by the suspect in the arrest scuffle, and one of them was hit by a bottle hurled by a bystander.

Less than two weeks earlier, a Homewood man and his sister were arrested and 16 pounds of marijuana worth $14,000 was confiscated.

Police were tipped to their alleged activities by residents of the area who have decided they will no longer tolerate drug users or sellers in their midst.

★ ★ ★

Of the Wylie Avenue incident, Sgt. Earl Buford, head of the Narcotics Squad, says: "Some residents in the area want to help police but there's another element that's trying to prevent us from doing our job."

What Sgt. Buford and his fellow officers need is cooperation from the average, law-abiding citizens.

They need information about drug dealings and assistance in identifying suspected peddlers.

What they don't need is obstruction from unruly crowds.

It's up to residents of drug hotspots, as the police call them, to choose which of the above two incidents they would prefer to see on the streets near their own homes.

THE CHRISTIAN SCIENCE MONITOR
Boston, MA, March 23, 1983

The illegal "drug culture" used to be a subterranean, outcast segment of American and European society. But research on both sides of the Atlantic shows the use and toleration of illegal drugs — marijuana, heroin, cocaine, and many others — spreading into all levels of society. The effects on health, work, safety, and personal relationships have often been found to be devastating. How can the Western world keep from becoming one big drug culture?

It will take nothing less than societies and individuals looking at what they are doing to themselves — and saying, "Enough!"

Is this a wildly unrealistic prospect when a relentless trend of drug abuse and acceptance seems to be in motion?

Not if the history of another devastating trend in human self-destruction is considered. For years, indeed centuries, human beings have abused their natural environment, harming themselves by harming their land, water, and air. How lonely the 19th-century conservationists seemed. How strong the movement to preserve the environment became when people finally saw what they were wreaking on the resources of their planet.

A similar turnaround can hardly be beyond possibility when the issue is preservation of human resources themselves from the encroaching environment of drugs.

Just how serious the challenge is may be gathered not only from the general run of news but from several recent studies. Last year, for example, the Council of Europe held a conference in Strasbourg on a virtual epidemic of drug abuse in a Europe that had once thought this to be mainly North America's problem. This week, in a roundup of the views of social scientists, the New York Times reports a growing social toleration of illegal drugs among older Americans even as their use among younger Americans remains on the decline.

In both Europe and America the resort to illegal drugs is linked to a climate in which pills and nostrums are assumed to be available for virtually every human ill. Some people go from seeking relief of pain to pursuing transitory pleasure. A disposition to handle problems with artificial means is fostered. It can be a short step to *illegal* artificial means.

The Council of Europe warned against treatment of addiction that "medicates the problem without solving it." In the atmosphere of a drug for everything it cautioned against dangerous models of parental evasion of responsibility.

In the US only 4 percent of the population had tried an illegal drug two decades ago. Now more than 30 percent of Americans over 12 have done so. Young people in America are still believed to use more drugs than those anywhere else in the industrial world. But studies have shown a decline each year for the past several years. Reasons are thought to be concern for health, peer pressure, and good grades for a tightened job market.

If young Americans can begin this kind of reversal, they should have the full support of their elders rather than the present ironic example of increased adult drug abuse and acceptance. Some adults indeed have been doing yeoman work in groups to reduce and prevent youthful drug abuse. There have been heartening instances of enlisting young people shoulder to shoulder with them.

All the necessary legal efforts to control the drug traffic will leave the problem unsolved so long as there is a willing market in a climate of social toleration. Cleansing the environment of these insidious agents of corruption will require more and more people marching shoulder to shoulder as they have done to say thus far and no farther in the destruction of the natural world.

St. Louis Globe-Democrat
St. Louis, MO, November 8, 1983

The good news, according to the director of the National Institute on Drug Abuse, is that the use of marijuana, cocaine and other drugs has leveled off nationwide. The bad news is that, even so, overall drug abuse remains alarmingly high.

"The levels of use by our young people are probably greater than in any other industrialized country," Dr. William Pollin, told the House Select Committee on Narcotics.

The evidence of leveling off comes from national surveys of high school seniors, households and drug treatment centers, Pollin said. He credited increased public awareness of the dangers of drug use and rigorous efforts to curtail supply and punish offenders for the stabilization.

"Until the late 1970s, there was a major debate in this country" about whether drug use was dangerous, he noted. "We really learned more about the health consequences of these drugs . . . and we finally began to communicate effectively that knowledge . . . "

Some congressmen disagreed with Pollin, saying they saw evidence that drug abuse was as bad as ever.

One thing is certain: Whatever the level of drug abuse, it is much too high for comfort. There should be no letup on the effort to educate the public on the dangers of drugs and on the drive against those who traffic in illegal narcotics.

The Orlando Sentinel
Orlando, FL, November 9, 1983

The volume of illicit drugs confiscated as they were being smuggled into this country increased dramatically last year — by 188 percent in captured cocaine and 83 percent in heroin. Chalk up that success to additional money poured into the drug war. Yet now the street price of drugs is falling and their purity is increasing. It is the inevitable market reaction to a war that is failing.

Those results don't surprise a lot of people. They don't believe the national drug epidemic can be controlled by trying to cut off the supply. The only way to win this war is by drying up the demand.

One effort along that line is a two-part national public television show that is tied to town meetings of parents and children. The purpose is to create public indignation about drug and alcohol abuse, much the same way that Mothers Against Drunk Drivers worked a successful campaign.

The second installment of *The Chemical People* will be shown at 8 tonight on Channel 24. Again this week, groups of parents and children will watch the show and then discuss the problem and what can be done about it. A list of these meeting places can be found on page 2 of the Local & State news section of today's newspaper. The goal is to use these meetings to launch task forces that can continue the fight.

Last week these meetings attracted as many as 3,000 people in Central Florida. That's hardly a crowd compared to the numbers at a Saturday football game, not when it is estimated that 17 percent of all high school seniors use cocaine and 3 million children under 17 are problem drinkers. But as Sheryl Hyatt of Kissimmee, one of the Central Florida project coordinators, put it, "It doesn't take a lot of people, just some concerned people."

And concerned we all should be. Drug and alcohol abuse among school-age children is a terrible thing. Each year thousands of youngsters die because of it. Thousands more are physically and psychologically ruined for life. Still more drop out of school and at some point become liabilities to society. The cost to the nation is in the billions of dollars.

No, we should not delude ourselves into thinking that a couple of television programs and some town meetings can, by themselves, solve the problem. But they can help lead to the realization that being "bombed" and "stoned" are not smart but plain dumb. Once public opinion is turned against those conditions, the free market system will take care of the rest.

THE INDIANAPOLIS NEWS
Indianapolis, IN, March 24, 1983

"Drugs are harmless" must have a sour sound for the nearly one-third of inmates interviewed in a survey who said they were under the influence of an illegal drug when they committed the crime that sent them to state prison.

The survey began by asking 12,000 state prison inmates around the nation about their drug use in general and ended by asking whether they were on a drug when they tripped into the clutches of the law. This procedure was aimed to minimize their temptation to make drugs an excuse for their crimes.

The Bureau of Justice Statistics, a U.S. Department of Justice agency, reported the inmates said half of all offenses were committed while they were under the influence of a drug — heroin in 20 percent of cases; about 25 percent of burglaries and 20 percent of robberies were committed while they were on marijuana, and 12 percent of robberies and 10 percent of larcenies were committed while they were on heroin.

The survey showed that heroin, which is used by 2 percent of the general population, was used by 30 percent of the inmates.

Half of the inmates had been daily drug users at some point in their lives and 40 percent had used drugs every day recently, the survey said.

Most of the daily use was of marijuana. Nearly 20 percent had used heroin daily and about 10 percent had used cocaine daily at one time or another.

Drugs are harmless? If they land the user in the slammer?

St. Louis Review

St. Louis, MO,
February 22, 1985

At a meeting of the international Commission on Narcotic Drugs last week in Vienna, Austria, a Vatican official issued a strong condemnation of drug abuse. Msgr. Giovanni Cierano of the Vatican Nunciature in Austria stated that drug misuse results from a moral and spiritual crisis in contemporary society.

Msgr. Cierano went on to mention that to a large degree the taking of drugs "challenges a human and cultural outlook that lacks sufficient ideals. It challenges paradoxically the permissive way of life, the materialistic mentality and the consumer society, all of which ignore essential elements and genuine aspirations of the human person."

We feel that there is much truth in this statement. Our society depends very much on drugs, both for good and for evil. The heart transplant operations would be impossible without drugs. Many of us have received drug prescriptions to relieve stress and get much-needed sleep. Our legislators are discussing the morality and wisdom of allowing beer and wine advertising on television. Many families would find it impossible to celebrate weddings or anniversaries without this same beer and wine. It is not the drugs which are the problem, but the use to which we put them that is the problem.

The Vatican official urged all who attended the meeting to take practical steps to meet the challenge of drug abuse. However, he also urged his audience to realize how much pain and anguish those who abuse drugs are trying to alleviate or avoid. He urged all to face the problem at its root. Drugs are one temporary way of answering the problem, but the problem remains. For many people unable to face up to the problems of living, the anguish of daily life is all too real.

Drug abuse is not a new problem, but it is a bigger problem now with more people having greater access to drugs and more means for obtaining them. Lent is a good time for all of us to look deeply at ourselves and our way of life. It is a good time to consider our goals, both materialistic and spiritual, and to come to terms with the challenges within our lives. Christ is the answer. Lent is a time in which the Lord encourages us, as He always has, to live not for ourselves but to serve others. It is a time to join our sacrifice to His in preparation for the eternities of Easter.

THE DAILY OKLAHOMAN

Oklahoma City, OK, November 11, 1985

THE movie industry has been accused of doing a disservice to American youth through the "quasi promotion" of drugs.

Before the filmmakers run and hide under the First Amendment cover, they should take stock of their product to see if the charge is true and, if so, clean up their act.

The accusation comes not from a conservative religious group, ridiculed by the liberal left in the entertainment world, but from a reputable educator.

Scott Thomson, executive director of the National Association of Secondary School Principals (NASSP), cites such films as "Easy Rider," "Private Benjamin," "Risky Business," "Fast Times at Ridgemont High" and "Animal House" as examples of promoting the drug culture. Earlier films, like Frank Sinatra's "Man With the Golden Arm," focused on the degradation of drugs, Thomson says.

The schools' drug education programs are ineffectual when placed against the overwhelming impact of the entertainment world, he argues. Strict self-policing by the industry might stave off demands for censorship.

The Salt Lake Tribune

Salt Lake City, UT, May 31, 1984

There is a tendency in the news and commentary business to call this or that problem of the moment a crisis and to demand prompt remedial action.

After living through the campus revolt-Vietnam War crisis, the energy crisis, the economic crisis and others, it is increasingly difficult to get excited about the next one. Those of the past seemed to have worked themselves out in due time, largely as the result of forces over which individuals and official agencies had little control.

It is in this frame of mind that we address the emerging illegal drug dilemma which, by many reports, is at or near crisis stage after two decades of steadily worsening conditions. The inclination is to conclude that this, too, will pass and that the frenzied "campaigns" against illegal drug traffic and use are understandable but futile. News reports of late tend to confirm this dreary assessment.

A recent story in The New York Times tells of surplus quantities of cocaine and heroin in the New York area which have forced prices down to a point that users of moderate means can afford the habit.

Another dispatch in the same newspaper details how the federal government is virtually powerless to prevent air delivery of cocaine by foreign suppliers. A third report begins: "On the seas and at 300 ports of entry along the nation's borders, federal law enforcement authorities say their limited resources enable them to seize only a small percentage of the illicit drugs entering this country."

And the General Accounting Office, conceding that the volume and street value of drugs seized "are most impressive," told Congress that "the seizures are dwarfed by the total drugs available. More drugs are entering the United States than entered five years ago."

This distressing state of affairs is what taxpayers have to show for millions of dollars spent by drug enforcement agencies in a losing battle to suppress the production, commerce in and use of marijuana, cocaine, heroin and sundry less popular controlled substances. And the agencies, pleading inadequate equipment and manpower, are crying to spend more.

Considering the immensity and diversity of the illegal drug trade and the huge profits to be derived from it, the amounts being spent on supression are indeed inadequate. But there is little reason to suppose that providing more money will produce significant reduction in this sinister traffic.

In the classic free trade sense, drug supply responds to demand and reaps enormous profit in the process. Official attempts to interdict the production and distribution of these widely and highly desired goods are foredoomed. Legalization would reduce the profit incentive but have the undesirable effect of increasing availability.

Curtailment of demand is the most obvious approach but also the most challenging. It requires changing the myriad societal conditions, attitudes and mores that make drug use attractive to large numbers of people.

These changes, we suggest, will eventually occur of their own accord. However, innovative attitude-altering measures, funded by money diverted from the hopeless interdiction effort, might speed that great day when the illegal drug crisis joins other once-feared but now half-forgotten terrors of the recent past.

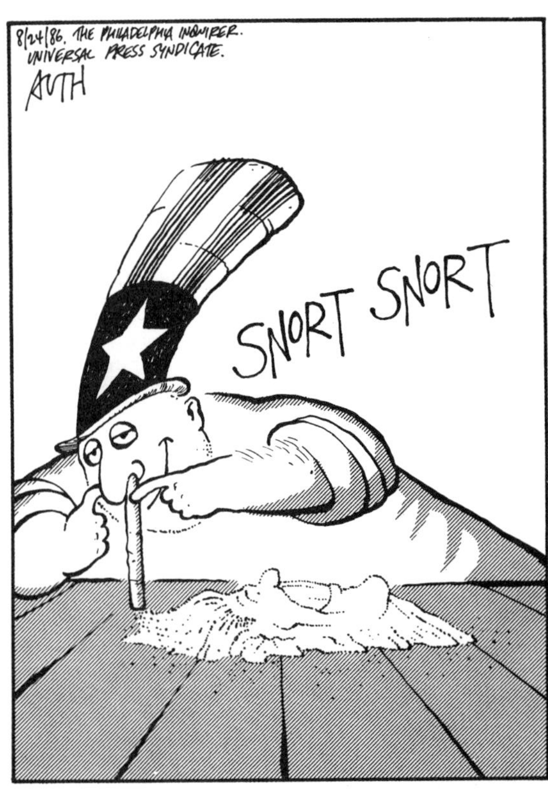

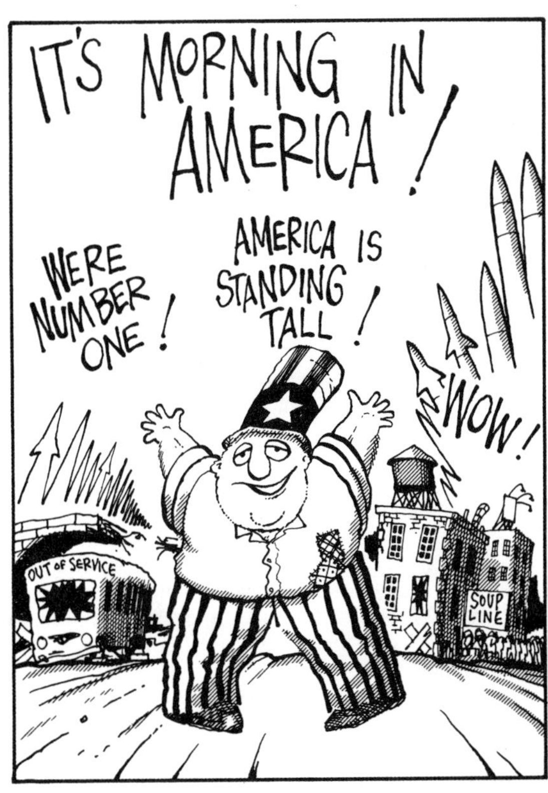

WORCESTER TELEGRAM.
Worcester, MA, July 26, 1985

Although public awareness of the dangers of drug abuse seems to be growing, there is an alarming trend in films and television toward glamorizing the use of marijuana, cocaine and other drugs.

Movies before the '60s portrayed drug users as junkies and losers, as in "The Man With the Golden Arm." That has changed in the '80s. A survey by Parade Magazine found 60 films, most made in the past five years, that show drug use in a favorable light.

The most obvious are the hardcore drug culture films. The 1969 box-office smash "Easy Rider" was an early film that glamorized pot, LSD and cocaine. Later, by the time of the Cheech and Chong films, characters were floating happily through clouds of marijuana smoke. Television's counterpart is the kind of drug humor that is a staple on "Saturday Night Live."

Another group of films, while not actively promoting drug use, shows drugs being used in a carefree, casual way by glamorous role models. Among these are some of the major box-office hits of recent years, including "Terms of Endearment," "Romancing the Stone," "Nine to Five" and "Private Benjamin." Many youth-market films, from "Animal House" to "Risky Business," depict heavy drinking and pot smoking as natural parts of growing up.

The survey identified comparatively few films with clear messages about the dangers of drug abuse, perhaps a dozen. And most in this category focused on heroin addiction or drug deals gone bad.

Despite the epidemic proportions of the problem, a proposed "substance abuse" rating along with the current PG, PG-13 or R ratings would be a dubious solution. Jack Valenti, president of the Motion Picture Association of America, takes a condescending attitude toward the "SA" rating proposal. He says that such a rating could open the way for a confusing mass of similar additions to satisfy various pressure groups — anti-abortion, animal cruelty, drunken driving and teen-age violence or suicide. He is right.

Government monitoring of film content, which would pose a threat to the industry's First Amendment rights, would not be an acceptable solution either. Government involvement is unpalatable even to actor Paul Newman, who became a vocal opponent of Hollywood's portrayal of drug use after the drug-related death of his son, Scott.

Some producers contend that the current spate of drug use in films merely shows life as it is. That rings hollow in view of the film industry's track record. Hollywood and glamorized lawlessness go way back. Too many Hollywood producers and performers, over the years, have used films to excuse, justify and promote their own corrupt and debased lifestyles.

Parents can help by taking the existing advisory ratings seriously. Producers could help by showing more self-restraint, but that seems unlikely.

In the hopped-up Hollywood fast lane, where a party isn't a party without a rich supply of cocaine, casual drug use seems just a normal reflection of life as it is. From a more normal perspective, it looks more like a case of pandering promoting.

The Birmingham News
Birmingham, AL, September 16, 1986

We need to get tough with drug dealers through effective law enforcement and strict penalties. We need to defend our national borders better against those who smuggle drugs into the United States.

But most of all we need to change our thinking about drugs. As a society, we need to stop tolerating this cancer. Our efforts to dry up the supply of drugs will come to naught if we don't slow down the demand.

That is why the Sunday night televised talk by President and Mrs. Reagan may help. Mr. Reagan has shown again and again he can communicate effectively with the American people. Maybe his efforts in the war on drugs will bring the level of awareness we need to truly change some public attitudes.

Almost as dangerous as the easy acceptance of drugs in some segments of our population is the apathy in other segments. "Many of you may be thinking: 'Well, drugs don't concern me,'" Mrs. Reagan said. "It does concern you — it concerns all of us because of the way it tears at our lives and because it is aimed at destroying the brightness and life of the sons and daughters of the United States."

Too often, parents think the drug problem can't touch their children. They're wrong. A recent survey of the top achievers in our nation's high schools revealed 27 percent of them knew classmates who use drugs.

Education Secretary William J. Bennett knows how devastating the problem of drug use is in our schools. His department is giving away a new handbook, *Schools Without Drugs*, which sets out clearly a parent's responsibilities in preparing a child to resist drugs.

Too often, employers think the drug problem will not affect their business. They're wrong. We must take steps, as the president has said, to create a drug-free work place in the United States.

If that means drug testing for some workers in law enforcement, safety and other fields, then such testing should be done to protect the innocent citizens who rely on those workers.

Too often, members of Congress believe they can make a problem go away by throwing money at it. They're wrong. We can't just appropriate huge sums to fight the war on drugs and then forget about it.

The drug epidemic is not a problem for government alone. It is a challenge for all of us.

We hope the Reagans made that clear Sunday night.

Cocaine Use Sweeps U.S. in 1980s

Cocaine, an alkaloid found in the leaves of the coca bush, affects the central nervous system and induces feelings of euphoria. Used since the time of the Inca empire, which flourished for hundreds of years in the Andean mountain region of Peru until the arrival of the Spanish in the 1500s, Inca priests and nobles chewed coca leaves in order to achieve and enhance their understanding of religious experiences. By the early 1900s cocaine had found its way, through patent medicines like Vin Mariani, into the lives of many people. A great deal of cocaine was produced for use in beverages. Coca-Cola contained cocaine until 1906 when the company, at the insistence of the U.S. government, removed the ingredient from the recipe. Both the Canadian government, in 1911, and the U.S. government, in 1914, put legal restrictions on the sale of the drug. Cocaine diminished greatly in popularity and it wasn't until the 1960s that it made a comeback. Its appeal was due in part to the public's acceptance of amphetemines, the effects of which are remarkably similar to those of cocaine. Because of the expense of cocaine, its use until recently was confined primarily to the upper strata of society, particularly to people in the sports and entertainment fields. But cocaine steadily gained acceptance among the young, college students, and many blue- and white-collar circles, as well. Although expensive, its popularity may have stemmed from the fact that people believed it to be nonaddictive.

There are several methods of taking cocaine. The most common is by "snorting" it into the nostrils. Another method favored by some heavy users is to inject the substance directly into the bloodstream. More recently, a process known a "freebasing" has become popular—and deadly. Freebasing involves heating ether, lighter fluid, or a similar flammable solvent, with cocaine—a potentially dangerous process that could lead to burns. (Richard Pryor, the comedian and actor, was almost killed in 1980 when he set himself on fire while freebasing.) The result is a purifed cocaine base which is smoked in a special pipe with wire screens. It is rapidly absorbed by the lungs and carried to the brain in a few seconds. The brief euphoria that results is quickly replaced by a feeling of restless irritability. The aftereffects of freebasing can be so uncomfortable that in order to maintain the high, users often continue smoking until they run out of cocaine or until they are completely exhausted.

Some 30% of all college students have at least sampled cocaine before graduating, according to a National Institute of Drug Abuse (NIDA) study issued July 7, 1986. The findings were also said to be valid for young Americans outside college. The survey found that 17.3% of college students had used cocaine at least once during 1985, a small increase over the 16.9% in 1980. The number of Americans killed each year by cocaine had risen to at least 563 in 1985 from as low as 185 in 1981, the NIDA reported July 10, 1986. But the number of cocaine users was thought to be stable. The figures, part of a NIDA survey, were unveiled by federal health officials at a Washington, D.C. news conference. "We're in a terrible siutation with cocaine," said D. Donald Macdonald, administrator of the Alcohol, Drug Abuse and Mental Health Administration.

Scientists now believe that cocaine is physically addicitive, *Time* magazine reported in its June 2 issue. As recently as 1982, researchers had reported in the magazine *Scientific American* that a dependency on cocaine was little more serious than one on salted peanuts—use was steady as long as there was a supply, but scientists thought a user did not miss the drug after it ran out. New research was said to indicate otherwise. Cocaine was thought to affect neurotransmitters, chemicals in the brain that allow nerve impulses to travel from one brain cell to another. Scientists believed that cocaine produced euphoria by stimulating a flood of these chemicals, but then made it impossible for them to be reused. The cocaine user would resort to more cocaine to combat the resulting depression, only to deplete his store of neurotransmitters even further. Eventually, doctors warned, the psychological effect on the brain could throw a user into a state of actual psychosis.

The Miami Herald
Miami, FL, September 3, 1983

THERE could hardly have been a worse piece of news to greet parents and teachers on the first day of school than *The Herald's* report on cocaine. A combination of dropping prices and rising purity indicates a glut, and that is bad news indeed.

The high price of cocaine traditionally has been a major obstacle to its use by young people. Few kids or wage earners could afford to develop a coke habit. That may change.

Undercover drug agents routinely negotiate to buy cocaine in bulk in South Florida. In 1981 they found $58,000 to $60,000 per kilo to be the going rate. Last year the average dropped to about $48,000. Now the kilo costs less than $30,000 — less than $100 for a gram — and is expected to drop further. Dealers almost certainly will use the lower prices to expand their once-adult market downward toward the youth who could not previously afford to buy.

That possibility demands a quick response from parents, educators, and other adults who are concerned about the welfare of the community's young people. For cocaine is dangerous — much more dangerous than marijuana, which itself is by no means harmless. Coke kills through overdose, through drug-induced accidents, and through degeneration of normal habits.

The danger of an influx of cheap cocaine to tempt younger potential users should add an even greater sense of urgency to the Drug Awareness Campaign that is now in preparation. Sponsored by the Junior League of Miami, Informed Families of Dade County, WTVJ-Channel 4, and *The Herald*, the community-wide program is scheduled for October. It will include a broad array of films, activities, literature, counseling, celebrities, and displays. The slogan is "Proud to Be Drug Free."

The key is assertive pride, the bolstering of individual resistance to pressure from the vocal minority of drug-using peers. That technique also figures in the U.S. Navy's anti-drug campaign, which uses the slogan "Not on my watch; not on my ship; not in my Navy." To that, young people might add: not in my car; not at my party; not on my team; not in my club; not at my school.

Abuse of drugs, including alcohol, is the major component in a shocking statistical fact about health-conscious America: The death rate for persons age 16-24, unlike the rate for any other pre-retirement group, actually is increasing. Technology has extended life expectancy, but no technology yet devised can save teenagers and young adults from the fatal consequences of their own abuse of dangerous drugs. Avoidable death has become an epidemic in the age group that otherwise is the nation's healthiest.

Into this explosive environment now is injected the unwelcome prospect of affordable cocaine. No development could symbolize better the importance of attacking the drug problem by reducing the demand as well as enforcing the law against suppliers. And demand can be reduced only by changing the social climate so that drug abuse is seen correctly for the stupid, self-destructive waste that it is.

The Pittsburgh PRESS

Pittsburgh, PA, December 23, 1983

If it were only a question of catching a few major smugglers and pushers, the Reagan administration's stepped-up war against the illicit drug traffic would rate a high chance of success.

Unfortunately, there is a giant market for such drugs. Thus, the outlook for controlling the smugglers and the pushers is dim.

This is especially true in the case of cocaine. According to law-enforcement officials, the immense profits to be made in dealing with this drug — together with widespread belief that it is no more dangerous than tobacco or alcohol — is luring more and more middle-class and upper-class Americans into the cocaine trade.

An estimated 10 million to 20 million Americans have tried cocaine, and the number of regular users is put at eight million. About six out of every 10 regular users eventually become sellers, both to support their own habits and because of the huge profits that beckon.

Businessmen, physicians, lawyers and bank officers — respectable people all — were among the alleged leaders of a smuggling ring that was cracked when 3,748 pounds of cocaine was confiscated in Florida last March, the largest such seizure to date.

In July, 106 persons, including businessmen and housewives, were indicted in Phoenix, Ariz., on charges of participating in a nine-state cocaine ring.

Yet arrests alone have not put much of a crimp into the cocaine traffic.

To wipe out this scourge, vigorous anti-smuggling efforts must, of course, continue. But we also need to improve education about cocaine's addictive and destructive effects and — most of all — ensure certain and severe punishment for those trafficking in it.

St. Louis Globe-Democrat

St. Louis, MO, September 20, 1983

To the surprise of virtually no one, a national survey among cocaine users has confirmed that cocaine is addictive. Moreover, it was found that almost one of four people who use the drug steal to support their dependency.

The survey was conducted with 500 cocaine users selected at random from among the first 50,000 people from 42 states who called a cocaine hot line. The hot line revealed some cold, hard facts about the dangers of using cocaine or any other drug.

"A vast majority (of cocaine users) use all of their savings, and almost one out of four states he was forced to steal from work for drugs," said Dr. Mark S. Gold, medical director for the national hot line and head of research at Fair Oaks Hospital in Summit, N.J., where the hot line is located.

The survey revealed that while most cocaine users admitted an addiction, free-base users of the drug found it more addicting than intranasal users, Gold said. Free-base users mix the drug with ether and a petroleum distillate to make a paste, then let the paste dry before they smoke it in a pipe.

"Three-quarters (of those) on free-base stated they preferred free-base to food, to their family, to their job and even to sex," said Gold, adding that more than 75 percent of the free-base users responded they "definitely" would experience withdrawal symptoms if they tried to quit the drug.

The survey found that 72 percent of the intravenous cocaine users also took heroin, with 75 percent saying they began as intranasal cocaine users before taking it intravenously, the doctor said.

To give an idea of the cost of the habit, Gold said the average free-base user responding to the survey said it cost $820 a week to buy cocaine. The average intranasal user, he said, spent about $436 weekly on cocaine.

The results of the survey should provide a sobering lesson to anyone who might think there's no harm in experimenting with drugs and getting a little high on cocaine or any other controlled substance. As the survey shows, taking a trip on drugs is not a free ride.

THE KANSAS CITY STAR

Kansas City, MO, September 20, 1983

The expense of cocaine use runs far beyond cost of the drug. Its purchase causes crime, some of it violent, some of it the white-collar type, that touches millions of Americans. Thus abuse of this drug and others extends to many people, most of whom have nothing to do directly with use of cocaine.

A recent sampling of abusers who called a drug hot line emphasized the problem. Nearly one in four seeking help admitted he or she stole at work to support acquisition of cocaine. These people are not victims of poverty. Indeed many are professionals who claim both a physical and psychological addiction to it.

Much more than a crime problem is involved here, however. While white-collar crime, which has been on the increase, is a target of the criminal justice system, drug use must also be treated as the social dilemma it is. The objective should be to curb the need for drugs. That in turn could reduce crime that accompanies abuse.

Programs are available in many jurisdictions to help addicts rid themselves of their drug habit. This effort recognizes that drug abuse is a significant social issue.

The crime fight and anti-abuse activities are intertwined by need. Both are necessary to make the streets, homes and businesses of this country safer.

The Houston Post

Houston, TX, September 22, 1983

The federal task forces assigned to the nation's war on illegal-drug smuggling appear to be gaining in the battle against marijuana haulers but are losing ground to cocaine traffickers. The situation calls for international and innovative approaches. The National Narcotics Border Interdiction System, headed by Vice President George Bush, reports that cocaine is being slipped into the country in such quantities that the underground market is saturated and dealers are slashing their prices.

Despite the fact that amounts of the drug seized in raids by the task forces have more than doubled since last year, cocaine is reported to be more available than ever. Seizures now average about 2,000 pounds a month but officials say the smuggling organizations are having so much success otherwise that they consider the amount they lose little more than overhead in their clandestine operations.

Rear Adm. D.C. Thompson, southeast regional coordinator of the interdiction system, said in Miami, "There is a glut on the market," and called it "a serious turn in the war on drugs." Other officials in Miami, hub of the underground network for distribution of cocaine in the United States, say the price of the drug there has dropped from last year's $60,000 a kilogram to as little as $25,000 now. In New York, the price is down from $75,000 a kilogram last year to about $30,000. In Los Angeles, the price has dropped by $10,000 since last month.

The methods used to intercept incoming bulky shipments of marijuana are not as effective against the cocaine smugglers who can hide a kilogram of the white powder in a space no larger than a football. Officials say a common method used by cocaine runners is to fly the powder from South America to the Bahamas, then carry it the short distance to Miami in high-powered speedboats.

Meanwhile, The sources of cocaine are expanding. Intelligence reports say that the coca crops are plentiful in the traditional growing areas of Bolivia and Peru and new cultivation is going on in Colombia, previously limited to cocaine processing and handling. One reason to expect more international help in the war on drugs is that the oversupply of cocaine is so great in the United States some dealers are turning to Europe for new markets. The illegal drug trade is costly to us all in terms of combatting it and the crime it generates. But the real tragedy is the scope of the demand created by the greed of a few.

The Kansas City Times

Kansas City, MO, March 12, 1984

The influx and influence of cocaine in this country is staggering. As a recent series in *The Kansas City Times* detailed, the fairly general and unpleasant consensus is that the problem is out of control.

Yet the drug is illegal. And its "recreational" use can cause both physical and psychological damage depending on the volatility of factors from amount and frequency to individual bodily response. As with other drugs, legal and illegal, what one person tolerates may harm another. Scientists who study substance abuse disagree on cocaine's addictive potential.

Such uncertainties alone would justify society, through its collective attitude and laws, to forbid cocaine. The verified deaths and lesser harm that can result make the stand of the majority — and cocaine abstainers are still in a majority — a wise one.

Yet it is discouraging, if not downright ludicrous, to examine what masquerades as battle between the law and drug traffickers. Stepped-up federal efforts to intercept cocaine in Florida may get 10 percent of the more than 60 metric tons annually reaching the U.S. Another pittance is seized on the streets. Nearly $700 million was spent on federal drug enforcement last year, about $100 million of it on the South Florida Task Force working the door to cocaine. Yet the trade booms.

There is a temptation to stop beating back a snow slide with a toothbrush by just making the drug legal. Then the country could collect taxes on the business and profits. For cocaine is big business. It supports smugglers and other criminals in high style, financing legitimate enterprises we all use once the money is laundered. Another extreme option would be for Congress to create a special foreign aid program and virtually support the economies in the countries of origin, starting with the farmers and middlemen in Colombia, Peru and Bolivia. Neither will happen.

Research psychologists know that high prices attract customers repelled by bargains, a principle partly at work in the drug mess. So perhaps it is time to stop hitting the national head against walls. It makes no sense to pinch pennies with children's school lunch allotments and watch the homeless accumulate in our big cities while pouring more and more dollars into an impossible crusade to stop cocaine trade and use. Doing the reasonable to express society's disapproval is one thing. Breaking the treasury is another.

Left alone, the high rollers, experimenters and emotionally immature may eventually learn that the world is not their oyster, even with the magic white powder. When they do, they can quit making fools of themselves and millionaires of two-legged skunks.

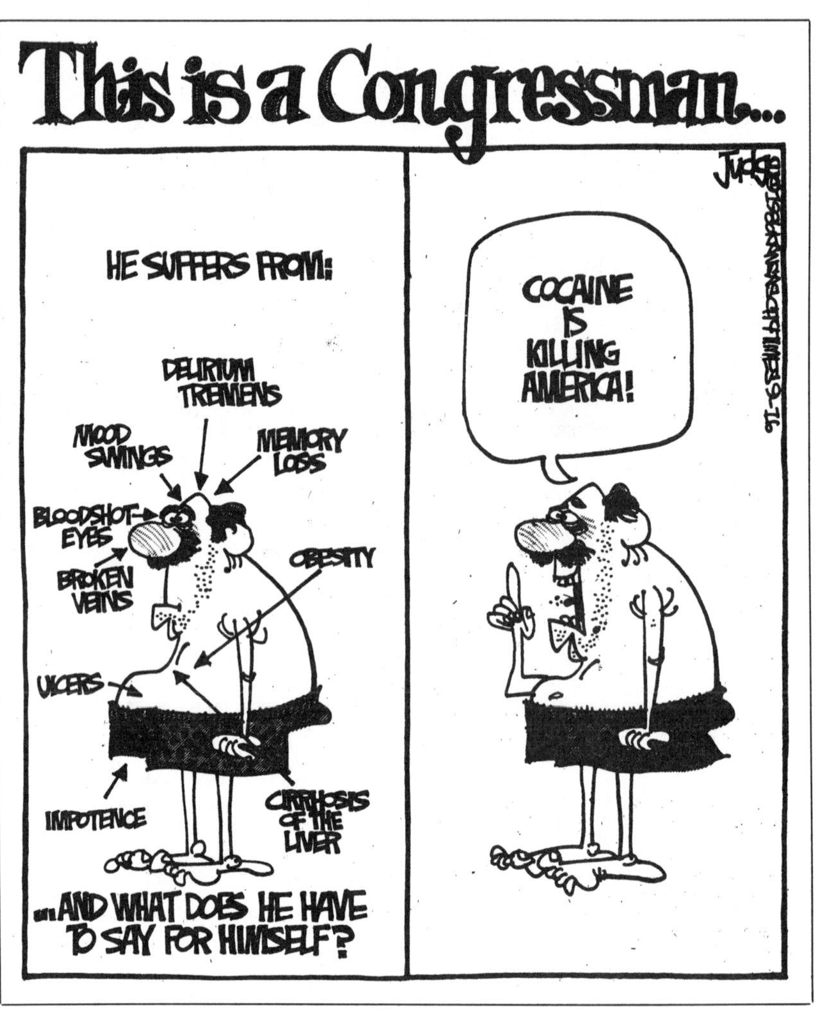

The News American

Baltimore, MD, November 19, 1984

Maryland law enforcement officials have known for some time that the state has a cocaine problem on its hands. Now, it turns out, the problem is causing state health officials just as much trouble.

Throughout the state, the number of persons using cocaine has shot up in recent months. The situation is being branded an "epidemic." The trend is alarming in terms of wasted human life, but health officials are also confronted with high and mounting treatment bills.

Many of the abusers — as many as 3,600 so far this year — cannot afford treatment at a hospital and are turning to the state's 55 drug treatment centers. A large number of them are indigent, but treatment is too expensive for even middle-class abusers.

The result is a virtual run on health clinics by abusers. The number of grave cases being treated at state centers is reported to have doubled in the last two years. In the words of a top health official, the state is getting "stuck" with the treatment cost.

Health officials have proposed the establishment of a 25-bed cocaine clinic as a stopgap remedy. The short-term treatment center — 28 to 35 days per patient — would be the first of its kind in the nation and would involve an estimated $150,000 start-up cost. Location of the center is yet to be determined.

Law enforcement and health officials predict that the cocaine problem is likely to get worse before it gets better in spite of stepped-up effort.

Gov. Hughes and the legislature would have to approve the proposal. The price tag will not be attractive. But both law enforcement and health officials predict that the picture will worsen before it gets better.

That means the tab on the present situation will not come down soon.

Fort Worth Star-Telegram
Fort Worth, TX, November 30, 1984

The recent explosion set off by drug traffickers outside the U.S. Embassy in Bogata, Colombia, should jar this nation and its hemispheric neighbors into a determination to wage total war against the cocaine culture.

The threats of the cocaine kingpins against U.S. diplomatic personnel in Colombia amount to nothing less than criminals openly defying the forces of law and order. The truly sad part of the whole affair is that the cocaine dealers have the wealth to hire assassins to carry out their threats.

They demonstrated as much in having Rodrigo Lara Bonilla, Colombia's minister of justice, killed last April. Bonilla was his government's leading opponent of the drug trade. His murder spurred the government of President Belisario Betancourt and the U.S. government to launch their most ambitious effort to wipe out the cocaine business in Colombia.

Scores of suspects have been arrested, cocaine processing laboratories have been raided, and homes, planes and estates of major drug dealers have been seized. Betancourt has agreed to extradite some of the drug kingpins to the United States.

The threats against U.S. citizens have been made in connection with the extradition promises. The Spanish ambassador to Colombia also has been threatened because his government is holding some drug traffickers who fled to Spain and the Spanish government intends to extradite them to the United States.

The drug dealers' boldness springs from their determination to continue in their highly lucrative business. The United States is their main market. Cocaine usage is booming. The demand is so great that they have been able to lower the price to bring it within reach of the American middle class. The results have been signficant increases in cocaine-related crime, death, injury and other forms of human misery.

The United States must join with Colombia and other countries where cocaine and other drugs are produced for illegal sale in this country to eradicate the sources of supply. Whatever it costs to get the job done will be money well-spent.

At the same time that the supply is being eradicated, major efforts must be made to catch the drug brokers in this country, educate the public against the use of such drugs and make it possible for persons who have become addicted to them to give them up.

The war against the drug culture must be two-pronged, one prong directed at the supply side and the other at the demand side.

WORCESTER TELEGRAM.
Worcester, MA, June 28, 1984

Worcester has had two jolting reminders that the drug plague is not restricted to Hollywood, New York and the other playgrounds of the rich and famous.

The first shocker was the Arnold Katz case, with its revelations of the criminal underside of the cocaine trade.

The second grim example came this week, when Gary E. Mosso and Jeffrey A. Sinnott were convicted of first degree murder and sentenced to life terms without parole at Walpole State Prison. Mosso and Sinnott, as well as the late Anthony S. Tamburro, were all caught in the tentacles of the drug octopus.

It is tragic beyond telling to see these young lives twisted, destroyed, wasted, poisoned. Although there are many other problems in life besides drugs, drugs can overwhelm all else.

A few years ago, there was considerable talk about legalizing marijuana, a less powerful drug than cocaine, hashish and heroin. But we don't hear so much of that sort of thing these days. Drugs are ravishing the lives and hopes of thousands of people, the John Belushis as well as the John Does. Most chronic drug users started off with marijuana.

For all the propaganda, there is nothing good about drugs, and that includes alcohol. Our society is only just beginning to address the problem of the substances that alter minds and moods to such devastating effect.

LAS VEGAS REVIEW-JOURNAL
Las Vegas, NV, November 29, 1984

An estimated 22 million Americans have tried it at least once, and its use is reported on the rise. One researcher calls it "the drug of choice of middle class America."

There's more bad news about cocaine: despite the largest federal law enforcement effort ever aimed at stemming its flow into the United States, the drug is so plentiful in this country its price has dropped by 50 percent in the past year. One drug enforcement official said a gram of cocaine sells for $60 to $70 on the street these days, often making it cheaper than an ounce of marijuana.

But there are two important distinctions between cocaine and marijuana: if you're caught dealing, the penalties are at least twice as severe for cocaine. And cocaine is classified as a narcotic drug. That means it's habit-forming, which all those "recreational" users out there ought to realize. In the Miami area, for instance, an average of two recreational cocaine users a month die from overdosing, according to police reports.

The illicit drug business in this country is booming, and the federal government is finding itself hard-pressed to curtail it. Smugglers are getting smarter at avoiding detection. And governments in foreign lands that produce drugs like cocaine don't seem to be all that eager to shut down drug operations. When there is big money involved, corruption has a habit of breeding.

Witnesses testifying this week before the President's Commission on Organized Crime told of the corruption in Colombia, a country believed to be the source of 75 percent of the U.S. cocaine market and 60 percent of the U.S. marijuana market last year.

One man said he recalled attending a round of parties during a month's visit to Colombia arranged by the country's cocaine kingpins. "We had national police, prosecutors, judges, political figures (attending), just about anyone who had anything to do with that region," he testified.

Another testified of the risks involved: 67 officers of the 400-member police force in Medellin, Colombia, have been "violently assassinated" this year by elements of the cocaine industry, the witness said.

It appears the Colombian government has been taking a harder line since April, when a minister of justice was assassinated, reportedly on orders of cocaine traffickers.

While the U.S. government has to be congratulated for staging an unprecedented assault on drug trafficking in this country, more has to be done, and least in two important areas:

— The administration simply must force foreign governments, especially the one in Colombia, to crack down harder on the production of cocaine. It seems rather incongruous that as the most powerful nation in the world we cannot eradicate the relatively few drug barons who shipped an estimated 71 metric tons of cocaine to the United States from Colombia last year.

— The administration must spend more to educate Americans about the perils of drug abuse. While it is encouraging that marijuana use among teen-agers appears to be dropping, Drug Enforcement Administration analysts say that heroin addiction is holding stable and cocaine use is spreading. The Reagan administration has about halved the amount of federal spending on drug abuse prevention and treatment programs.

According to a Wall Street Journal article, law enforcement officials unanimously concede that their best efforts will not shut down the drug trade unless U.S. demand or foreign supplies dry up.

THE BLADE
Toledo, OH,
August 24, 1985

FOR those under the impression that taking cocaine is a kind of glamorous recreational pastime which carries no price tag beyond the cost of the substance, consider what baseball player Tim Raines had to say about his "problem" of three years ago:

"I struck out a lot more; my vision was lessened. A lot of times I'd go up to the plate and the ball was right down the middle and I'd jump back, thinking it was at my head."

Or another player, Lonnie Smith: "I think it slowed me down, not just running but my mental thinking. I wasn't as alert. Look at my defense. It seemed like I was averaging two or three errors a game."

These and other players in recent press accounts have acknowledged the obvious: Their performances suffered, as did those of their teams, when they were taking cocaine. That fact was reflected in a statement from the president of the Montreal Expos, who said that the drug was the reason that his team did not win a pennant in 1982.

These disclosures have been greeted by the usual head-in-the-sand attitude by the players' union, which continues to oppose across-the-board drug testing for players.

Although the incidents involving Smith, Raines, and others occured several years ago, it is well known that drug abuse is still a problem — and, in fact, may be growing. As long as baseball and its players, as well as participants in other sports, wink at illegal activities of this kind, they will open themselves to public cynicism and loss of popularity.

The candor from the players who have conquered cocaine is a reminder that major league baseball has a drug problem. It is one that will not go away until the players themselves insist on stamping it out.

Houston Chronicle
Houston, TX, September 25, 1985

Recent government studies confirm that the United States has become a society that is widely influenced — and profoundly damaged — by cocaine abuse. Those studies refute any idea that use of cocaine is a relatively harmless, though highly illegal, recreation.

As one researcher said, "Now, we know the truth." Emergency-room admissions and deaths associated with cocaine have tripled in the last few years.

The studies are reassuring in their finding that cocaine is not a serious problem among high school students. This may stem from the extensive drug education efforts. Another factor may be the high price.

Cocaine abuse seems to be concentrated in young adults, but for this group the numbers are staggering. Surveys indicate that one in four Americans between the ages of 18 and 25 have at least tried cocaine. Technically, this makes 25 percent of young adults felons. In Texas, possession of even minute quantities of the drug is punishable by two to 20 years in prison.

The physical toll paid by cocaine users is now known; the damage to society as a whole in crime and corruption cannot begin to be measured. Even so, little doubt can remain that cocaine has become a devastating scourge that cries out for national attention.

THE TAMPA TRIBUNE
Tampa, FL, December 14, 1985

Vice President George Bush was in Miami this week riding around in the U.S. Customs Service's new, one-of-a-kind anti-smuggling power boat, Blue Thunder. But in the real world it is still raining drugs.

It has been nearly four years since the federal government began an intensive drug war conducted by a Miami-based task force of federal customs and drug enforcement agents formed by the Reagan administration and led, nominally at least, by Vice President Bush. The past year was the best ever for agents, who seized 25 tons of cocaine in southern Florida and the Caribbean; that was more than double the 1983 total.

But the price of a kilogram of cocaine (2.2 pounds) is now $30,000, about half what it was before the task force arrived.

U.S. Senator Lawton Chiles, who guided much of the drug war legislation through Congress, said recently: "With all of the efforts, when you look at the bottom line, the price of coke is lower and it's more available than when we started."

Miami and Dade County remain the hub of the drug trade, primarily because of their location and Latin population. A group of Colombian families run the drug rings, although one of the biggest South American godfathers is Bolivian. Hillsborough law enforcement agencies say that they have seen an expansion of the cocaine trade in the area within the past year, as measured by Colombians moving to Tampa — and by the confiscation of 700 pounds of the drug from a boat that docked in Clearwater Wednesday.

The drug deals may be made in New York or Los Angeles but the money passes through almost every corner of southern Florida. What people see on the TV series, "Miami Vice", is not just so much video fiction.

The deals are made and the cocaine manufactured — a relatively new and dangerous development — in inner city neighborhoods, middle-class suburbs and exclusive enclaves. (The volatile chemical ether is used in refining coca leaf paste into cocaine.)

But it's made in those places because people in those same settings all across this country create a demand for the powerful stimulant, once throught to be only psychologically addictive but now known to create a strong physical dependency.

The supply has risen to meet that demand. Thus the price has fallen. In the early 1980s, when it was clear that the cocaine market was no passing fancy and profits were fancy indeed, South Americans planted thousands more coca shrubs on the slopes of the Andes.

U.S. agents are fighting hard and even some South American governments are paying less lip service to our government's demands to get tougher with their citizens. But the war can only be an aggressive holding action as long as there is a market for cocaine. As the United States' government learned in the late 1970s when it and the Mexican government combined to eradicate the Mexican marijuana crop, cultivation of the plant became domestic, springing up in northern California counties whose lumber-based economy had fallen apart. And it sprung up, too, in the palmetto and pine scrubland of central Florida.

It is as Colombian government officials tell U.S. representatives: "It would be easier for us if your citizens didn't create the demand." Success in this war will not come by attrition. It will come when users discover they can get high on living without cocaine.

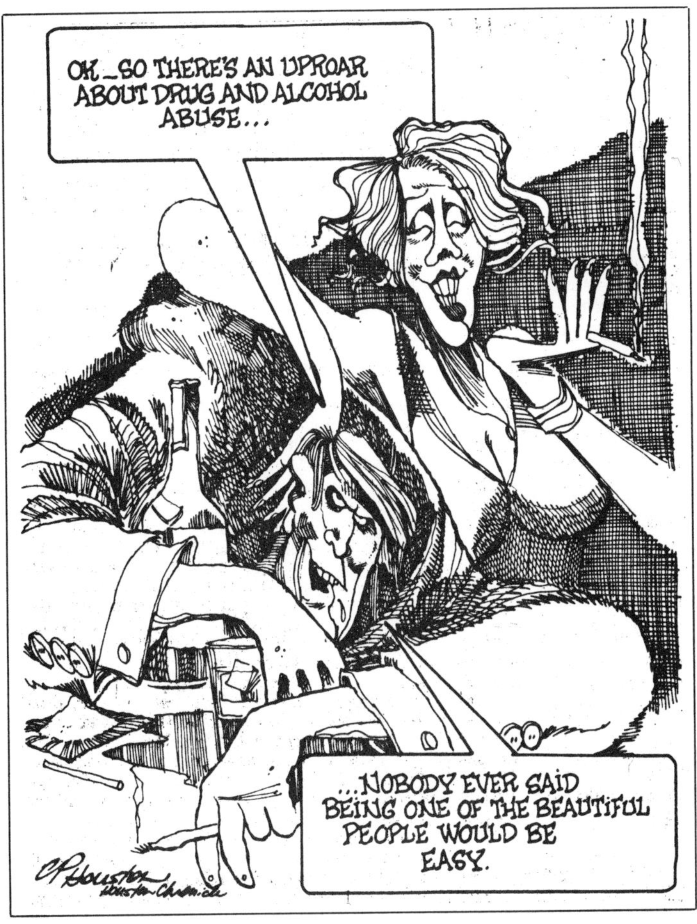

The Hartford Courant

Hartford, CT, September 17, 1985

In a sad but reassuring spectacle, former students at Choate Rosemary Hall in Wallingford are going to federal court to plead guilty to taking part in a cocaine-smuggling ring at the exclusive preparatory school. So far 12 have appeared, and more are expected, including the supposed ringleader.

No one who admires Choate can be happy about this affair. The dark spots on the school's reputation will take a long time to fade, and its ability to attract high-caliber students may suffer as a result.

But it's good to see that the law is being enforced, especially when it means taking the well-to-do to court. For a while, as the Choate affair simmered, there was no sign that local, state or federal authorities were doing anything about information suggesting that Choate students paid for a trip to Venezuela to bring back cocaine.

The two who allegedly made the trip, Derek Oatis of Meriden and his girlfriend, Catherine Cowan of Little Rock, Ark., were arrested in April 1984 at John F. Kennedy International Airport when customs agents found cocaine in his luggage. But even five months ago — nearly a year after the arrests — no one, including U.S. Attorney Alan H. Nevas, would indicate that an investigation of other former Choate students was under way.

The silence, and the lack of further arrests, left the public to suspect that the double standard that's so often evident in criminal cases — one for white-collar crooks, another for everyone else — was again at work.

Although that may not have been true in this case, it was in several others recently. Two of the most prominent have been the E.F. Hutton & Co. check-kiting scheme and Eli Lilly and Co.'s failure to report deaths linked to Oraflex, an arthritis drug.

The Justice Department let Hutton off with a $2 million fine; Lilly's penalty was $25,000. In neither case were corporate officials prosecuted, except for Lilly's former chief medical officer, who pleaded no contest and was fined $15,000.

Such protectiveness has prompted the Senate Judiciary Committee to investigate the Justice Department's handling of white-collar crime, and its hearings will come none too soon. A double standard for prosecuting is incompatible with justice.

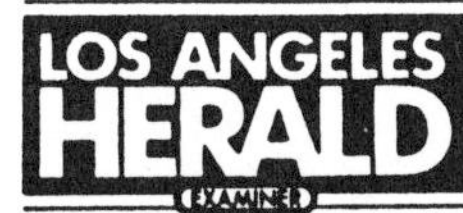

Los Angeles, CA, September 22, 1985

A killer is on the loose. Its name: cocaine.

A series of drug-abuse studies just released by the federal government debunks the myth that cocaine is primarily a high-class recreational drug used by jet-setters, professional athletes and beautiful people. Instead, the reports lay it on the line: Cocaine can be a vicious health threat and is powerfully addictive.

Documentation is found in the fact that emergency-room admissions associated with cocaine use tripled between 1981 and 1984. So, too, did the number of deaths. Although addiction to the drug is not the inevitable outcome of heavy usage, often it is — more often than for other drugs.

Increasingly, cocaine's victims are the young. Two researchers who released results of surveys that have been going on for the last decade reported that about one in every six high-school seniors experimented with the drug in 1984. One in every four young adults has tried the drug.

Although daily use is uncommon among high-school students, the fact that experimentation among them is on the rise is a matter of great concern; those who start in high school tend to increase their usage later. Even in high school, lifestyles are freer, cash more available. Thus, the habit grows.

How many lives will have to be destroyed before society gets the message? How many sports heroes will be forgiven and let back on a team after they dally with drugs, thus setting heaven knows what example for the young? The message is clear and ugly: Americans, particularly young adults, are at tremendous risk once they tread a now-familiar path that starts with heavy marijuana smoking, often leads to experimentation with cocaine and ends in an addiction that can be deadly.

The Campaign Against Marijuana and the Battle for Legalization

The belief that the nationwide upsurge of criminal behavior was closely linked to the growing use of marijuana was originally encouraged by Harry Anslinger, commissioner of the Federal Bureau of Narcotics. He conducted a personal campaign, felt by many to be primarily an effort to gain political power, against the "killer weed," which resulted in state legislation banning marijuana and the passage of the 1937 Marijuana Tax Act. While it did not actually ban marijuana on a federal level, the bill outlawed the nonmedical, untaxed possession or sale of the drug. Anslinger's campaign was based on the contention that marijuana was "criminogenic," that is, causing criminal behavior. By the time the La Guardia Commission report, which cleared cannabis of its criminogenic charge and testified to its relative harmlessness, was released in 1944, the stereotypes fostered by Anslinger and such propaganda films as *Reefer Madness* were strongly imbedded in the psyche of the American people, who were too preoccupied with World War II to pay much attention to it. During the 1955 Senate committee hearing, Anslinger testified that marijuana use inevitably led to heroin addiction, a false allegation that apparently stuck in the public mind. Despite the negative press, marijuana use continued to spread. Encouraged during the 1950s by the "Beat Generation," represented by such authors as Jack Kerouac, marijuana found a broad new audience: the American middle class and intelligentsia. In the 1960s it gained even more popularity on college and high school campuses, becoming almost a symbol of American youth and the gap that separated people from their parents against the backdrop of the Viet Nam War.

The National Organization for the Reform of Marijuana Laws (NORML), a volunteer citizen action group was founded in 1970 to seek changes in U.S. laws regarding marijuana. NORML lobbies for legislative reform of laws, collects and disburses educational material and provides speakers for interested groups in an effort to end criminal penalties for the possession, use, and cultivation of marijuana. An organization of 25,000 members, NORML brought legal action against the Federal Drug Enforcement Administration to make marijuana legally available for medical uses, and was instrumental in the passage of legislation which now allows marijuana to be used as medicine in 33 states.

THE TENNESSEAN

Nashville, TN, January 14, 1985

A Washington group has conducted a study and found that marijuana was Tennessee's most valuable cash crop last year, exceeding legal cash crops such as tobacco, cotton and soybeans.

Tennessee was the eighth largest marijuana producer in the nation according to the National Organization for the Reform of Marijuana Law (NORML), with a crop estimated at $525 million in street value. In all, the group said, Americans harvested a record $16.6 billion worth of pot last year, with an estimated 30 million Americans using the drug regularly.

Since NORML is interested in legalizing marijuana, its report might be suspected by some as calculated to show that it is useless to try to outlaw the crop — that the output keeps on increasing in spite of the laws against it. Tennessee narcotics officers estimate that the amount of marijuana harvested in the state last year was worth about half of what NORML said it was. But that still makes pot the No. 1 cash crop in the state last year.

It is doubtful if NORML will produce much sentiment for the legalization of marijuana in Tennessee. However, it seems that the growers of pot are becoming more and more adept at skirting the law and in finding new ways to grow the plant without detection.

The Washington report said that in the past year increasing amounts of marijuana have been grown in personal "victory gardens," in basements, closets and other hidden places where they can't be seen from helicopters and the public streets. It seems that many marijuana users are cutting their risks by growing pot for their own consumption instead of for sale. This makes it even more difficult for the authorities to make headway against the problem.

It is difficult to know how to proceed when millions of people seem determined to flout the laws against the use of marijuana. Happily, the use of some types of drugs in the schools is down. It should be the focus of any anti-drug program to prevent addictive drugs from falling into the hands of school-age children.

This suggests that the greatest effort and most money allocated for drug prevention should go for education and for saving those not yet hooked from a lifetime of drug dependency.

The Courier-Journal

Louisville, KY, November 29, 1983

THE NEWS of Kentucky's superior ranking in the marijuana-growing world is a little like being told your high school class just voted you "most likely to go to prison." There's not much honor in the distinction.

Since it's illegal to grow pot and the authorities get a little tetchy if they catch you heading toward the cannibis patch with a hoe and watering can, there is understandably little information available on how much of the weed is under cultivation. But the guess experts say the state's marijuana crop is worth anywhere from $500 million to $1 billion or so.

The high end of that estimate would make it the state's most valuable cash crop; burley, the legal smokable leader among farm commodities grown in Kentucky, earned farmers only $900 million last year. Of course, burley is selling for around $1.77 a pound while the same amount of prime Kentucky Lucky goes for nearly $2,000.

Even in a bad year — which last year was, for legitimate and illegitimate farmers alike — the marijuana growers still made a hefty, untaxed bundle. But farmers are farmers, no matter what the crop; as the pot business grows in Kentucky, California, Hawaii and across the country, illegal plot plowers might soon expect to be treated as such.

Just imagine: Pot PIK. President Reagan's Payment In Kind plan to induce farmers not to grow crops by paying them off in the crops they didn't produce could take on a whole new dimension. Since less is more, marijuana can be produced on fewer acres; to protect growers, the land obviously would have to be organized into a marijuana base system modeled on the state's tobacco bases.

And the Department of Agriculture would have to come up with price supports to protect marijuana farmers. As it does for the dairy industry, the USDA might buy all the surplus pot growers could grow, then store it in government warehouses. When the warehouses bulged, the pot could be given away to poor people along with the free cheese and butter that are already being distributed. What with marijuana's questionable health effects and all that saturated fat from the dairy products, the poor then might not always be with us.

To save itself from being buried in marijuana, which grows in crannies more mundane crops spurn, the government would of course have to begin paying farmers not to grow it. And to protect U.S. producers from unfair foreign competition, Congress would have to slap an import quota on foreign-produced pot, while exploring the export market for U.S.-grown weed.

Kentucky State Fair would have a new exhibit. And the next time the Soviets wanted to buy U.S. grain. . . .

The Honolulu Advertiser
Honolulu, HI, April 12, 1984

Is Hawaii the nation's top producer of what may be the number one crop in the country — illegal marijuana?

Part of the problem is that nobody knows for sure just how much marijuana is grown here or elsewhere in the nation. But some of the current educated guesses make interesting and worrisome reading.

A REPORT in the Washington Post the other day said pot may be pushing corn as the number one cash crop in American agriculture. Others suggest it's already on top. Reported the Post:

"The Department of Agriculture doesn't monitor marijuana production, but one group that does, the National Organization for the Reform of Marijuana Laws (NORML), puts the value of the 1983-84 pot crop at $13.9 billion — a figure it calls conservative, rather than high, as it were.

"In contrast, the USDA's farm income figures for 1982, the latest year available, indicate that American farmers earned $13.4 billion for their corn..."

The Post quoted NORML's latest report as ranking California first with a $2 billion crop; Hawaii next at $1.6 billion; Oregon and Kentucky tied for third at $600 million each, followed by North Carolina at $550 million.

But in testimony to a congressional committee this week, Michael Lilly, this state's First Deputy Attorney General, reported that Hawaii feels it is the nation's number one producer.

REGARDLESS of who's first, the essential point is that marijuana presents Hawaii with what Lilly calls our most serious drug problem — and an uncertain contribution to the economy.

Our marijuana industry is more trouble than it is worth for the community in general when you add up the cost of Green Harvest and other irradication, confiscation and enforcement efforts around the state. Marijuana cultivation has also made many of Hawaii's mountains and valleys dangerous places for the average person to go, a social cost.

Still, Lilly's testimony indicated Hawaii has a relatively good record in trying to deal with the problem, accounting for more than half the marijuana confiscated in the five Pacific states.

But efforts here and elsewhere are still running behind the growth in production. The Post report quotes a federal drug official as saying that the 3.8 million marijuana plants destroyed last year may be only 10 to 15 percent of the national crop.

MARIJUANA is considered by many to be Hawaii's largest cash crop. As such, here, as nationally, it is part of a large underground economy that contributes to the legal economy, although to what degree is debatable.

Estimates are that pot is used regularly by some 30 million Americans (out of 230 million). No doubt most users are otherwise law-abiding persons.

For such reasons various groups have suggested marijuana be legalized, regulated for health and taxed. Others, seemingly a majority, are opposed. They cite health uncertainties and arguments that society already has too many drugs too easy to get.

It makes for an interesting argument. But the fact is marijuana is not going to be legalized nationally soon. And Hawaii as a state can't act alone, making itself a legal production center for a drug illegal elsewhere in the nation. In fact, national legalization might be the downfall of Hawaii as a major marijuana center, since other states would get in the business in a big way.

THE RESULT is a dilemma as the nation sorts out its attitudes and its options on marijuana.

It seems to call for a mixture of some toleration toward limited individual use and new and tougher enforcement efforts against large commercial producers and dealers, which is what we are getting, albeit not in the degrees some may want.

Portland Press Herald
Portland, ME, October 17, 1983

The time was in Maine when growing marijuana was basically a cottage industry. No longer. This harvest season suggests marijuana has become a major industry all across the state.

The other day, for example, sheriffs seized about 1,000 pounds of marijuana at a Lincoln County farm. The pot was extremely high grade with a retail value of about $2 million.

From evidence secured in raids throughout Maine it's becoming clear that marijuana farming here is a fulltime occupation utilizing the latest agricultural techniques. Earlier this month police raided a farm in Belgrade and claim to have discovered a modern irrigation system linking more than 75 plots.

Increasingly, marijuana farmers are producing an extremely high-grade product, far higher in potency than the usual home-grown variety.

It's doubtful if growing marijuana in Maine has exceeded the smuggling of pot into the state (that continues to be a major enterprise), but the marked increase in marijuana farm busts makes clear that the state's problems with marijuana are increasing.

Aside from increased law enforcement, there seems little the state can do to attack the problem. The laws, which provide for a civil penalty for casual marijuana use but major penalties for possession of large amounts, seem adequate and reasonable.

Unhappily, there's big money to be made in smuggling and growing marijuana. And so long as the potential rewards are great, there will always be those willing to run the risk.

The Seattle Times
Seattle, WA, January 9, 1985

ACCORDING to the National Organization for the Reform of Marijuana Laws (NORML), marijuana grown illegally in the United States continued in 1984 to achieve increasing importance as a cash crop.

Marijuana farming last year, says NORML, produced a harvest worth an estimated $16.6 billion. If the figure is accurate, it means that marijuana crops now are worth considerably more than hay or soybeans (valued at about $11.5 billion each) and are approaching the $19.5 billion listed by the Department of Agriculture as the value of last year's national corn crop.

The federal Drug Enforcement Administration contends that NORML's figures are vastly exaggerated. More likely, the agency says, domestically grown marijuana is worth somewhere between $8 billion and $10 billion. Regardless of whose statistics are right, it's clear that homegrown marijuana is a huge and growing business.

One reason for the expansion of domestic growing operations is the high cost of varieties imported from places such as Colombia and Mexico, principal suppliers of the U.S. market.

Demand remains high despite persuasive medical evidence of a direct link between marijuana use and serious health problems, not to mention the drug's effect on behavior.

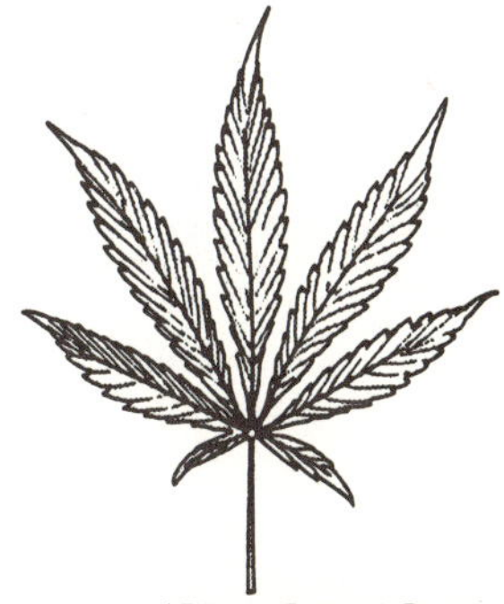
Editorial Research Reports

Leaders of NORML argue that the best hope of keeping marijuana out of the hands of adolescents lies in government regulation of its production and sale. That would amount to legalization, a step strongly opposed by law-enforcement officials.

But if the value of the domestic crop continues to rise, the case for legalization may well grow stronger on economic grounds. With harvests yielding billions of dollars, government regulation could produce huge tax revenues applicable to reduction of state and federal deficits.

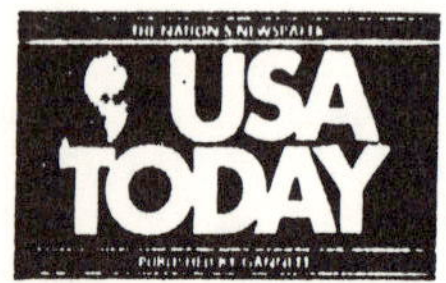

Washington, DC, August 9, 1985

They moved in on Monday, 2,200 strong — a joint effort by federal, state, and local law enforcement officials. It was the USA's biggest crackdown on marijuana growing.

This week, the task force destroyed 342,635 plants, some worth as much as $3,500 each.

So far, 175 people have been arrested. Authorities destroyed 20,000 plants in California and 40,000 in Michigan. In just one Ohio county, pot worth $2.6 million was found.

Led by U.S. Atty. Gen. Edwin Meese, authorities are trying to raise the risks and costs of growing pot — marijuana is now the nation's second biggest cash crop.

Some argue that these raids are just a publicity stunt, grandstanding that won't affect the marketing of marijuana. They say the only way the government can control the drug is to make it legal, and then regulate and tax it.

But legalizing marijuana would be a mistake.

That would send a clear signal to millions of people, including millions of teen-agers, that smoking dope is OK.

It isn't. On Thursday, two experts who've studied the drug reported that marijuana use among the USA's young is "a huge problem" responsible for a range of troubles, including moodiness, apathy, bad grades, and vandalism. They estimated that 130,000 high school seniors will get stoned every day in school this fall.

Those who want to legalize marijuana often minimize its health risks.

The surgeon general has said young people who use marijuana may disrupt the development of their nervous and reproductive systems. Researchers know marijuana contains a lung irritant linked to emphysema and a carcinogen linked to lung cancer. Its intoxicating element damages the liver, the lungs, and the brain.

All these chemicals stay in the body and accumulate. The damage adds up, from one marijuana cigarette to the next. Even so, some ignore the evidence — just as they ignore the surgeon general's findings about ordinary cigarettes.

Do we really want to make it legal for people to hurt themselves with yet another mind-altering drug?

Studies show that about 5 percent of high school seniors use marijuana — half the number who smoked in 1978. But what would happen to that welcome trend if we legalized pot? Its use would surely increase, and so would the damage it does.

If it were legal, marijuana would be merchandized and widely marketed, like soap or perfume or liquor. Young minds would soon see smoking dope as something "the beautiful people" do.

We have enough trouble with alcohol abuse and the damage it does. Do we really want another drug on the market that could destroy more lives?

Of course not. Legalizing marijuana is no way to win the war against drugs — it's the way to lose it.

THE DAILY OKLAHOMAN

Oklahoma City, OK, December 30, 1985

THE federal government is so big that sometimes it gets crosswise with itself. One agency may push a program that conflicts with official administration policy, and Congress may even pass laws that counteract each other.

One case in point is the tobacco subsidy offered by the Department of Agriculture, while the U.S. surgeon general warns of the link between cigarette smoking and lung cancer.

Another example surfaced in a ruling by the Internal Revenue Service that the National Organization for the Reform of Marijuana Laws is a "public charity." That means contributions to NORML's campaign to legalize pot are tax-deductible.

That, of course, runs directly counter to the Reagan administration's campaign against marijuana use. It also tends to undermine efforts by some congress-members, notably Oklahoma's Rep. Glenn English, to get the U.S. Drug Enforcement Administration to step up the war against marijuana growers.

Advocates of "decriminalizing" marijuana have contended no evidence exists that it causes permanent damage to the health of users. They have argued that, since so many Americans use pot, we might as well quit arresting them because that breeds disrespect for the law.

But for several years increasing scientific evidence has shown definite bad effects from long-term use of marijuana. The complicated chemical makeup of cannabis saliva, from which marijuana, hashish and hash oil are made, impairs the brain, reproductive systems, the lungs, body cells and the heart.

People who believe in NORML's aims have every right to contribute to the organization. But taxpayers in general should not be asked to subsidize efforts that run counter to official public policy and would be so destructive to the long-term health and welfare of the nation's young people.

THE COMMERCIAL APPEAL

Memphis, TN, July 29, 1986

THE National Organization for the Reform of Marijuana Laws (NORML) became known in the 1970s as an advocate for teenagers threatened by harsh prison sentences for possessing small quantities of marijuana. Now it has discovered a new clientele: big-time international cocaine dealers.

According to the Washington Monthly magazine, seminars in which high-priced lawyers share tips about how to defend drug smugglers and distributors now produce about one-third of NORML's budget.

The group's national director, Kevin Zeese, admits, "If I were to name one thing that really pulled NORML out of debt, it would be these drug defense seminars." A Key West conference last December attracted about 200 lawyers who paid $475 apiece.

Zeese claims, "The only way to stop drug traffickers is to legalize drugs. NORML wants to put the traffickers out of business." We reject that logic. Would deaths like that of Len Bias be less likely or less tragic if the substances that cause them were legal?

But even on its own terms, NORML's actions are inconsistent with its professed philosophy. If one sincerely believes that the way to stop the traffickers is to repeal narcotics laws, one should concentrate on just that rather than on helping individual traffickers stay out of jail.

That is why some of the organization's own veteran activists are now among its angriest critics. According to the Washington Monthly, they believe that by 1983 "NORML's lawyers were no longer in a position to change the drug laws since their livelihood depended on them."

NORML's new agenda is entirely legal: Every accused criminal, even the most repulsive, is entitled to a defense lawyer. But for the sake of honesty its leaders should drop their idealistic rhetoric.

The Augusta Chronicle

Augusta, GA, September 19, 1986

Richmond County has come a long way since 1976, when Commissioner Norman Simowitz, running for the state Senate, ran on a platform which included the legalization of marijuana!

On Wednesday, in the same chambers where Simowitz used to preside, three Republican County Commission candidates unveiled a bold, innovative local proposal to coincide with the national war on drugs.

Incumbent Jack Padgett Jr., along with Lee Neel III and Herb Beckham, are calling for the creation of a local drug "prevention and eradication" task force. Sheriff Charles Webster, they say, wholeheartedly endorses the idea.

Resources would be allocated, say Messrs. Padgett, Neel and Beckham, to assemble a team of experts who can look into the local drug problem and prepare an educational campaign. The ultimate goal: Fight the upsurge of illegal drug use, especially cocaine.

The task force would consist of four to five individuals with $100,000 to $125,000 allocated for salaries, and Padgett will propose adding the funds to the county's 1987 budget.

There is money currently available in county coffers for creating such a task force, and taxes need not be raised. Its creation should become a bipartisan concern.

The force would be a perfect entity for schools and other community groups to work with in battling drug pushers and combatting drug abuse.

The Register

Santa Ana, CA, January 14, 1986

Last week's announcement by the National Organization for the Reform of Marijuana Laws that what used to be called "the weed with roots in Hell" was the Number One cash crop grown in America last year should serve as a reminder of the futility of our current pogrom against marijuana growers.

The federal government, in combination with various state and local governments around the nation, spent millions of the taxpayers' dollars last year in an effort to eradicate the domestic marijuana crop. Law enforcement officers descended on rural areas in helicopters and military vehicles, wearing flak jackets, wielding M-16s, terrifying local populations — and for what?

The announcement by NORML suggests that they didn't even make a significant dent in the marijuana crop. The most significant accomplishments of the war on drugs included wholesale violation of the civil liberties of hundreds of rural residents, most of whom were innocent of any wrongdoing, and the diversion of law enforcement resources away from the investigation and prosecution of real crime.

Also, of course, the drug-enforcement officials earned salaries. This fact may help to explain the otherwise inexplicable passion with which the American people cling to their useless and counterproductive drug laws.

These laws may have little or no appreciable effect on the availability of drugs in our society. They may be utterly ineffective at achieving their goals of protecting us from drug-related crime and from drug-related threats to the public health. They may be counterproductive in the sense that they actually make matters worse than they would be otherwise. But there are at least two groups in the population who do benefit from these laws.

The first of these groups is organized crime, which enjoys what almost amounts to a government-protected monopoly in the drug field, and is enabled thereby to charge exorbitant monopoly prices for its products.

The second group is what Michael Sonnenreich, the former head of the National Institute on Drug Abuse, calls "the drug abuse industrial complex," the network of lawyers, doctors, psychologists, counselors, law enforcement professionals and corrections officials whose jobs depend on illegal drugs remaining illegal.

It is the drug-abuse industrial complex that lobbies most passionately and indefatigably for the preservation of our drug laws, and for constant increases in the resources we devote to the drug enforcement effort. It is the drug-abuse industrial complex that feeds the mass media the distortions, half-truths and outright lies about the effects of drugs on individuals and society that keep the public bamboozled into believing the war on drugs is worth fighting in the first place.

In fact, that war is not worth fighting. It is merely a pretext for unjustifiable government intrusions into our personal lives, a prescription for increasing instead of decreasing the problems caused by drug use, and a welfare program for professional meddlers who might otherwise be unemployed.

THE SACRAMENTO BEE

Sacramento, CA, August 4, 1986

There may be some law enforcement justification for the annual CAMP (Campaign Against Marijuana Planting) raids, scheduled to start today, into Northern California marijuana fields. But given the far more urgent and dangerous threat of cocaine, crack and the synthetic drugs being manufactured in this state, do those raids really represent the best use of already-scarce resources?

The CAMP raids, a paramilitary drive against marijuana fields, drying sheds and distribution points, involves state, federal and local agencies. It has a budget of nearly $3 million for personnel, helicopters, fixed-wing aircraft and other equipment. At $30,000 per person, that money would be sufficient to hire 100 full-time additional officers to go after the drug labs and distribution networks which, according state law enforcement officers, could — and should — be shut down if the investigatory resources were available.

There's no doubt that large-scale marijuana growing in California's northern counties has brought with it rural violence between competing distributors or against innocents — campers, hikers — who wander into those marijuana patches. Obviously, people legitimately using public lands should be protected and law enforcement affording such protection maintained. But what happens in a month in the marijuana fields hardly measures up to what occurs in a day in the drug wars on the streets of Oakland or Los Angeles. Nor are the collective medical dangers of the product remotely comparable to those of crack, cocaine, heroin and the synthetic drugs now on the market.

The promoters of CAMP talk about the large numbers of marijuana plants destroyed in past raids, but that probably does little more than raise the price a little in San Francisco and shift some of the business to an even tougher mob importing drugs from South America. Almost as perverse, the legitimate effort to dramatize the dangers of those things to the community is seriously undercut when major, well-publicized campaigns are being mounted against a drug that almost everyone acknowledges is far less of a hazard.

There appear to be signs that such concerns are now being voiced within the law enforcement community. The more quickly those concerns are translated into policy, the better. CAMP makes for nice publicity — now and then a public official can get his picture taken with a flak jacket marching into a marijuana patch. But in the context of a larger drug enforcement effort, it's probably a misplaced effort.

THE DENVER POST

Denver, CO, April 7, 1984

THE WASHINGTON Post, falling for yet another wild guess disguised as a statistic, recently reported a claim by the National Organization for the Reform of Marijuana Laws that the nation's illegal pot crop this year has a market value of $13.9 billion.

The article breathlessly noted that the figure would be enough to make marijuana "the No. 1 cash crop in American agriculture," surpassing corn sales of $13.4 billion. The comparison is silly, of course, since it pits the supposed retail or "street value" of the illegal weed against the wholesale corn price.

Still, it's obvious the government hasn't succeeded in shutting down the pot traffic by harassing the growers. The tongue in our cheek suggests it's time the government got really nasty with pot farmers — by trying to help them.

Government has been "helping" agriculture massively for 50 years — during which time the family farm has neared extinction.

Instead of spraying paraquat on marijuana patches, the U.S. Department of Agriculture should simply pay pot farmers not to grow pot, as it already pays dairy farmers not to milk their cows.

Maybe it could compensate the pot farmers for the pot they don't grow with the weed it seizes from smugglers. It could call such a program PIP, for "payment in pot."

But that's just the beginning. As a legal industry, the pot growers could be forced to run the full bureaucratic gantlet of OSHA, EPA, FDA, affirmative action, wage and hour laws, windfall profits, Social Security, IRS and the rest. A paltry $13.9 billion wouldn't feed those bureaucratic locusts for long.

Hurling the full firepower of federal benevolence into the war against pot would be reminiscent of that village in Vietnam. We could say we had to help the pot industry in order to destroy it.

THE ARIZONA REPUBLIC

Phoenix, AZ, August 7, 1985

IN saying that "those who choose to use a banned substance should accept the risk," U.S. Interior Secretary Donald Hodel makes a strong case for reconsidering the use of a weed-killer such as paraquat on marijuana fields on public lands.

While it might be argued that paraquat is controversial, so is marijuana. Its use — and abuse — has been the subject of many a debate.

There can be no argument, however, about the illegality of growing marijuana, and this is the point that Hodel stressed during a visit to Phoenix as part of a fact-finding tour of national parks in five Western states.

Hodel's comments came in connection with what lawmen called the first nationwide raid on marijuana growers. Dubbed "Delta 9" and coordinated by the federal Drug Enforcement Administration, the three-day effort resulted in the eradication of more than 100,000 cultivated marijuana plants across the country.

In Arizona, the search-and-destroy mission netted an estimated 440 plants, 400 of them along Clear Creek east of Camp Verde. The drive fell short of its goal of 1,000 plants, authorities said, largely because harvesters had beaten lawmen to another 400 plants near Snowflake.

The extent of the marijuana problem was shown when it was reported that U.S. marijuana growers harvested a record $16.6 billion worth of the drug in 1984, making it the nation's second most valuable agricultural product. Last year's corn crop was worth $19.5 billion, according to the U.S. Department of Agriculture.

Much of the marijuana is cultivated on public lands by growers who, with large illicit profits at stake, go so far as to rig booby traps and threaten visitors to national parks with bodily harm.

Cultivated plants aren't the only problem, though. In the course of the nationwide raid, it was reported that an estimated 7 million wild marijuana plants were discovered in northern Indiana, where they are said to be common.

The spraying of paraquat to eradicate marijuana in Georgia and Kentucky was halted in 1983 by a court order until paraquat's impact on the environment could be determined. Opponents of the spraying argued that paraquat affects other wildlife and foliage and poses a health hazard to marijuana smokers.

What about the hazard posed by smoking "untainted" marijuana that hasn't been treated with a herbicide such as paraquat? The drug hasn't exactly been given a clean bill of health.

U.S. Attorney General Edwin Meese accurately describes marijuana as "a gateway narcotic" that leads users to harder drugs.

If the United States ever hopes to close that gate, efforts to put marijuana growers out of business must be continued. A new look should be taken at the environmental impact of paraquat and the feasibility of using it or some other herbicide on marijuana fields.

As for the use of marijuana, its impact on society has been well documented.

the Charleston Gazette

Charleston, WV, August 16, 1985

THE average time for murderers to spend behind bars is four years, eight months, reports an article in *USA Today.* Rapists spend three years, six months, while those who are guilty of assault spend an average of two years, two months.

Contrast these terms spent in jail with the terms handed out to marijuana dealers and smugglers. The average sentence is 10 to 15 years and many convicted of crimes linked to narcotics and other drugs receive life sentences.

Some states, New York in particular, impose harsh sentences in hope they will serve to deter the dope pusher and discourage the illegal traffic.

But this is the stuff out of which opium dreams are made.

So long as the profits to be realized from sales of marijuana, cocaine, heroin and other mind bogglers are so huge, willing couriers and sellers will be found to accept the risks of apprehension, prosecution and imprisonment.

What law enforcement authorities ought to realize — and don't — is that more persons profit from the illicit drug traffic than are caught, convicted and put away.

What law enforcement authorities further ought to realize — and don't — is that the harder they make it for the drug traffic to flourish, the more the stuff will cost and the bigger the profits for everybody.

Every couple of years somebody in the Justice Department or the Federal Drug Administration gets a brilliant idea: crack down on drugs.

Forgotten is the crusade initiated three years earlier that deflated within less than six months.

Over the years these wars on drugs have had no impact on the amount of proscribed substances brought into the country. Had the wars been successful, they wouldn't have to be repeated every time some flea-brained sheriff or federal district attorney is stunned by the thought that he can achieve what nobody else has been able to achieve.

Is a solution to America's vast and continuing illegal drug problem available?

Probably not.

Societal problems, like drug addiction (which includes, let's not forget, alcoholism and dependency upon tobacco), syphilis, rabies, drunken driving, polluted streams and air, are neither readily nor easily resolved, and often when they are resolved, the determining agent was unrelated to the problem itself. Example: rabies, which had been a curse for human beings for centuries, ended when Louis Pasteur discovered a treatment for hydrophobia and subsequently a vaccine was perfected to inoculate animals against the deadly virus.

One tentative answer is the legalization or the decriminalization of all drugs, plus close supervision of drug addicts. Clearly profit must be removed from the manufacture of, the trade in and the sale of drugs, if society is to get a handle on the problem. The lone realistic way to accomplish this is through legalization.

The History of Cannabis in Medicine

Cannabis has been used medicinally for centuries. The earliest known written reference occurs in a Chinese pharmacological treatise dating from 2737 B.C. and attributed to the emperor Shen Nung who, according to tradition, was the first to teach his people the medicinal value of cannabis. The *United States Pharmacopeia* listed it as a recognized medicine in 1850 and it appeared in the list until 1942. During the latter half of the 19th century, American doctors used cannabis in the treatment of pain, convulsive disorders, hysteria, asthma, rheumitism and labor pains. Even Queen Victoria's personal physician prescribed it for a wide range of disorders and discomforts. Cannabis preparations were on the shelves of every pharmacy and were widely prescribed until medical use of the plant was prohibited in 1937. But in 1939 New York Mayor Fiorello La Guardia appointed a committee to study the use of marijuana, particularly in New York City. By 1944 the committee had cleared the drug of the "criminogenic" charge, testified to its relative harmlessness, negated the charge that its use might lead to the use of opiates and even suggested that it might be helpful in the detoxification of morphine addicts.

As of January 1987, 33 states had enacted legislation authorizing programs of legal access to tetrahydracanabinal (THC) for victims of cancer and glaucoma. Recently discovered possible medical applications of THC include relieving pressure on the eyeballs in the treatment of glaucoma, and opening constricted bronchial airways in the treatment of asthma. Its most widespread use has been as an antimimetic for the nausea of vomiting induced by chemotherapy. Cannabidolic acid, a cannabis alkaloid, is a topical antibiotic. Various studies have shown that while cannabis preparations tend to be unstable, vary greatly in strength, are insoluble in water and have an onset of action that is lower than other drugs, they have the advantage over other analgesics, hypnotics and sedatives in that they do not lead to the development of either physical dependence or tolerance; they have extraordinarily low toxicity and lead to no disturbance of vegetative functions. Furthermore, from what we know about other classes of drugs, it is altogether possible that when new congeners of the various cannibinol derivitives are developed—if indeed some have not already been—many or all of these problems will be overcome. Equally likely is the possibility that medical uses already known will be enhanced and new ones discovered.

Portland Press Herald
Portland, ME, August 16, 1983

Law enforcement agencies too often seem unable to to curb illegal street corner sale of marijuana. Yet ironically the federal government has been remarkably successful in preventing the legal use of marijuana for medical purposes.

Maine and a number of other states have approved laws permitting the legal use of marijuana to ease the suffering of cancer patients undergoing chemotherapy or for use as a treatment for glaucoma. But the laws are generally useless since it's all but impossible to obtain federal approval to use the drug.

The federal restrictions have literally forced some cancer patients to the streets to purchase pot in order to alleviate the side effects of chemotherapy. Not long ago a state legislator was forced to buy marijuana illegally in order to aid a cancer-ridden relative.

Given the abundance of medical evidence that marijuana has been found effective for cancer patients undergoing chemotherapy who do not respond to standard anti-emetics, as well as a treatment for glaucoma, it's small wonder that 54 House members have signed on as co-sponsors of a bill to ease federal restrictions on the medical use of marijuana.

Unhappily, the federal Drug Enforcement Administration opposes the bill on the grounds that the existing law already makes marijuana available. Technically, that may be true. But from a practical standpoint the red tape is virtually overwhelming. The application process may take months; that's too long for many sufferers to wait.

Any number of drugs, including all sorts of opium derivatives which are far more dangerous than marijuana, are now routinely administered by physicians. Considering the widespread illegal sale of pot, it's little short of cruel to unnecessarily withhold marijuana from those who would benefit from its legitimate medical use.

The Providence Journal
Providence, RI, August 18, 1983

Marijuana, in the view of some physicians, may have practical medical uses. It is said to benefit some people some of the time, principally those with glaucoma or who suffer severe nausea after taking anti-cancer drugs. It's logical that physicians should be allowed to prescribe marijuana under carefully controlled guidelines.

But the only legal way now permitted by federal drug authorities is so involved and time-consuming — the application for experimental use is 68 pages long — that few doctors are eager to put themselves and their patients through the fuss.

Admittedly, much still has to be learned about the therapeutic use of marijuana. It seems to work for some people while having no benefit for others.

Rep. Stewart B. McKinney, R-Conn., is convinced that federal restrictions deprive some likely beneficiaries of medical relief. He proposes to amend the Controlled Substances Act and let physicians write marijuana prescriptions for designated medical uses. Because these uses are still experimental, they would presumably be resorted to only when more orthodox therapy fails.

Mr. McKinney's bill, the first ever submitted on this topic, has drawn 54 co-sponsors. His argument is attractive and his measure deserves more than the cold rejection given by the Drug Enforcement Administration, which said that people can already get marijuana legally on an individual basis. Sure they can. In Rhode Island, their fate depends on a patient qualification review board set up by the Department of Health. In the program's first year, only 21 patients were allowed to receive marijuana — actually, a pill containing its active chemical ingredient, THC (tetrahydrocannabinol).

Mr. McKinney says the red tape is so restrictive that patients turn to illegal sources, sometimes on referral by the doctors themselves. This is a wholly absurd way of providing health care. The medical quality of marijuana acquired on the street is unknown; the ingredients are not measured and classified; and dangerous impurities may be present.

The congressman from Connecticut in no sense condones drug abuse or seeks to liberalize the use of marijuana as a "recreational" outlet. His bill is of limited application, is solely humanitarian and should be given thoughtful consideration.

San Francisco Chronicle

San Francisco, CA, August 16, 1983

IF A DOCTOR must fill out a 68-page application and send it along for approval by as many as five different government agencies in order to gain access to marijuana for medical research in relief of cancer patients, this government is running much too uptight in fear of criticism by anti-marijuana moralists.

Representative Stuart B. McKinney, R-Conn., is sponsor of a bill to enable doctors to prescribe marijuana to patients who are in need of the drug: it counters the nausea of chemotherapy and the pressures in the inner eye of glaucoma sufferers. How does the Reagan administration justify its opposition to opening up this legal access to marijuana, when it is so useful in making cancer therapy bearable? Current law classifies the drug as having "no accepted medical use," which is belied by merciful experience. McKinney's bill to open up marijuana for legal medical prescription to the legitimate needs of cancer and glaucoma victims should have Congress's consideration.

San Francisco, CA, March 27, 1986

TEN YEARS AGO, people would doubtless have scoffed at the idea that marijuana could be the source of physical and psychological damage. This weed was supposed to be a "natural" phenomenon, something grown in the bosom of the green earth — and so without the harmful effect of laboratory-created substances.

But the latest scientific report card on marijuana, particularly the potent strain resulting from more sophisticated growing techniques, is an ominous one. Dr. Sidney Cohen, a professor of psychiatry at UCLA, after a survey of the latest findings, has come to these cautionary conclusions:

The active ingredient in marijuana, known as tetrahydrocannabinol, or THC, causes changes in the reproductive systems of test animals; marijuana smoking amongst pregnant women can affect fetal development adversely; extensive lung damage has been documented in chronic smokers; THC has impaired the immune systems of test animals, and marijuana aggravates the problem of drunken driving.

GRANTED some researchers are reluctant to draw direct connections between animal studies and the effects on humans and say more human studies are needed. But because the effects of marijuana smoking are more subtle than other drugs, that kind of research can take years before it is conclusive.

These new studies constitute a warning bell that must be listened to. There is the potential for tragedy here.

The Seattle Times

Seattle, WA, March 16, 1984

A FEW years ago in Olympia, it was hard to find a legislator who would sanction the legal use of marijuana in easing the suffering of cancer and glaucoma patients. But then, that was in an era before state government had lapsed into its present almost-anything-goes approach to raising revenues.

In a state that now relies increasingly on booze and big-stakes gambling to help pay its bills — the Lottery Commission has just voted to go ahead with its get-rich-quick Lotto game (rich if you can beat the 1-in-3.8 million odds) — it was only natural that somebody would suggest taxing what may be one of the leading cash crops of all time, marijuana. A bill imposing a $20-an-ounce tax on the sale or use of pot and other illegal drugs got an amazingly big 35-10 vote in the Senate the other day.

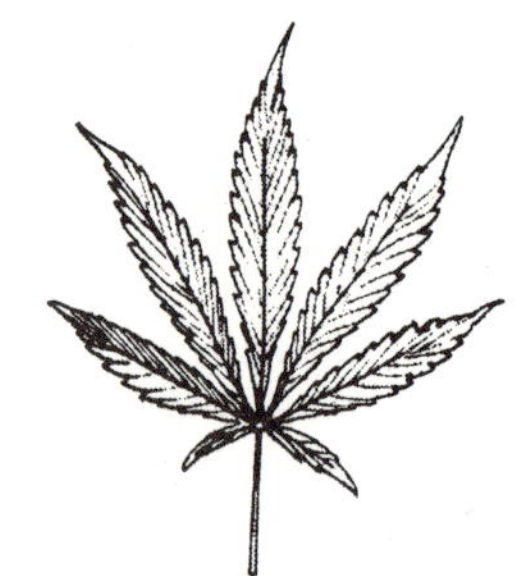

Editorial Research Reports

We can only guess what may be coming next. A state tax of some kind on prostitution?

Some who voted for the measure may have reasoned that there's not much difference between the state's cashing in on illegal drugs and its sales of other substances with an equal potential for harm through its monopoly liquor stores.

Yet the state got into the liquor business originally on the same premise that it is using in its proposal to tax marijuana — as a control measure. And few would argue that "control" of liquor here has curbed the rampant use and abuse of alcohol.

The Senate bill is, of course, bad business and ought to be killed outright. Noting that the measure in effect would surround illegal drugs with an aura of official recognition, Sen. Dan McDonald, R-Bellevue, put the issue in cogent perspective.

"This is a very cynical way to get at a real problem," McDonald said. "What will a kid think when a pusher comes around and shows him a joint with a Washington state tax stamp on it?"

Portland Press Herald

Portland, ME, September 24, 1983

The U.S. Constitution's guarantee of religious freedom doesn't give members of any church the right to break the law. That was decided by U.S. District Judge Edward T. Gignoux in the marijuana smuggling trial of an Ethiopian Zion Coptic Church member in Portland last year and reaffirmed this week by a jury in Springfield, Mass., following the trial of the same man on new pot charges.

The defendant, David Nissenbaum of Monson, Mass., was free on bail pending appeal of his five-year sentence in the Portland case when he was found guilty of marijuana trafficking, cultivating and possession in Springfield. In both cases, he argued that marijuana is a religious sacrament of the Coptics and that church members shouldn't be prosecuted for importing, growing or using the drug.

But Gignoux and the Massachusetts jury disagreed. Gignoux noted that the Constitution protects religious beliefs, but not religious practices, especially when those practices violate the law.

What if, for instance, a church wanted to revive the ancient religious practice of human sacrifice? Should church members be immune from prosecution on murder charges? Of course not.

Our laws are designed to preserve the public peace, health and safety. No one is exempt from obeying them in the name of religious freedom. If they were, the laws would be rendered meaningless.

Members of any church are free to believe whatever they wish. They are not, however, free to do whatever they wish when those actions are illegal and threaten the welfare of other segments of society.

EVENING EXPRESS
Portland, ME, August 31, 1983

It has now been five years since the Maine Legislature enacted a law which permits the prescribed use of marijuana for medical purposes. Many other states have passed similar laws.

It is a medically proven fact that marijuana is often effective in controlling the acute nausea that sometimes can make chemotherapy for cancer such an ordeal. The drug has also proved useful in delaying or preventing blindness in glaucoma cases.

Yet, patients who could find the drug useful as a treatment for the effects of these diseases continue to be denied access to legal marijuana. It is a cruel prohibition that cries for remedy.

The problem lies principally with the federal government which seems bent on erecting every sort of roadblock to the medical use of the drug.

The U.S. Drug Enforcement Administration, for example, is currently fighting against passage in Congress of a bill to ease federal restrictions on the use of marijuana for medical purposes. The DEA argues that the measure is unnecessary since laws already on the books make marijuana available to cancer patients and others.

But while that is true, the fact is government regulations are so restrictive as to make it virtually impossible for those who could be treated with the drug to obtain it readily.

It makes no sense. Physicians routinely prescribe drugs far more potent than marijuana to ease the suffering of their patients and to effect cures.

Considering the fact that illegal pot is readily available to millions of Americans on the street, it is absurd for federal bureaucrats seemingly to go out of their way to prevent its legal use by those who could truly benefit from the drug.

The Miami Herald
Miami, FL, August 25, 1983

CANCER is one of the ugly but widespread realities of our time. Chemotherapy treatment for it is ever more successful, but one unfortunate yet common side effect of that is a debilitating, persistent nausea.

Several studies show that a mild drug helps to counter and control the nausea accompanying chemotherapy. Unfortunately, Federal law prohibits doctors from prescribing this drug except under the most extraordinary circumstances.

The same mild drug has been proven to arrest the pressures in the inner eye caused by glaucoma, a disease that often leads to blindness. Like chemotherapy patients, however, those who suffer glaucoma are prohibited by Federal law from having access to this drug through routine medical prescription.

The drug in question ironically is easily obtained and popularly consumed in virtually every community in the nation — illegally. It is marijuana.

Rep. Stewart McKinney, a Republican from Connecticut, is sponsoring a bill in Congress that would permit doctors to prescribe the use of marijuana for limited medical purposes. His proposal is endorsed by 54 congressional co-sponsors, though the Reagan Administration opposes it.

The idea should become law. Medical doctors now are empowered to prescribe far-stronger drugs — morphine, for example. Morphine is a proven antidote to intense pain. Despite the danger of addiction, the law properly does not prohibit morphine use by doctors when, in accordance with accepted professional judgment, the drug is needed. The same rationale should apply to marijuana. Or to heroin or any other scientifically proven drug, for that matter. Hostility and fear generated by *abuse* of a drug should not result in punishment of seriously ill patients who would benefit from its properties.

Obviously, any law that would legalize any use of such drugs must be drawn rigorously to avoid unintended distribution of the substances. In addition, before marijuana can be prescribed, it must be produced under lab conditions that comply with the procedural safeguards enforced by the Food and Drug Administration. Medically prescribed use of marijuana should of course be governed by the rules that apply to other prescription drugs that hold the potential for abuse.

The law should not stand between medical knowledge and its ability to ease illness and pain, however. Mr. McKinney's humane bill deserves to become Federal law.

Newsday
Long Island, NY, August 21, 1983

If marijuana can help cancer patients overcome the extreme nausea associated with chemotherapy, why shouldn't doctors be readily able to prescribe it?

And why shouldn't marijuana and its derivatives be available to glaucoma victims if it can help preserve their eyesight?

Part of the reason is marijuana's classification in federal law as a Schedule I drug, one of "no accepted medical use." The classification is plainly wrong.

A variety of studies have established that marijuana has at least some medical usefulness in treating cancer and glaucoma patients, even if it is not the drug of choice for everyone.

No one says marijuana is a panacea, and not everybody likes it. It may carry as much risk to the heart and lungs as tobacco and may produce as much disorientation as alcohol. But those are not sufficient reasons to keep it entirely off limits. All medications have potentially harmful side effects; physicians must always weigh deficits against benefits.

Those benefits have received enough recognition to warrant reclassifying marijuana as a Schedule II drug, one with a high potential for abuse but for "currently accepted medical use with severe restrictions."

Marijuana is already available in some places for the technical purpose of research. Twelve hospitals in New York State are allowed to dispense marijuana on a limited and experimental basis. But for most cancer and glaucoma patients, it's legally beyond reach.

An effort to ease current restrictions and allow marijuana to be prescribed for limited medical uses is under way in Congress, and it deserves support. The bill's sponsor, Rep. Stuart McKinney (R.-Conn.), argues that "kids can get this stuff readily on the street corner and people who really need it can't get it if they want to stay within the law."

Sick people shouldn't be denied medicine their doctors feel they need, and they shouldn't have to go to pushers to get it.

Medical Uses of Heroin Debated

Heroin is a central nervous system depressant which also relieves pain. Developed in 1898 by the Bayer Company in Germany, it was originally considered a better analgesic than morphine, a more efficient cough suppressant and a nonaddictive cure for morphine and opium withdrawal symptoms. It took some 12 years for the medical profession to realize that heroin was at least as addictive as morphine. The Harrison Narcotic Act of 1914 was the first attempt to control the medicinal use of heroin. Its manufacture in the United States was prohibited and law enforcement agencies were made responsible for its control by 1924. The dangers involved in heroin use became recognized worldwide; by 1963 heroin was used medically in only five countries and manufactured legally in only three.

But, as heroin was replacing morphine and opium on the street and the international black-market, with underground laboratories and well-organized operations, grew rapidly, the medical uses of heroin were ignored and even shunned. The United States House of Representatives September 19, 1984 rejected a measure that would have permitted physicians to prescribe heroin to ease the pain of terminally ill cancer patients. The bill was defeated by a vote of 355 to 55 after an emotional debate. Opponents, including the Reagan Administration and the American Medical Association, argued that the heroin would be diverted for illegal use and that recently approved painkilling drugs were as effective as heroin. They also suggested that the measure would send the wrong message to domestic drug abusers and foreign drug suppliers. Sponsor Henry Waxman (D, Calif.) and other proponents of the bill argued that alternatives to heroin were not as effective as claimed. Many cited personal experiences with cancer victims who had died in great pain. Supporters also said that the amount to be used in the proposed program—about 15 pounds (7 kilograms) a year—would be too small to pose a law enforcement problem. They also pointed out that Great Britain and many other nations had long permitted the use of heroin for terminally ill patients.

According to a National Institute of Health panel in May 1986, patients suffering from pain were likely to be treated with either too much or too little medication. According to the experts, cancer patients or post-surgery patients often did not get enough painkillers, while victims of chronic pain frequently ran a risk of addiction from too-lavish dosages. No firm count was given of all people affected, but one panelist said up to five million post-surgery patients might receive too little medication. The panel called for more research in fighting pain and for better programs to teach pain management to health professionals. It also endorsed pain-fighting techniques that did not use drugs, such as physical therapy, relaxation techniques and biofeedback.

The Detroit News

Detroit, MI, February 11, 1983

Once again, Congress has before it a bill to allow physicians to administer heroin to terminal cancer patients who suffer intractable pain.

There are several thousand cancer patients who will die this year after suffering terribly. Heroin is the most effective pain reliever available. Yet physicians are forbidden to prescribe it. The basis for the prohibition is the drug's addictive quality, and the danger that it may be diverted from medical use to the streets.

It is true that heroin is ordinarily an appalling blight not only on the lives of those who become addicted, but also on the lives of those who may be victimized by the crimes of addicts. Government has a legitimate interest in limiting heroin's use.

But surely the *one* circumstance in which the drug has a positive value ought to be recognized by law. Heroin's addictive quality is of no consequence to a dying patient. And the danger of diversion is rather a red herring considering the current availability of the drug on the streets.

Other controlled substances are routinely dispensed through hospital pharmacies, and diversion doesn't seem to be an insuperable problem. Heroin is available for cancer patients in several other nations.

Terminal cancer patients are not a large constituency, but one of the marks of a humane society is concern for the special needs of small groups. This bill rates prompt enactment into law.

DESERET NEWS

Salt Lake City, UT, January 9-10, 1984

Should doctors be allowed to prescribe heroin as a pain reliever for dying cancer patients?

Because heroin has such negative connotations, the first knee-jerk reaction is to reject anything to do with the illegal drug. Yet the issue deserves a closer look.

The question keeps coming up nearly every year as bills are introduced in Congress to legalize this strictly limited use of the drug. But they fail to make much progress because of opposition by various medical and drug groups.

A measure now in Congress seeks to authorize the Department of Health and Human Services to set up demonstration programs using heroin with terminal cancer patients who aren't helped by other drugs.

Such a research program ought to be allowed simply on humanitarian grounds. An estimated 8,000 cancer patients die in agony each year because morphine and other pain-relievers are ineffective for them.

The argument for heroin is that it is more potent and more easily administered than morphine and has fewer unpleasant side effects.

A Utah doctor who deals often with terminal cancer patients said heroin produces euphoria, which could be a great help to many dying patients who are sick and miserable even while being kept pain-free with the usual drugs.

And while heroin is powerfully addictive, that is hardly a concern where someone is dying and needs relief from pain.

Some opposition has come from the American Medical Association, claiming that heroin is no more effective than other drugs, such as morphine. But the AMA objections appear to be based more on the reputation of heroin as an illegal drug than on significant medical reasons.

Doctors in at least 39 other countries do not agree with the AMA stand. In those places, including such nations as Britain, heroin is routinely used to relieve pain of terminally-ill patients, usually cancer victims.

Certainly, tight controls would have to be applied to any heroin use, and agreements reached on what constitutes a "terminal" patient. But a pilot program to test the drug's effectiveness deserves a chance.

The Washington Post
Times Herald

Washington, DC, March 26, 1984

CHANCES are that Congress won't accomplish much in this presidential election year, but there is one piece of business that it should not fail to complete. It should pass legislation—with an impressive and growing bipartisan list of sponsors in both houses—that would legalize the carefully controlled use of heroin in the treatment of cancer patients dying in intractable pain.

One of the curiosities of medical practice in this country is that hundreds of billions are spent to prolong life, but relatively little attention is paid to making sure that patients survive in a tolerable degree of comfort and alertness. Modern medicine keeps promising better painkillers, and new methods of administration may offer patients more continuous relief from currently available drugs. But—as experts testifying recently before Chairman Henry Waxman's health subcommittee strongly asserted—many patients now die in needless agony because they are denied access to heroin, the one drug that could relieve their pain.

Heroin has come into increasing use as a painkiller in Great Britain in recent years because of its demonstrated superiority in treating certain cancer patients. Heroin acts faster than morphine and other widely used painkillers, and it can also be administered in smaller doses—an important consideration in treating emaciated patients. Moreover, unlike other potent drugs, it does not make the patient comatose, depressed, nauseous or hallucinatory. As a result, patients are able to remain alert, communicate with other family members and, because anxiety and depression are relieved, may also live longer.

Heroin was banned from medical practice in this country in 1924 because of fears that it would be diverted to illegal street use—an unwarranted fear that still motivates opponents of the proposed legislation. Since only very small quantities of the drug would have to be kept by hospitals—most cancer patients do not suffer intractable pain—the same precautions used to guard other street-valuable drugs would be adequate to prevent misuse. To be on the safe side the proposed legislation adds still further controls.

Right now hundreds, perhaps thousands, of cancer patients are racked with pain while their families watch in despair. In testifying before the Waxman committee, Dr. Allen Mondzac, chairman of the D.C. Medical Society's Cancer Committee, noted that "right now, in America, we know of a drug which is the most potent, effective, soluble and rapidly active narcotic ever created. It is not available. I do not understand this." Neither do we.

THE MILWAUKEE JOURNAL

Milwaukee, WI, September 9, 1984

Heroin: The word is synonymous with ravaged lives, crime and social decay. So sinister is heroin's reputation that the drug is not legally available for a legitimate, humane purpose: relieving pain among terminal cancer patients.

Rep. Henry Waxman (D-Calif.) has introduced legislation allowing doctors to prescribe heroin for dying cancer patients when conventional pain remedies are ineffective. The measure, which will come up for a vote in the House soon, deserves to pass. It offers a compassionate, socially responsible way to ease the agony of people for whom drug dependency is not an issue.

Opponents, including the Reagan administration, fear that even limited authorization of heroin will encourage its abuse. But the Waxman bill sets up a system of strict safeguards. For example, the drug would be stocked only by a limited number of hospital pharmacies and hospices. In Great Britain, which has a similar system for distribution of heroin to the terminally ill, theft is not a problem.

The Waxman bill envisions a trial period of four years and calls for a review of heroin use every three months. That approach strikes a sensitive balance between two valid interests: protecting society and relieving human suffering.

The Wichita Eagle-Beacon

Wichita, KS, April 12, 1984

Mention of daily use of heroin almost inevitably conjures up images of pain and suffering. But ironically, there is a context in which heroin is not a causative factor, but can be an alleviating one. Even heroin, the prototypical scourge of drug addiction, may have a beneficial purpose in some instances.

That is so in the easing of intractable pain for terminally ill cancer patients — patients whose suffering may be so intense that no other analgesic drug will make it tolerable. None of the prospects associated with inevitable death are pleasant to contemplate. But prolonged agony should not be one of them, if there are means available to counteract it.

Those means are available in Britain, where the hospice movement has helped cultivate more reasonable, realistic attitudes toward coping with impending death. Heroin treatments of patients in extreme pain, unable to swallow other types of medicine, supplanted morphine treatments several years ago. Such treatments are not yet approved in the United States. Bills have been introduced in both houses of Congress that would legalize the limited use of heroin in such unfortunate circumstances.

The question of narcotic addiction becomes a moot point in those cases. Certainly, one can't assail the prescription of heroin to ease insufferable pain as drug "abuse." Rather, that represents probably the only positive use to which this drug, which has degraded and ruined so many lives, can appropriately be put: to make those whose lives are coming to an end comfortable in their final days.

The Augusta Chronicle

Augusta, GA, July 25, 1984

The medical benefit of heroin as a pain reliever for terminally ill cancer patients is not clear. Some studies conclude that other, more conventional drugs do the job as well; others, that heroin indeed blunts agony more effectively. In any case, Congress should approve pending legislation (H.R. 5290) making injectible heroin available to some hospitals.

There are simply more good arguments for approval than against. Heroin is not, say, laetrile. Its narcotic properties are indisputable, and it would not seduce patients from legitimate treatment. The only persons for whom it would be prescribed would be, sadly, those near death. What harm could it do?

It is hard to believe, too, that heroin would not be the best pain-deadener for at least some patients. Everyone is physiologically and psychologically unique. Drug A may work better on Mr. Smith, Drug B on Mr. Jones. Those in intractable pain should have as wide a narcotic variety as possible. (Some physicians, skeptical of the heroin option, point out that a neurologist can snip a nerve if things get horrible. Often, however, that means paralysis, and many patients understandably want to depart this life "whole.")

Moreover, as columnist William Buckley Jr. has written, heroin is now available only to those who abuse it. It is ironic that on many inner-city streets today, slimy little pushers are selling a few minutes of euphoria to junkies, while doctors and nurses can't impart the same sensation to writhing cancer victims. Shouldn't this be changed?

Painful death is a universal possibility. Science has a limited power to mitigate that circumstance. Science has been put to far worse uses.

Richmond Times-Dispatch
Richmond, VA, April 13, 1984

For seven years, the National Committee on the Treatment of Intractable Pain has urged Congress to pass a bill allowing the use of heroin for dying cancer patients whose horrible, body-wracking pains cannot be relieved by medicines currently available to hospital pharmacies and physicians. For seven years, the cautious instincts of politicians have prevailed and the pleadings of this private organization composed of medical personnel and other professionals, as well as cancer patients and their families, have gone unheeded.

Amazingly enough, however, a bill authorizing the medicinal use of heroin under tightly controlled conditions has reached first base in Congress during this presidential election year, when politicians normally are cautious to a fault. Sponsored by Rep. Henry A. Waxman, D-Calif., the "Compassionate Pain Relief Act" won unanimous approval of the health subcommittee of the House Energy and Commerce Committee March 21 and was reported to the House floor without objection April 5 by the full committee. (Third District Rep. Thomas J. Bliley Jr. of Richmond is among the co-sponsors.) A "historic first" is how Judith Quattlebaum, the national committee's president, views the legislation's emergence, at long last, from a committee. Hawaii Sen. Daniel K. Inouye, a Democrat, has a companion bill with 19 co-sponsors, one of whom is Virginia Sen. John W. Warner, a Republican.

Despite bipartisan support, getting this controversial legislation through a campaign-conscious Congress against such formidable opponents as the Reagan administration and the American Medical Association will be no cinch. But were this to occur, it would be a wonderful thing for some 8,000 to 40,000 terminally ill cancer patients whose pains are not relieved by other drugs. In the name of mercy, it ought to happen. And soon.

For the past 60 years since heroin was outlawed for medical use in the United States, most physicians have relied on morphine to relieve intractable pain. But increasingly massive amounts of morphine are required for some patients, and the injections themselves only add to the extreme pain. Heroin, which is derived from morphine, has the advantage of being water-soluble and more potent; it can be administered in smaller doses. It also conveys to the dying patient a feeling of well-being. The experience in Britain, one of 47 countries where medicinal use of heroin is legal, has been that the mind of the cancer victim remains alert enough to work crossword puzzles, and that as late as the day before death, the patient is able to converse coherently with his family, Ms. Quattlebaum informs us.

Street heroin has wrecked countless lives, and the federal government is right to fight the illicit trade relentlessly. But fears that medicinal heroin will wind up adding to woes in the street do not appear to be rationally based. Little diversion from hospitals has been reported in Britain, and the Waxman bill lays down even stricter conditions than exist there. And even if every single ounce of medicinal heroin were somehow to be re-routed to the streets, it has been estimated that the illicit volume would expand by only 2.8 percent.

That threat's not nearly large enough to justify withholding this possibility of blessed relief from people who are dying in terrible pain. Washington ought to muster enough election-year political courage to pass this humanitarian measure.

THE INDIANAPOLIS NEWS
Indianapolis, IN, April 20, 1984

The use of heroin for special pain relief is drawing more support in Congress.

Legislation to provide the drug for terminally ill cancer patients has been passed by the House Energy and Commerce Committee and now goes before the entire House of Representatives.

Sponsored by Rep. Henry Waxman, D-Calif., the bill would authorize the secretary of health and human services to set up a four-year pilot program. The drug would be provided only through a doctor's prescription, through hospital and hospice pharmacies.

The Reagan administration and the American Medical Association oppose the proposal, partly out of fears about the potential abuse of the program, as well as the addictive nature of heroin.

The trouble with those fears is that heroin is already very available on the street corners of most American cities. Opposing this measure won't stop the illegal heroin trade; approval of the bill can hardly add to the already abundant traffic.

Support for the principle behind this legislation can be found in interesting places, including the Bible, in the book of Proverbs. Kings are told not to drink beer and wine, "lest they drink and forget what the law decrees, and deprive all the oppressed of their rights."

But those who are close to death should be given pain relief: "Give beer to those who are perishing, wine to those who are in anguish; let them drink and forget their poverty and remember their misery no more."

Waxman's bill ought to be approved by the House of Representatives. And the Reagan administration should drop its opposition to this sensible proposal.

THE SAGINAW NEWS
Saginaw, MI, November 20, 1984

A great deal can be done to relieve the dying, those who have no hope of recovery, and are in horrible pain.

Doctors and nurses, hospices, friends and family care.

But does Congress?

Too many of its members seem to care more about the political effect of spurious arguments that easing the agony of the terminally ill will somehow damage society at large.

Just before adjournment for the campaign, the U.S. House voted, 355-55, to deny the legal prescription of heroin for the dying. The arguments of compassion failed against the fears of lawmakers from drug-abuse centers such as Florida and Harlem that hospital heroin would somehow spread drugs to the streets.

Maybe the fears are justified. Those areas have done little to control a trade which has made too many "investors" filthy — and we use the word advisedly — rich.

But the National Committee for the Treatment of Intractable Pain, many of whose members have watched loved ones suffer without relief, has effectively met every argument during its 10-year battle. Yet it has, for the time being, lost again.

Maybe it's too much to expect people up for election to vote for anything smacking of approval of heroin use. So for a while longer, the desperately sick will be denied a substance which, however subversive for the young and living, could ease their passing.

It's not a pretty topic. Even the American Medical Association opposes this one legalized use of heroin. It may be that doctors fear that if the drug does find its way into the streets, they would be blamed.

But the American Nursing Association supports it. Surely safeguards can be worked out. Surely hospitals can control distribution. Most surely of all, we should do whatever is necessary to comfort the dying in their final moments.

England and many other civilized nations accept that humanistic principle. The Canadian Medical Association has called for restoring medicinal use of heroin. Can it be that national drug abuse has so anesthetized our own sensibilities that we cannot see any legitimate use for drugs?

So much more the reason to get rid of the cocaine and heroin peddlers.

In the meantime, a new Congress may finally grant that the dying need not suffer quite so much, and approve the Compassionate Pain Relief Act — for pure mercy's sake.

THE INDIANAPOLIS NEWS
Indianapolis, IN, March 24, 1984

Pain relief for terminally ill cancer patients is the objective of sensible legislation recently approved by a subcommittee in Congress.

The bill, sponsored by Rep. Henry Waxman, D-Calif., would allow heroin to be used for pain relief for patients in severe pain.

Approved by the House Energy and Commerce's Health Subcommittee, the legislation would provide a strictly monitored five-year program to dispense heroin for cancer victims. A patient's doctor could prescribe the drug, but a hospital medical review board must also approve the prescription. The heroin would be provided through supplies confiscated by the government.

The idea has gained support from the experience of 47 other countries, where heroin is used for this pain-killing purpose, and not just for cancer patients. The legislation in Congress would limit its use to cancer alone.

The proposal in Congress has been opposed by the Reagan administration and the American Medical Association. One of the main fears, of course, is that heroin is addictive and harmful.

But it's also readily available on the street corners of many American cities. Legalizing it for limited pain-killing purposes is not going to create any boom in the heroin traffic in the United States. Opposing this measure will do nothing to slow down this traffic.

As columnist William Buckley Jr. has noted: "The irony is that anybody in a major city can acquire the knowledge necessary to buy heroin from a dirty little pimp, but licensed doctors may not administer the identical drug to men and women — and children — literally dying from excruciating pain."

The Reagan administration would do well to back off from its shortsighted opposition to this measure. And Congress should move ahead to approve it.

THE RICHMOND NEWS LEADER
Richmond, VA, March 30, 1984

For 60 years, the American medical profession has been denied the legal use of one of the most potent painkillers known to man: heroin. In 1924, to reduce heroin addiction on the streets, heroin was banished from the list of legal drugs.

Since then, the incidence of certain kinds of cancer has grown, but doctors have not been able to use heroin to ease the suffering of their patients. For seven years, various groups — notably the National Committee on the Treatment of Intractable Pain — have tried to win congressional approval for the use of heroin under carefully controlled conditions. But Congress has been reluctant to act, (a) fearing that legalized heroin would increase illegal drug traffic and (b) hesitating to approve the use of a drug known to be highly addictive.

A few days ago, a House health subcommittee unanimously approved a bill to permit the use of heroin for cancer patients in a five-year program subject to numerous safeguards. The measure enjoys bipartisan support in both houses, and the outlook for passage this year may be good — despite opposition from the Reagan administration and the American Medical Association. Apparently growing concern for the 8,000 or more Americans who suffer intractable pain during terminal cancer each year is providing momentum for a bill that should provoke little controversy.

One doctor says, "We know of a drug which is the most potent, effective, soluble, and rapidly active narcotic ever created. It is not available. I do not understand this." He is not alone. Heroin is used routinely in almost 50 other countries to treat intractable pain. It makes little sense to worry about heroin addiction for a cancer patient in agony. The small amounts needed to treat them do not threaten a huge explosion in heroin trafficking. Illegal heroin is readily available to addicts on the streets now, while cancer patients who would benefit from it are denied its legal use.

Some doctors believe other painkillers can be equally effective, although heroin does not cause many of the virulent side-effects of some of the stronger narcotics. Heroin does not put a patient in a stupor or render him a vegetable in his final days. It permits him relief not only from pain, but also from anxiety, and allows him some dignity in dying. Anyone who read the late Stewart Alsop's vivid and depressing description of the pain suffered by his fellow patients in a cancer ward must wonder why doctors should be denied the use of a highly effective drug to ease such suffering.

Modern medicine in recent years may have made quantum leaps in cancer treatment, but many Americans still die in needless pain from cancer that can be neither treated nor cured. The U.S. seems to be held in thrall to a baseless fear about the use of a "bad" drug for a humanitarian purpose. Marijuana — which also has medicinal benefits for some conditions — suffers from the same reluctance to admit that some "bad" drugs may be put to good use.

All doctors may not choose heroin as a drug in easing pain for cancer patients, but certainly heroin ought to be available as an option if other drugs fail. The House subcommittee has taken a constructive step in advancing heroin toward legal use under narrowly defined circumstances. Now both the House and Senate can stop dissembling about drug addiction and illegal drug traffic, and follow suit.

The Pittsburgh PRESS
Pittsburgh, PA, March 16, 1984

The medical establishment in the United States apparently believes something that its counterparts in some 39 other countries do not: Heroin has no therapeutic value.

In these other countries, heroin is widely used to relieve intractable pain in dying patients, especially cancer victims.

Doctors in Britain may prescribe heroin not only to treat cancer but also for heart attacks, pain after surgery, childbirth, severe burns and other injuries, and even to maintain drug addicts.

Few people in this country advocate such liberal use of this powerful drug. But surely there is a case to be made for utilizing it to ease the last days of terminally ill cancer patients.

Yet year after year, bills to legalize this severely limited medical use of heroin have languished in Congress.

The American Medical Association says that heroin is no more effective than other available drugs, such as morphine. The National Institute of Drug Abuse opposes heroin because of its "addiction potential." Pharmacists are afraid that legalized heroin would fall into the wrong hands.

The addiction argument is ridiculous in view of the fact that we are talking about dying people. The safeguarding of hospital supplies of heroin should be no more a problem than with any other drug used in illegal traffic.

As for the AMA's position, morphine and other pain-relievers are ineffective in as many as 8,000 cancer victims who die each year.

Heroin, a derivative of morphine, is more potent and more easily administered than morphine and has fewer unpleasant side effects.

A bill now in Congress would authorize the Department of Health and Human Services to set up demonstration programs for cancer patients who aren't helped by currently available drugs. The heroin would come from illegal supplies seized by drug enforcement agencies.

We can't think of anything that would better qualify as a "human service" than diminishing the pain of cancer patients, as well as that of their loved ones who must watch them suffer.

'Designer' Drugs Hearings Held

The Senate Budget Committee September 18, 1985 held hearings on the phenomenon of so-called "designer" drugs. Committee member Lawton Chiles (D, Fla.) declared that the custom-made narcotics threatened to "revolutionize the way drugs are used and sold in our country." Chemists designed the drugs to have much the same properties as illegal narcotics but subtly different chemical structures. The chemical differences would be enough to evade the law, since banned drugs were legally defined by their chemical structure. Committee witnesses testified that the drugs could be made at low cost and in massive quantities by using readily available chemicals and equipment. Designer drugs had been the subject of many news stories. Most of the drugs were said to be used by heroin addicts and to have been derived from fentanyl, a surgical anesthetic. Fentanyl is about one hundred times more potent than morphine. One such variant was reported to be 3,000 times stronger than heroin. It is usually used intravenously as a preoperative anesthetic, for brief anesthesia or for post-operative pain. In terms of drug abuse, anesthesiologists and nurse anesthetists have been known to self-administer the drug to provide sedation and sleep. Compulsive use can become a possibility. Fentanyl is also the basis for the manufacture of "China White," a slang term for a designer drug. Because of its potency, overdose is a possibility. Other designer drugs include an imitation of the painkiller Demerol. Several of its users were reported to have lost motorcontrol, their symptoms resembling those of advanced Parkinson's disease. Creation of designer drugs was said to date from 1979 or 1980 and to be concentrated in California. Officials in that state said 87 of 90 reported deaths linked to the drug occurred there.

Houston Chronicle

Houston, TX, December 30, 1985

The Senate has approved and sent to the House legislation that would close the loophole in drug laws that permits producers of so-called "designer drugs" to spread their mischief around at a lucrative profit while escaping, at least temporarily, the penalties that threaten peddlers of regulated drugs.

These "designer drugs," created by underground chemists, are meant to provide the effect of regulated drugs and are extremely dangerous because of the unknowns involved. The legislation would make it easier to prosecute those who make and sell "designer drugs."

Sen. Strom Thurmond, R-S.C., who introduced the bill, called the unregulated drugs "a frightening and eminent threat" to society, and he is right. These made-to-order drugs have been involved in some bizarre incidents, and their profitability assures their spread if strict laws are not passed to control them.

The Des Moines Register

Des Moines, IA, July 15, 1985

A new California fad that, like others have done, seems to be spreading eastward, is the creation and use of "designer drugs."

This is the name given to chemical formulations that produce about the same effects as heroin, cocaine and other illegal drugs but are beyond reach of narcotics laws because these laws define controlled substances by their molecular structure, and the "designer drugs" have a slightly different mix of molecules than the drugs they mimic.

Not only are they not illegal, but some of them appear to be more dangerous than the originals. Many are easily compounded by anyone with a fair working knowledge of chemistry, with rather inexpensive equipment, and from fairly easily obtainable raw materials. They often can be altered to keep them ahead of any additions to the drug laws.

Legislation has been introduced in Congress, with the backing of the Reagan administration, to ban, not only the specifically defined drugs banned by the Controlled Substances Act, but drugs designed to produce similar physical or psychological effects.

It is questionable how effective existing drug laws are. Moreover, a case can be made that, just as adults are free to exercise their own judgment about using such "respectable" but harmful substances as alcohol and tobacco, the government ought not try to tell them they can't use other things that make one feel good but harm the mind or body.

But as long as there are legal efforts to control such drugs, it makes sense to amend the law in such a way as to get them all.

The Courier-Journal

Louisville, KY, August 4, 1985

"DESIGNER DRUGS" — the legal chemical relatives of illegal substances — have much in common with the ever-changing chameleon. Just as those lizards alter their colors to evade predators, so have chemists kept one step ahead of the law by making minor changes in their concoctions. Such trickery couldn't be used to skirt the law if Congress were to enact a proposed ban on production and distribution of these drugs.

So far, law enforcement officials have been engaged in a losing battle against designer drugs. Underground chemists can produce potent and previously unknown drugs as quickly as the government can outlaw them. Minor changes in molecular structure can render an illegal substance legal.

The proposed law would eliminate the need to scramble to implement an emergency ban, like the one that took effect July 1 for the hallucinogen called "Ecstasy," every time some chemist changes a molecule. That process can take up to three months. Instead, the law would ban the production or distribution of substances that are similar in structure or effect to drugs already prohibited by the Federal Controlled Substances Act.

The proposal, as a Drug Enforcement Administration official acknowledged, is headed into uncharted legal territory. Drug laws usually must define precisely what is being prohibited, so it is uncertain how judges would rule on legal challenges to legislation that banned substances not even invented yet.

But there's good reason for a degree of vagueness in the law: This approach may be the only effective way to stop makers of these substances from avoiding prosecution by constantly altering their formulas. And even though useful therapeutic benefits are attributed to some designer drugs, such affects in a few cases seem to be outweighed by the harm caused in many more.

For instance, synthetic heroin, used by an estimated 20 percent of California's 100,000 heroin addicts, can be 3,000 times stronger than the real thing and pack an especially deadly punch when used by novices. Users of one variety of synthetic heroin have developed Parkinson's disease, a malady characterized by tremors and paralysis, and brain damage. In one study, the drug MDA caused a 40 percent reduction of activity in certain brain cells two weeks after it was used.

Besides hurting individuals, drug use takes a toll on society by reduced efficiency in the workplace, costly medical treatment and crime.

Use of these substances can't be effectively combatted as long as tinkering with a few molecules can produce a new, equally potent variation that is above the law. The Justice Department's plan is a wise strategy for this new front in the war against drugs.

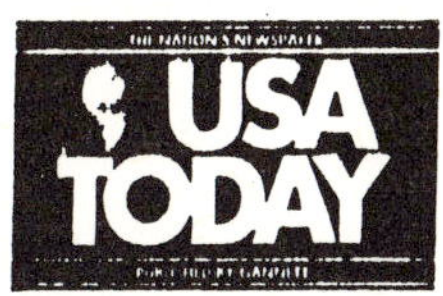

Washington, DC, July 29, 1985

Kim Romero's arms and legs are stiff and painful. She tires easily and mumbles. She has all the symptoms of Parkinson's disease. But she's a victim of "designer drugs."

Three years ago, the Watsonville bookkeeper and six other Californians took MPTP, a deadly copy-cat drug that looks, sells, and feels like heroin, but packs thousands of times the punch.

In a way, these seven are lucky. Sometimes, designer drugs kill.

More than 100 users have died since 1979 from MPTP and other "designer drugs." Doctors are watching at least 200 drug users for symptons of Parkinson's disease.

So far, designer drugs have been more prevalent on the West Coast. But law enforcement authorities — who have enough trouble dealing with drugs being smuggled into the USA — fear the homespun chemicals will spread east.

Their fear is well-founded.

A basement entrepreneur can make a $2 million batch of designer heroin by buying $500 in chemicals. All he does is tinker with the molecular makeup of a common surgical anesthetic. By the time law officers make that illegal, he has altered the formula again.

Authorities have been fighting a losing battle against these copy-cat drugs. They need all the help they can get. A newly introduced Senate bill — backed by the Justice Department — could provide one more weapon by outlawing the manufacture, distribution, or possesssion of designer drugs.

Critics say the legislation is too broad, that you can't outlaw something that hasn't been invented. Obviously, the language of a designer-drug law should never stifle invention and creativity, such as legitimate research.

But if we do nothing, we run the risk of current drug laws losing all meaning. Eventually, copy-cat chemists may be able to duplicate all of the drugs we've outlawed.

And the costs to our public health system are sure to soar, as Parkinson's diesase and other unforeseen effects take their toll.

Few took it seriously when PCP, a designer drug called "angel dust," started cropping up in Los Angeles in the mid-60s. Now, PCP — which causes almost demonic behavior in users — has spread its destruction throughout the USA.

That's the risk we now face with designer drugs. Imagine hundreds, maybe thousands, of drugs as dangerous as PCP.

Some suggest that laws intended to control drugs have failed and a designer drug law will, too. They suggest we don't need any laws against drugs, even the most deadly. That's absurd. A sane society should provide all the weapons needed to fight the drug war.

And a law against designer drugs is a crucial weapon. Failure to provide that weapon in the fight against designer drugs would be a design for disaster.

THE COMMERCIAL APPEAL

Memphis, TN, July 30, 1985

THE already terrifying narcotics scene is being made even worse by "designer drugs."

Kitchen chemists are beginning to turn common chemicals into cheap synthetic drugs capable of severely damaging nervous systems and causing death. An estimated 100 persons have died from the potions and many more have developed permanent paralysis or trembling, according to testimony before a congressional committee.

These drugs are similar to standard illegal narcotics but have slightly different chemical formulas. One congressman said, for example, that a few hundred dollars worth of chemicals could be turned into millions of dollars worth of synthetic heroin.

Since most federal and state anti-narcotics laws define illegal substances by their chemical formulas, designer drugs technically are legal.

There is an urgent need for Congress and state legislatures to come up with legislation that would cover these new formulations. Widespread manufacture of such diabolic drugs could produce misery too horrible to contemplate.

Sunday News Journal

Wilmington, DE, December 29, 1985

BY STRANGE coincidence, during the very week that Delawareans were reading about Michael C. Hovey, the Du Pont Co. chemist charged with manufacturing and distributing 3-methyl fentanyl, the U.S. Senate voted to close loopholes in the controlled substance law.

Manufacture, distribution and possession of specifically named substances such as heroin and cocaine have long been illegal. Unfortunately, trafficking in and use of these and other illegal drugs have continued, but when the violators are apprehended, they can be prosecuted and often are convicted.

But there are other substances, at least as dangerous and addictive as heroin and cocaine, that can be synthesized in laboratories. Popularly known as designer drugs, these chemicals have been appearing on the street recently with devastating effect. More than a hundred deaths since 1984 have been attributed to 3-methyl fentanyl, largely because of the extreme potency of this compound in the most minute quantities.

At first, law enforcement officers were helpless in dealing with synthetic substitutes because none had been named specifically in the controlled substance law. Then, as the new drugs and their potential became understood, they were added one by one to the list of illegal substances under provisions of the 1984 Comprehensive Crime Control Act.

The 3-methyl fentanyl allegedly made and distributed by Mr. Hovey became part of the prohibited drug roster on April 28. This makes prosecution of Mr. Hovey possible.

But another compound, p-fluoro fentanyl, which agents from the Drug Enforcement Administration are reported to have also found in Mr. Hovey's home, is not yet listed as a controlled drug. Hence Mr. Hovey or anyone else can at this moment go scot-free when making or selling this and other unlisted synthetic drugs that mimic heroin and other addictive narcotics.

This troublesome situation of the law falling behind the imaginative and relatively simple synthesizing of dangerous drugs can be corrected by the Controlled Substance Analogs Enforcement bill that the Senate passed shortly before adjourning for Christmas.

The proposed law would make it a crime to knowingly or intentionally manufacture, possess or distribute a "controlled substance analog" for human consumption. And the analogs instead of being cited by name and formula are described as having a chemical structure "substantially similar" to controlled substances listed in schedules I and II of the Controlled Substances Act, or as being designed to have effects "substantially similar" to those produced by controlled substances from schedules I and II.

These definitions of the term controlled substance analog avoid the trap of naming specific chemical formulas that can all too quickly be overtaken by slightly altered formulations that enable drug manufacturers and distributors to escape prosecution.

At the same time, the bill treads carefully so as not to inhibit legitimate research. Intent to manufacture and distribute an illicit substance must be established; also the substance must be intended for human consumption; and work done in compliance with FDA regulations is exempted.

The Controlled Substance Analogs bill had bipartisan support in the Senate Committee on the Judiciary, chaired by Sen. Strom Thurmond, R-S.C. Delaware's Sen. Joseph R. Biden Jr., the ranking minority member on the committee, worked for passage of the bill, which was approved by voice vote in the Senate.

The next move is up to the House committee headed by Rep. William J. Hughes, D-N.J. We urge the committee to act positively and promptly.

Passage of the controlled substance analog legislation is an essential tool in the fight against drug abuse. And, unlike other tools such as the hiring of additional drug enforcement agents, there is no cost involved nor any foreign policy issues to be considered.

'Crack' Explosion Alarms Nation; Crack, Cocaine Effects Compared

About one million Americans had tried "crack," a cheap, potent form of cocaine that some experts rank above heroin in danger, the National Institute of Drug Abuse (NIDA) reported June 13, 1986. Crack had been known in parts of the United States for as long as three years. But in the last months of 1985 and the first half of 1986, its use is said to have exploded. By one count, the drug could be bought and sold with relative ease in Los Angeles, Detroit, New York and 14 other major American cities. U.S. Attorney Rudolph Guiliani said crack accounted for up to half of all drug cases the federal government had prosecuted in New York since October 1985. Crack's sudden expansion in use met an outburst of public fear and anger. Newspapers, magazines and television graphically painted its dangers. Churches and community groups mounted grass-roots campaigns to harass dealers and warn away potential users. The widespread alarm also stoked growing public anxiety over cocaine itself. Figures on who used crack were sketchy. Many in the public were most concerned for teenagers and even younger schoolchildren were reported to have fallen victim to the drug. But preliminary findings suggested that most users were men aged 20-35, most often with incomes that were comfortable or better. About half were said to be black, and the majority lived in cities. But police reported that the drug was already spreading to the suburbs. While cocaine is sold as a powder, crack is available as solid chips and lumps, making it easier to ingest, with a more powerful effect similar to freebasing.

Crack is stronger than cocaine. The process by which it is created gives it a degree of purity that outstrips cocaine by 70% or more. A crack dealer boils down a mixture of cocaine, water and baking soda and allows it to harden. It is then sold off a few milligrams at a time for $10-25. While inducing a comparable effect, crack is more economical to use than cocaine. Yet crack's strength also means that an addiction could ultimately cost more than might a dependency on cocaine or even heroin. Regular users of either cocaine or crack become ensnared in a cycle of chemical highs and lows. But crack's cycle is faster and, because of that, its grip is stronger. Addiction is quick. Experts estimate that cocaine dependency requires three to four years of use. Crack addiction is said to take six to ten weeks. A user can expect grave health effects. Heavy use could bring on emphysema-like symptoms in the lungs, and the circulatory system could accelerate drastically. The body's blood vessels constrict, but blood pressure and heart rate climb. The result is sometimes coronary attack. Long-term use is believed to bring on changes in brain chemistry that produced paranoia and even psychosis. New research findings suggest that all cocaine, including crack, could have a devastating physical effect on the brain.

The News and Courier
Charleston, SC, June 1, 1986

Crack — described as a drug dealer's dream and a user's nightmare — has not yet become widespread on the streets of Charleston and North Charleston as it has in other metropolitan areas of the country, but authorities are certain this new scourge is on the way. The drug, an almost pure form of cocaine that is smoked instead of snorted or injected, is cheap and the high it produces is intense. Users invariably want more. Some addicts say they became hooked after using crack only once. The psychological and physical consequences of taking the drug are numerous and severe.

The nation is being put on notice about the dangers of this drug and its sudden appearance in the United States. Numerous newspaper, magazine and television reports have focused recently on the seriousness of the problem. The best way — perhaps the only way — to insulate the Charleston community from this highly addictive form of cocaine is through public awareness. Parents should educate themselves and their children about crack. Civic clubs should seek out qualified speakers to address the issue. Churches should join in this effort. The time to act is now.

The Star-Ledger
Newark, NJ, July 3, 1986

Last month, a 22-year-old college basketball star who had just signed a contract with the Boston Celtics that would have made him an instant millionaire overdosed on cocaine and died of cardiac arrest. Over the past weekend, a 23-year-old pro football player died from a lethal dose of cocaine that induced a fatal heart attack—24 hours before he was to be married.

These two drug-related deaths have attracted national publicity because they involved sports celebrities—and no doubt there will be more from that sector. But there will be a lot more deaths from cocaine overdosing that will remain virtually anonymous—mere statistics on police blotters—because the victims are ordinary citizens.

Nevertheless, they share a common mortal link: They are—or they will be—victims of the sharply rising addiction to cocaine, the "in" narcotic that not too long ago was widely accepted as a recreational drug, along with marijuana. Statistics now starkly reveal that cocaine has become a killer drug.

The deadly implications of cocaine use were clearly evident in the deaths of two well-conditioned athletes, Len Bias, University of Maryland basketball star drafted by the Celtics, and Don Rogers, who played for the Cleveland Browns. Their tragic fates should serve as a chilling social commentary on the mortal ravages of the Drug Age that had its insidious origins in the 1960s.

There is more than enough grim evidence to sustain the morbid finding that cocaine no longer can be casually regarded as a "recreational drug." The New Jersey medical examiner, Dr. Robert Goode, aptly noted that it should be viewed in a more ominous, contemporary vein as "recreational poison." Deaths related to cocaine use are expected to double or even triple because of the escalating use of the drug in all its forms.

Cocaine—and more recently, its more potent form, crack—has been taking a sharply increasing share of the illicit drug market. It is up to 30 percent, with half representing crack. A key reason for the rapidly expanding sale of cocaine is that it has become more available—and cheaper.

The illicit trade in cocaine has become big business, a multibillion-dollar industry, which has been wryly characterized by Peruvian President Alan Garcia as "Latin America's only successful multinational." And it is purely a matter of supply and demand.

Even the most vigilant law enforcement will not appreciably stanch the floodtide of illegal drugs moving across our borders. Drug pushers only thrive because there is a market for their illicit product. For drug abusers, the increased number of drug-related deaths could be a forbidding preview of their future.

Herald *SYRACUSE* American

Syracuse, NY, July 13, 1986

Federal officials this past week released statistics that should surprise no one who has read a newspaper lately: Compared to five years ago, three times as many people are dying as a result of using cocaine.

The evidence is all around us. In the last month, we have seen University of Maryland basketball star Len Bias and Cleveland Browns football standout Don Rogers added to the gruesome tally. Their cases are of the type that makes national news, but every city has its casualties. The drug is everywhere. Estimates vary, but virtually everyone with an informed opinion pegs the number of regular cocaine users in this country well into the millions.

Yet no one openly encourages it. On the contrary, everyone who speaks out voices emphatic opposition to it. In just the last week, National Football League Commissioner Pete Rozelle unveiled a plan to have every player routinely tested for drug use. And Education Secretary William Bennett has threatened to cut off federal aid to colleges that fail to combat drug use on campus (as if it weren't already proscribed).

First lady Nancy Reagan has made it a personal crusade, and the White House says the president has plans for a campaign of his own. Our own U.S. Sen. Alfonse D'Amato this past week demonstrated how easy it is to buy "crack," a variety of cocaine, on the streets of New York. And former Syracuse University basketball star Tony Bruin, after being sentenced to five years probation on a cocaine charge, vowed Thursday to spread the word to the community's youth about the dangers of the drug.

It's not as if this deadly peril is being kept a secret. The message is clear — cocaine is a killer.

So what is it that inspires people to use cocaine? If there were one, simple answer to that one, there would be no cocaine problem.

For many, it's an escape from the torment in their lives, a few moments of euphoria to mitigate the pain — or the monotony — of their day-to-day existence. But that doesn't apply to someone like Len Bias, who had the world by the metaphorical tail — success, money, fame — yet risked it all and lost it in an uncautious moment.

Why would Bias do it?

Why do millionaires crave more and more money? Why do happily married men cheat on their wives? Perhaps the answer is to be found in the title of the old song, "Is That All There Is?" — the fundamental human urge to seek the next plateau. And off the edge of that last plateau so often lies disaster.

Given the opportunity — and in the case of cocaine, that opportunity is all around us — people will engage in self-destructive behavior for the smallest of reasons, or for no reason at all. The solution — if there is to be a solution — would seem to lie in minimizing the opportunity.

Authorities tell us that cocaine is cheaper, more potent and more available than ever before. Despite doubled and redoubled efforts by law enforcement at every level, every community is inundated with this garbage. No amount of official effort is able to put a dent in the trade, it's just too lucrative for those engaged in it. It's merely a handy target for candidates' righteous outrage at election time.

The cocaine business is flourishing for two reasons: 1) People want it; and 2) the people who don't want it, tolerate it. Too many people are simply looking the other way when they encounter the use of cocaine and other illegal drugs. Nothing, it seems, can stir them out of their lethargic attitude.

There are no quick fixes to this problem. No amount of urine testing, police stings, political posturing, celebrity deaths will change anything as long as the public mindset is largely apathetic. If the same kind of public energy could be mustered in the fight against drugs as, for example, the anti-abortion movement, or the anti-Vietnam war crusade, some slow progress might be realized.

But despite all the recent publicity, no popular groundswell on such a scale is apparent. Drugs, for the most part, remain "somebody else's problem." Until they are perceived as the national scourge they are, drugs are likely to remain tucked conveniently away in the back of the public consciousness.

And the death toll will continue to climb.

Wisconsin State Journal

Madison, WI, August 1, 1986

The deaths of Len Bias, a young basketball star, and Don Rogers, a promising professional football player, brought home in shocking terms the message that cocaine can kill.

Medical professionals and others familiar with the drug were already painfully aware of its deadly effects. Sadly, it took the sacrifice of two healthy athletes to galvanize public attention.

Until the Bias-Rogers incidents, how many people were aware that cocaine has claimed more than a score of lives in Wisconsin? (Twenty-one deaths between 1980 and 1985 were related to cocaine, state figures show.)

So far as we know, most of the people who supplied those 21 fatal fixes are alive and well. Some probably remain in the cocaine supply "business," not really caring that their illegal actions could lead to even more deaths.

The Legislature recently toughened state laws dealing with cocaine possession and sales, but those changes did not address the question, "How should society deal with someone who supplies an illegal drug that kills someone else?"

Two state legislators, Republican John Merkt of Mequon and Democrat John Medinger of La Crosse, think they have the answer: treat them like killers.

They have proposed broadening the definition of second-degree murder to include deaths from cocaine and other drugs. Such cases probably would be tough to prosecute under Wisconsin's current second-degree murder law, which defines "conduct imminently dangerous to another" but also requires evidence of "a depraved mind" for a finding of guilt.

The state manslaughter law does not fit the bill, either, because it applies to killings in the heat of passion, in self-defense or in defense of another person.

Merkt and Medinger will present their proposal today at a meeting of the state Council on Alcohol and Drug Abuse. While rewriting a criminal statute is no minor undertaking, it is an idea the council should endorse.

If drug dealers know they are facing the possibility of a lengthy prison sentence every time they sell a gram of cocaine, the chilling effects on this despicable market could be significant.

The News and Courier

Charleston, SC, July 14, 1986

It was just a matter of time before the cheap and highly addictive form of cocaine called "crack" would show up locally. The question was how quickly police would act.

Now we have the answer. Following up on a tip last week, the police sent an undercover agent to a migrant camp on John's Island. By time the bust was over, nine farm workers had been charged and crack with an estimated street value of $15,000 had been seized.

County police Capt. Ronald R. Perry explained that the police are "sending a message to dealers that crack is dangerous, and we're doing everything in our power to see that they go to jail." Magistrate Randell McIntosh, who set a total bond of $150,000 on the first suspect, sent the same message when he said that crack "is too potent for me to extend any kind of charity ... "

All but three of the eight who were arrested in the bust are being held in lieu of bonds ranging from $100,000 to $5,000.

The message from local police, judges and juries should be clear: Charleston county is not the place for dealers in crack. Their crimes will not be tolerated.

The Union Leader

Manchester, NH
August 10, 1986

A woman, the mother of two grade-schoolers, was watching a TV report on the deadly "crack" cocaine and those who push it to young and old alike.

Turning to a companion, the woman said, "I think they should kill the drug-pushers."

She is not alone. President Reagan said the same thing last week. It's a sentiment shared, we think, by millions of Americans.

There's a force alive in this country today that, if harnessed and correctly channeled, can put a huge dent in our drug problems.

It is the force of rage felt by reasonable, responsible Americans as they watch criminals literally getting away with murder and their friends and children destroying themselves and, in the process, tearing at the very fabric of society.

Surely, it is a time to shout, "Stop!"

But this must be a unified effort, led by elected officials and community leaders at all levels. It must be done by example and by deed. It must be led by officials unafraid of the criticism of the social tinkerers and self-proclaimed civil libertarians who don't care to protect the rights of the law-abiding majority.

Surely these leaders must sense that the majority is on their side, that common sense dictates a fair, clear and firm approach to those who are wreaking destruction through drugs.

That common sense was evident in a random Union Leader poll of New Hampshire teens one day last week. Dozens of teens were asked what they thought of drug testing in schools, along with the seizure of automobiles used by teen drunks. The response seemed overwhelmingly favorable.

Colleen Mahoney, a 16-year-old junior at Merrimack High School, gave a typical response.

"As far as testing, if you don't have anything to hide, you don't have anything to worry about. Those who are using drugs are interfering with the learning process."

The death penalty for drug pushers? Yes, indeed. And for the mob kingpins who finance them, too.

Suspension from school for students on drugs? Again, yes. Offer help, of course. In fact, demand rehabilitation before re-admitting the student. But let all know that drug use can't and won't be tolerated.

It's time to act. The people demand it.

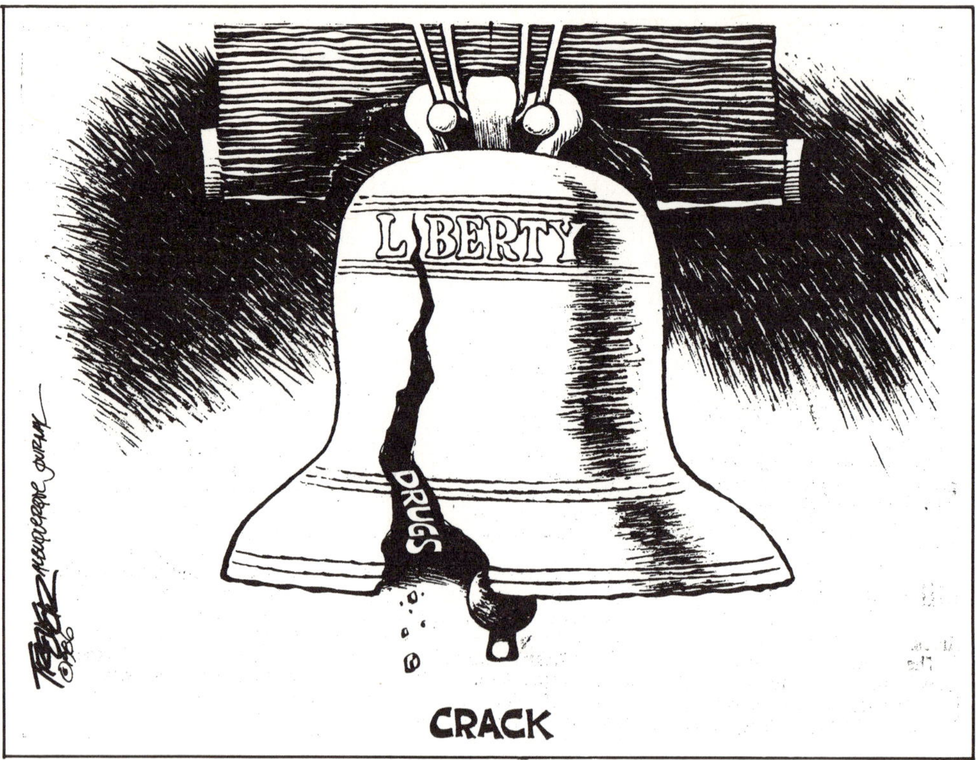

The Evening Gazette

Worcester, MA, June 18, 1986

Crack: A highly addictive cocaine derivative that renders many users violent and paranoid.

Crack, sometimes called rock, was little used on the East Coast 18 months ago. But it has hit New York City and Boston, creating psychotic reactions in users that haven't been seen since the heyday of LSD. The Worcester Police Department has made its first seizure of what appears to be a small amount of the substance. Something must be done to rid the streets of the narcotic.

Crack is one of the deadliest forms of illegal drugs in use. A 16-year-old New York City youth calmly walked into a police station and told the lieutenant at the desk: "I want to report that I killed my mother." Two days before, the mother had caught him smoking crack and during the fight that erupted, the youth stabbed her to death in a drug frenzy. It was only after his supply was gone that he turned himself in. It was the eighth violent crime blamed on crack in the New York City in the past four months.

Police Chief Thomas Leahy says that Worcester doesn't yet have crack houses, spots that serve high school students and young adults in New York. They're similar to opium dens that once catered to wealthy Chinese addicts. But crack houses have been found as close as Boston. A young man carrying 1,051 vials of crack in a duffel bag — worth about $26,000 — was arrested in Boston as well. The state police laboratory first pronounced that crack had been found in Massachusetts last December.

Heroin users who switched to crack say it is far more addictive and more dangerous to the user. Unfortunately, it is attractive to young people, affluent or poor. Victims as young as eight years old have been reported. In a recent sweep of street dealers in New York City, 18 of the 44 arrested were selling crack within a half block of a school. One expert on addiction calls it "the fast food of drugs."

In an age where parents worry constantly about what lies in wait for their children, crack is just one more monster to contend with. Drug Enforcement Administration officials are clearly worried that it will become the "drug of choice." The effect will be devastating to society should that occur.

The Pittsburgh PRESS

Pittsburgh, PA, August 10, 1986

Local and federal law enforcement officials in New York City have come up with a new wrinkle in the battle against "crack," the potent cocaine derivative.

They began confiscating cars driven by persons coming into town to buy the illegal drug.

A 16-year-old federal law allows the confiscation of property used in drug transactions. Heretofore, the measure has been used mostly against drug dealers. But officials decided to start using it against buyers as well.

During a four-day period, 30 cars were taken in Manhattan, mostly from young persons living in middle-class suburban communities. Police Commissioner Benjamin Ward issued a warning:

"If you come to New York to buy crack, bring carfare and be prepared to take the bus back."

Other areas would do well to follow New York City's lead. If a person stands to lose his wheels, he might think twice about running out to buy a dangerous drug for a momentary high.

The Des Moines Register

Des Moines, IA, July 15, 1986

Will the coincidental deaths of two prominent athletes from cocaine within a week do what the cocaine deaths of two — or 200 — unknowns could not do? Will they call enough urgent attention to the fatal unpredictability of cocaine to have a real effect on reducing use of the drug?

Maryland basketball star Len Bias may have been using his first cocaine to celebrate being drafted by the Boston Celtics. It hasn't been established yet whether Cleveland Browns' defensive back Don Rogers was a previous user or merely tried some at a pre-wedding bachelor party.

But neither man apparently took an unusual dose. The coroner who examined Rogers said the cocaine level in his blood would not necessarily have been fatal in another person, because individual tolerances differ widely. Rogers' blood contained 5.2 milligrams of cocaine per liter; Bias' blood, 6.3 milligrams. Fatal doses have been known to range from less than 1 milligram to about 21 mg.

Considering how widely the drug is used, this obviously is not literally a "Russian roulette" situation — one chance in six you spin to the chamber with the bullet. If it were, casualties would number in the thousands daily, and cocaine use would dry up.

But, as Bias and Brown have shown, one does take a chance of triggering an unforeseeable and instantly fatal reaction. The fear of that should scare away some number of potential users who otherwise would shrug off the serious — even fatal — effects that come years down the road.

But how many? How many of you cigarette smokers, who now shrug off the knowledge of greatly increased chances of early death from cancer or heart attack, would stop cold turkey if it could be shown (as it has *not* been) that an occasional unpredictable reaction to one cigarette might kill you instantly, next year — or next smoke?

The Honolulu Advertiser

Honolulu, HI, September 19, 1986

Given its accessibility on the Mainland, it was inevitable that a highly addictive smokable form of cocaine called "crack" would eventually make its way to Hawaii. Indeed, Honolulu police recently uncovered five "crack houses" where this illegal drug is being made and sold.

What isn't yet inevitable, however, is that this form of cocaine will become as insidious here as it is in some communities. By taking grassroots action, Hawaii still has an opportunity to prevent the spread of this drug and to come to grips with the larger problem of cocaine and other illegal substances.

DURING TODAY'S national outpouring of sentiment against all illegal drugs, crack has been seen mostly as one element of a larger problem. That it is. But it's also important to view crack on its own — as a new, potentially deadly substance.

Because it's relatively cheap and induces a fast "high," crack is much more than simply another drug fad. What many users may not realize is its addictive properties and that it can cause serious medical side effects.

Socially, meanwhile, excessive use of, and craving for, this form of cocaine can lead to crime, delinquency and problems at work and school.

For the past two decades, Hawaii's history with illegal drugs has centered mostly on the growing and smoking of marijuana. But from all indications, crack and other forms of cocaine pose even more harmful risks to users and to society, partly because they're so highly addictive.

There are a number of ways to deal with this pernicious drug. One is police work, to root out suppliers and dealers. But it's in Island schools, homes, youth and athletic clubs and other institutions that the war against crack will be won or lost.

Parents, teachers, social workers and others can play a role in the crackdown against crack by being aware of the drug's existence, and of users' symptoms. Then, the task is to educate our youth as to why crack shouldn't be smoked.

PREVENTING THE spread of this dangerous substance in Hawaii won't be easy. Yet, if there's a hopeful sign, it's that most residents are supportive of educational and legal actions to crack this problem before it veers out of control.

DAILY NEWS

New York, NY, August 3, 1986

"The city's murder rate—fueled by bloody crack-related killings—has continued to soar upward after five years of decline."

"Police cited the crack epidemic in releasing new figures that show sharp increases in violent crime and theft."

"Feds kill 1, nab 3 in drug chase."

"A dozen cops swooped down on a drug-plagued Manhattan neighborhood yesterday and nabbed a dozen dealers—but a short time later, it was back to business as usual."

"Child beaten to death; suspect was high on crack."

DISPATCHES FROM THE WAR ZONE. Did you miss them? There will be more. Tomorrow. And every tomorrow after that. Until the enemies—the drugs, the dealers—are vanquished.

This war will not be settled by treaty. It's a war to the death. Right now, too many innocents are dying. Children, lured by playground pushers with their vile little vials of dope. Cheap dope. Buy it for song: A dirge.

The cops send out their special units. They sweep the human jackals, the dealers, off the streets. The squad cars leave—and the dealers, more dealers, arrive. A lot of those who are carted away, arrested, just take little rides on the judicial merry-go-round. Around a few turns for a few hours, eyes out for the brass ring.

Consider the case of one, arrested three times in six months. His sentences were 90 days, 30 days and probation. In *that descending order.*

Madness? Yes. Is it any wonder the good people of this city—the victims of the muggers who need a fix, the parents of the kids with plastic vials in their pockets or needle marks in their arms—are going crazy? Or simply losing hope?

SWIFT, STRICT JUSTICE is only part of the answer to their desperate pleas, their present despair. In this war, a comprehensive battle plan is needed. Not scattershot hit-and-miss efforts, speeches full of sound and fury signifying nothing but political ambitions, or opportunism.

What would happen if all the money spent on anti-drug press releases and stamps to mail them out was redirected to the actual cause? Of course, that's a fantasy.

Proposals were offered in New York last week by city and federal officials: More judges, tougher penalties, deportation of illegal aliens convicted of drug offenses, stepped-up border patrols and increased Coast Guard surveillance. Excellent proposals, but just that. Ideas. Words. The people have had it with words. They want action.

Yet more flailing, failing action will be worse than nothing. What's needed is a fully coordinated, centrally planned, comprehensive war plan. Then war—all-out war. It must be planned and paid for. It will have to be lobbied for. It will take a task force of prosecutors, elected officials, law enforcement personnel, community activists, big business—all working *together*.

The people overrun by pusher punks and junkies can do only so much—picketing, protesting, teaching and safeguarding their children. They can take only so much. They are at the breaking point—between rage and resignation.

They deserve better. A lot better.

THE ATLANTA CONSTITUTION
Atlanta, GA, June 20, 1986

Sen. Lawton Chiles (D-Fla.) thinks Congress should act immediately to give law-enforcement agencies help in combating the wildfire spread of the dangerous new drug known alternately as "crack" and "rock." He is right. The problem is serious. Crack, a highly refined form of cocaine that offers the intense high of free-basing without the potentially explosive distilling process free-basing requires, is almost instantly addictive. It can cause severe depression and paranoia. And doctors say frequent use can cause serious brain damage.

It's mind-altering effects have been blamed for at least five homicides in New York City in which users, apparently suffering extreme paranoia after coming down from a crack high, killed relatives or friends. It has contributed to a sharp rise in violent crimes in that city, and has led to a 48-percent increase in the number of people seeking help for cocaine addiction.

To make matters worse, it is also cheap. A fix sells for as little as $10. That has made it popular with teenagers and even schoolchildren.

Chiles has proposed legislation that would elevate crack to "Schedule I" status among illicit narcotics, putting it in a class with those drugs considered by the federal government to be the most dangerous. It deserves the honor. The change would allow for stiffer penalties against those found guilty of possessing or distributing it. Under current law, crack dealers get an undeserved break. They face relatively small fines and must be arrested several times before stiffer penalties can be imposed.

Chiles would also make it a felony to employ minors in the manufacture or distribution of the drug. That would double the current penalties for such offenses, which would mean that first offenders could face up to 20 years in prison. That may be excessive, but Chiles' point is important: Crack dealers routinely use minors in their operations to hustle customers on the street, to sell to other youngsters and to act as lookouts.

Again, Chiles sounds an important alarm: A rapidly growing national problem needs sustained national attention. His colleagues should be all ears.

The Afro ⊛ American
Baltimore, MD, July 19, 1986

All too often, it takes a tragedy to spark action, and the recent deaths, by overdose of cocaine, of two top athletes brings to the fore, action in the war against drugs.

The myth has been promulgated for years, that cocaine use was non-addictive. Reports from the U.S. Public Health Service indicate that not only is the drug addictive, but it can kill — even on first use.

First Lady Nancy Reagan joined the war against drugs quite some time ago, and now President Reagan plans to join in, and give a series of anti-drug speeches in the crusade.

The new menace on the street, the drug "crack," has alerted anti-drug officials, and brought into focus a concerted attack on this new threat.

There are about 300 bills pending in Congress to tighten drug controls. The tragedy has struck, and hopefully now, we will begin to see more action. Meanwhile, the toll-free Cocaine Hotline, 1-800-662-HELP, is there for those who need help.

Chicago Defender
Chicago, IL, July 30, 1986

There's a new group joining the army against the illicit use of cocaine and we think the organization is greatly needed. It is called the Cocaine Prevention/Advisory Group. Its formation was recently announced by Chicago Department of Health commissioner, Lonnie C. Edwards.

One of the great things about this new effort is that the group will be made up of representatives from treatment and prevention programs which are already in place. It will also have members from various Chicago community organizations as well as adolescents recruited from the schools and numerous youth establishments.

There are several positives to this. First of all, the group can act as an umbrella coalition where members regularly share anti-drug information in quick and effective ways. Such knowledge can then be disseminated by the members of CPAG among their own particular groups. It can then be used to increase the anti-narcotics educational awareness of users and potential abusers.

The group also will be able to make positive contributions to the residential adolescent substance abuse treatment program which will be opening in September at the Department of Health's Chicago Alcoholic Treatment Center (CATC).

New types of drugs are hitting the streets. Currently the average city may have designer drugs, crack (a new and deadly type of cocaine), and numerous other forms of illegal drugs pushed on its residents. These new narcotics demand the use of new anti-drug strategies by authorities. Old ways and methods may prove ineffective in fighting against the current threat of these new and deadly drugs.

Crack is a particularly bad health threat. It is reported that: it can addict the consumer after two or three tries; the "high" from it is more intense than the average cocaine high, lasts for five or 10 minutes but is usually followed by severe depression, guilt, and feelings of worthlessness and; when the user tries to relieve the negative feelings by smoking more crack, the short high returns, followed by the long nightmare of bad feelings. It's a vicious, crippling and deadly cycle. Some people, not knowing the potency of the drug, have had strokes and heart attacks as a result of using it.

There's no doubt about the fact that drugs and the industry which distributes them are serious blights on society. It's also a fact that the major method of dispensing drugs in the United States comes from organized crime. To reduce its effectiveness, anti-drug elements have to be better organized. Their flows of information, methods of counseling and preventing the dispersal of drugs must be well-formed and functional. This is necessary whether the anti-drug organization is a medical, law-enforcement or advisory group.

"I firmly believe that in working together we can provide our young people with the help and support they need to resist the pressures they experience to use drugs," said Doctor Edwards. We agree. In fact, such action may be the best chance our young people have.

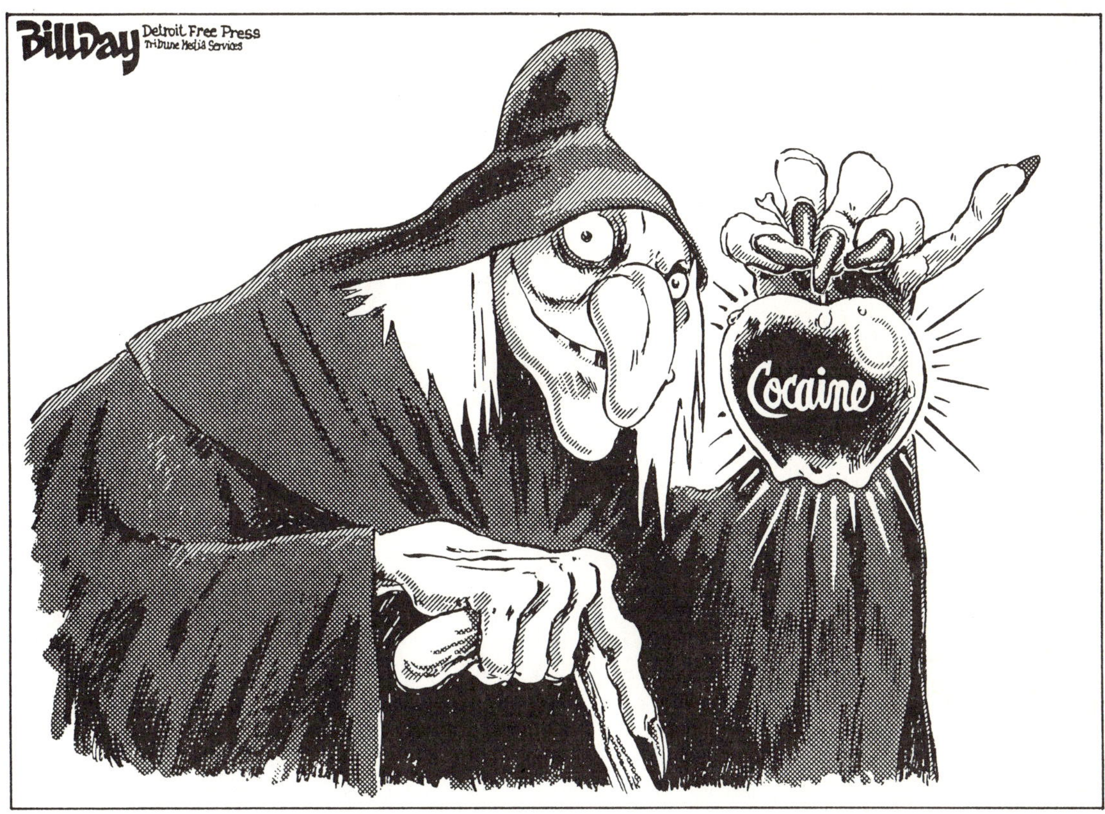

The San Diego Union

San Diego, CA, June 27, 1986

The nation is justifiably shocked by the sudden, cocaine-induced death of Len Bias. After all, here was a gifted young athlete who was about to achieve most of his childhood dreams. He had just been selected as the Boston Celtics's first-round draft choice. He had also signed a multimillion-dollar contract with Reebok shoes.

Moreover, Mr. Bias was a devout Christian who came from a close-knit family. He had reportedly warned his brother about the danger of drugs. And most everyone who knew him generally recalls a shy, sensitive person not given to making rash decisions.

Why would such a special young man jeopardize his future and, indeed, his life by ingesting pure cocaine in the early morning hours of June 19? Was Len Bias led to believe that snorting cocaine was a socially acceptable way to celebrate his moment of glory?

Whatever the case, this All-American basketball player is yet another casualty in the drug epidemic that is ravaging this nation.

The insidious epidemic destroys thousands of young victims each year. Thousands more are condemned by drugs to a life of poverty, crime, and despair. And the problem is getting worse.

An estimated 20 percent of Americans 18 to 25 years old have either used cocaine or use it on a regular basis. According to the most recent government data, approximately 5,000 Americans are daily trying cocaine for the first time. In fact, cocaine abuse has reached such alarming proportions in this nation that it is now the most common drug-related cause of persons being admitted to hospital emergency rooms.

This deadly drug is so plentiful on American streets that the price of pure cocaine has plummeted within the last few years. And the purer the cocaine, the more dangerous it is to the gullible young person looking for a quick and stylish high.

That certainly appears to have been the case with Len Bias, whose cruel death ought to shock the younger generation and parents into facing the grim facts about drug abuse. Chief among them is that anyone who fools with cocaine is flirting with death.

We would hope that the untimely demise of this talented young man will prompt a nationwide campaign that deals with the drug crisis. Such a campaign should heed the words and warning of Donald Brown, a San Diego Charger rookie and close friend and former roommate of Mr. Bias. "He was not another dumb, drugged athlete who got burned, but a man who made a mistake."

Would that our young, in particular, ponder the meaning of Len Bias's fatal mistake and then say *no* to drugs.

Detroit Free Press

Detroit, MI, July 11, 1986

THOUGH THIS nation's community leaders and police forces are right to mount a campaign against cocaine in the wake of the tragic deaths of star athletes Len Bias and Don Rogers, neither hysterics nor moral polemics will persuade people of its danger.

Scare tactics often backfire, becoming dares to thrill seekers. In our society — which tolerates an alcoholism rate linked to 100,000 deaths a year — heated words about cocaine would be taken by many as plain hypocrisy.

Ronald Siegel, a drug expert at the University of California in Los Angeles, estimates that 24 million people use cocaine daily across the country. Its use is widespread in the office suites and party palaces or our cities. It is also proliferating on city streets in the more potent but less expensive form of "crack." While Mr. Siegel claims that there are one or two cocaine deaths a day nationwide, it is impossible to know just how frequently cocaine use contributes to death.

The best strategy against the cocaine threat is a steady program of education. Two decades ago, reports about so-called bad trips on LSD tempered the early enthusiasm of some over that drug; so did the news of heroin overdoses give would-be addicts pause. There is no quick fix for the cocaine epidemic. If a real sense of danger can be conveyed in credible ways to present and future cocaine users, something worthwhile will have been accomplished.

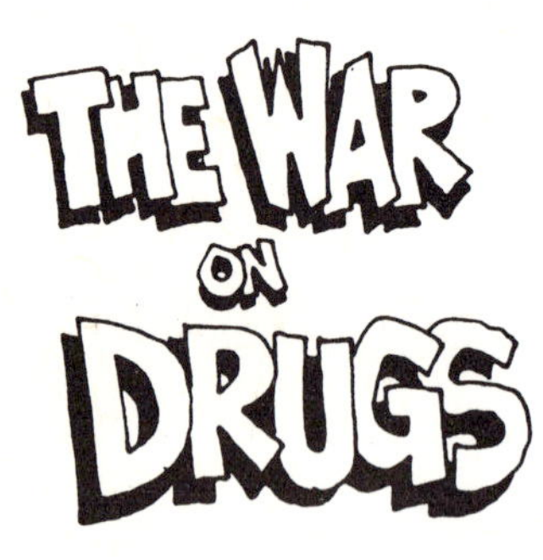

THE WAR ON DRUGS
AUTH
9/14/86. PHILADELPHIA INQUIRER
UNIVERSAL PRESS SYNDICATE.

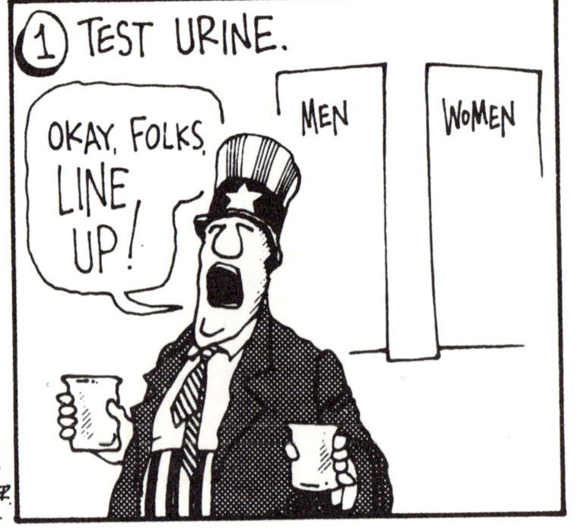

1 TEST URINE.
OKAY, FOLKS, LINE UP!
MEN
WOMEN

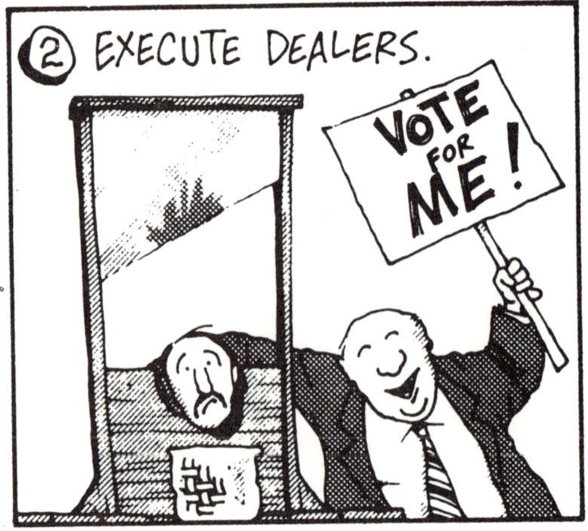

2 EXECUTE DEALERS.
VOTE FOR ME!

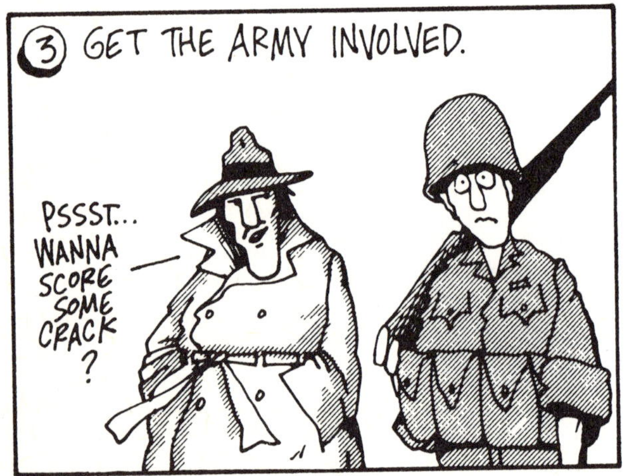

3 GET THE ARMY INVOLVED.
PSSST... WANNA SCORE SOME CRACK?

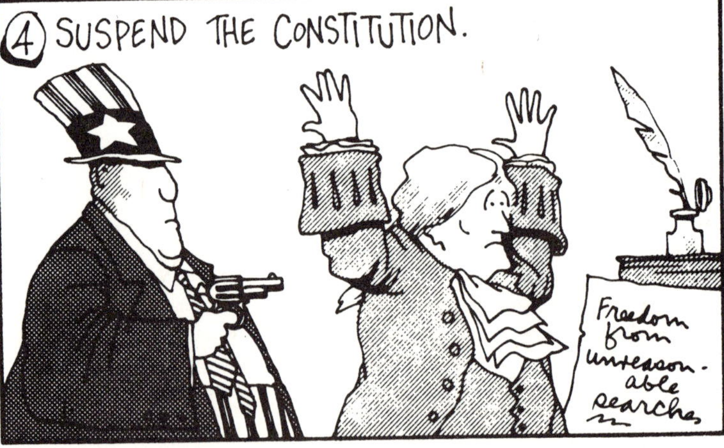

4 SUSPEND THE CONSTITUTION.
Freedom from unreasonable searches

Part II:
Law Enforcement and the Reagan Administration's Drug Wars

The first law in the United States to regulate narcotics was the Harrison Narcotics Act. Passed in December 1914, it became effective in 1915 and was designed primarily to channel the flow of opium and coca leaves and their derivitives and to make their transfer a matter of record. Forms issued by the Collector of Internal Revenue were required for all transfers of the drugs between manufacturer, wholesaler, retailer and doctor. A tax was also levied on the narcotic. Under the law the only way an unregistered person could legally possess one of these drugs was when he obtained it through a prescription.

The Comprehensive Drug Abuse Prevention and Control Act of 1970, more familiarly known as the Controlled Substances Act, is the legal foundation of a federal strategy aimed at reducing the consumption of illicit drugs. The Controlled Substances Act brought up to date and consolidated all federal drug laws since the Harrison Narcotics Act of 1914. The Drug Enforcement Administration (DEA) of the Department of Justice is responsible for enforcing the provisions of the act.

A drug user needs a vast amount of money to support a habit—usually more than he has access to by legal means. The typical categories of crime indulged in by drug users to support their habits are: theft, drug dealing (buying and selling), confidence games, pimping, prostitution, gambling and forgery. Studies conducted by the National Institute of Drug Abuse (NIDA) have found that many drug users commit more than one type of crime to maintain their habits, although they tend to focus on a particular activity. It has also been found that those addicted to drugs at a younger age tend to commit crimes more frequently later on. The seriousness of crimes involved grows greater with age. Among youthful addicts there are more muggings and purse snatchings; older addicts commit robberies. Everyone is a victim in crimes that involve drug abuse: the business community, the addict and the non-addict are all hurt. While it cannot be generalized that all addicts are criminals, there is an undeniable connection between crime and addiction. Supportive measures by the courts, treatment and rehabilitation, along with correction, parole and probabtion would certainly help to reverse the criminal trend.

There is a massive involvement of organized crime in drug trafficking largely because it is extremely lucrative. Illicit retail drugs sales in 1980 were estimated by the United States government in 1986 to be $70 billion, a figure nearly equal to the combined profits of the 500 largest industrial corporations in America. Drug money is often "laundered" or passed through legitimate businesses, some of which are fronts in major enterprises, before it is put back into the drug trade.

To combat organized crime and drug trafficking, the Reagan Administration has recently reorganized the DEA and brought the Federal Bureau of Investigation (FBI) into the fight. In addition the Navy and Coast Guard are cooperating in interdicting smuggling operations. The DEA was established in 1973 to replace the Bureau of Narcotics and Dangerous Drugs and enforce the controlled substance laws. To this end, it investigates and prosecutes individuals involved in the growing, manufacture or distribution of controlled substances destined for illicit traffic in the United States. In order to expand its facilities and become more efficient, the DEA began working with the FBI in 1982 when Attorney General William French Smith announced the groups would have concurrent jurisdiction of the federal drug laws.

The Reagan Administration's battle against drugs does not stop with law enforcement mobilization. Reagan himself has sounded a massive publicity campaign since his second press conference in 1981 when he said, "It is my firm belief that the answer to the drug problem comes through winning over the users to the point that we take the customers away from the drugs." Since then, Nancy Reagan has made the drug tragedy her pet project, pushing the point with her "Just Say No" crusade in the schools and pressing the entertainment industry to deglamorize the treatment of drugs in films, television and music.

Reagan Launches New Antidrug Campaign

President Ronald Reagan vowed a new drive against drug trafficking in an October 2, 1982 radio message to the nation. "We're making no excuses for drugs," he said, "hard, soft or otherwise. Drugs are bad; we're going after them." That message was followed by the announcement two weeks later of an Administration program to fight narcotics trafficking by organized crime. Reagan proposed that 12 new regional task forces, modeled on the one operating in south Florida and headed by Vice President George Bush, be established in large cities. Their task would would be to focus on distribution networks rather than on street sales and local sellers. The teams would be comprised of agents from several law enforcement agencies, including the Federal Bureau of Investigation (FBI), the Drug Enforcement Administration (DEA) and the U.S. Customs Office. The plan, to be put into effect in January 1983, would cost an estimated $130 million to $200 million. Reagan's speech did not mention how the plan would be financed, but Administration officials said funds would be shifted from the budgets of other federal agencies. Administration officials October 14 said about 900 new FBI agents would be hired under the proposal. The Reagan Administration in January, 1982 had announced an expanded role for the FBI in narcotics cases. Under the Administration proposal, 200 new assistant U.S. attorneys and a supporting staff of 400 would also be hired. The plan also called for creation of 1,260 additional places for inmates at the 11 federal prisons. At the unveiling of the plan, Attorney General William French Smith said that illicit retail drug sales in 1980 had totaled more than $79 billion—an amount roughly equal, he said, to "the combined profits of America's 500 largest industrial corporations."

St. Louis Globe-Democrat

St. Louis, MO, October 16–17, 1982

President Reagan's $200-million war on drug trafficking and organized crime is going to make life miserable for thousands of "fat cats" who until now have been able to increase their illicit drug trade and other criminal activities every year.

Promising to "end the drug menace and cripple organized crime," Reagan said his new program will blanket the nation with federal narcotics task forces in 12 cities, including one to be based in St. Louis.

Administration officials said the drug enforcement task forces will infiltrate drug rings, concentrating on long-range investigations aimed at breaking up networks rather than street pushers. Although Congress will have to approve permanent financing for the new program, the administration plans to get it started by transferring funds from other programs.

Under the Reagan plan, up to 700 new agents for the FBI and the Drug Enforcement Agency will be hired, along with 500 other law enforcement officers and prosecutors in other federal departments.

These new agents will replace the most experienced crime-fighters, who will used to staff the task forces.

The size of the task forces indicates how formidable they intend to be. Each will consist of 52 federal investigators, 20 federal prosecutors, 50 enforcement officials from outside the Justice Department and 20 clerical and paralegal employees. Reagan also said he would call for increased coordination among federal agencies in the all-out war on drugs and enlist the support of the nation's governors as well.

St. Louis Circuit Attorney George Peach has made a good suggestion — that the new Reagan program also include strong emphasis on anti-drug education programs for young people. As Peach says, "We have to convince people not to use drugs in the first place." It is the tremendous demand for drugs of all kinds that makes the illegal drug business so lucrative and so many hoodlums willing to risk the heavy penalties they face if they are caught.

The Dallas Morning News

Dallas, TX, October 18, 1982

ALTHOUGH a proposed crackdown on drug dealing was an important part of President Reagan's address on crime this week, seven other parts of the campaign deserve attention.

Most coverage centered on the announcement that President Reagan wants to expand the current blockade in South Florida with a $200 million program that would set up task forces in Houston and 11 other cities. That's understandable because the drug epidemic is at the heart of most of the country's crime. In 1980, as Atty. Gen. William French Smith points out, illicit drug sales equaled the combined profits of the Fortune 500.

Rather than continue to surrender the battle to the crime chieftains and drug subculture because it is so extremely difficult to combat them, the administration plans to make it hot for the merchants of addiction. The new initiative looks promising because it is aimed at the top levels of the drug trade, the Cosa Nostra drug families, the Colombian smugglers, the powerful motorcycle gangs.

But the President also correctly pointed out that drug crime is part of a climate of lawbreaking that must be changed as well. Street crimes such as drug-pushing and white collar crimes such as bribery are not unrelated. All prosper in a climate of neglect and indulgence. The same atmosphere nurtures the street criminal, the drug pusher, the mobster, the corrupt policeman and public official.

The President's answer is to mobilize the counter-attack on a national, regional, state and local level. In addition to the drug task forces, he is proposing a blue-ribbon commission similar to the Kefauver Committee of the 1950s, to lead a region-by-region analysis of organized crime's influence, in order to expose and eradicate the crime networks.

Third, the nation's governors will be asked to lead state reforms for better enforcement of local laws against racketeering and illegal gambling, a vital source of revenue for organized crime.

Fourth, a cabinet-level committee of all federal law-enforcement agencies will review interagency programs and intergovernmental efforts to improve cooperation.

Fifth, a special training program will be established through the Departments of Justice and Treasury, to help train local law-enforcement officials.

Sixth, a new legislative offensive to reform criminal statutes dealing with bail, sentencing, criminal forfeiture, the exclusionary rule and labor racketeering, will be made in the 1983 Congressional session.

Seventh, the Attorney General will be asked to submit a yearly report on the status of the fight against organized crime and drug trafficking.

And eighth, increased expenditures will be allocated for prison and jail facilities so fewer criminals will be released simply because there is no room in overcrowded prisons.

There's no cure-all promised, just a desperately needed start. As the President observed in his speech at the Department of Justice, we live at a turning point, one of those critical places in history where time and circumstance unite the sound instincts of good people to make a difference in the lives of future generations. It is time to turn the battle around.

The Courier-Journal

Louisville, KY, October 13, 1982

EVERY MODERN president eventually declares war on America's drug problem, and some cynics have noted that the "eventually" often seems to correspond to election time. So it was no surprise when, 30 days before next month's congressional elections, President Reagan announced that he had "taken down the surrender flag and run up the battle flag" in a new war on drugs.

As Hamlet once muttered, "Words, words, words." And some of the words are even the same. When Mr. Reagan first announced, on June 24, that he would assemble officials of various federal agencies for some coordinated planning on the subject, he said — you guessed it — "We're taking down the surrender flag that has flown over so many drug efforts; we're running up a battle flag."

Whether this battle flag will become more than a tattered metaphor from a tired or unimaginative speechwriter remains to be seen. So far, the apparent result of the coordinated planning has been presented to the public as a jumble of sometimes conflicting words.

Thus, several days after Mr. Reagan's October 2 pledge to unveil a battle plan, one group of administration insiders told newsmen that the emphasis would be on reducing the demand for illegal drugs. Other sources, meantime, were saying that the war would continue to be fought on the enforcement front — hitting at the *supply* of drugs, rather than demand.

Small wonder that Delaware Senator Joseph R. Biden, a critic of anti-drug efforts in both the Carter and Reagan administrations, commented that no campaign — even a so-called coordinated one — could possibly work without a coordinator. But President Reagan *has* a coordinator, Dr. Carlton Turner, appointed simultaneously with that first announcement in June.

That raises several intriguing possibilities. Could it be that Dr. Turner has not yet been introduced to Senator Biden, who is a member of the Judiciary and Intelligence committees and a staunch advocate of anti-drug measures? Is Senator Biden, a Democrat, (1) aware that Dr. Turner was named to the White House staff, but (2) more interested in making political hay? Or is the Reagan drug effort still so understated that it qualifies — in Senator Biden's words — as "minuscule."

If the problem weren't so serious, the nation could afford to tune in tomorrow for the answers to these and other questions about the President's drug campaign. But the battle flag is flying, which must mean that action is afoot. Or a-planned. And at least, as the cynics say, until November 2.

Herald News

Fall River, MA, October 16, 1982

President Reagan is having his most controversial season right now, but there will be few on either side of the political fence who will oppose his plan to fight the traffic in drugs.

The President is proposing a new program that will divide the nation into 12 regions, each with its federal task force to help solve the drug problem.

According to Justice Department officials, 1500 agents will be assigned to the task forces, and the money to pay for the program will be taken from the appropriations from other anti-crime projects.

This last provision is the only one which will arouse much, if any, dissent.

A new program designed to make real inroads in the amount of drug traffic is important enough to deserve its own appropriation rather than funding taken from other projects.

Drug traffic is destructive enough in its own right to warrant a very considerable federal outlay, but over and above the destructive potential of drugs, the traffic is very closely tied in with organized crime groups.

The disruption of the drug network will inevitably have a disastrous effect on the operations of organized crime.

For that reason the war on drug traffic and the war on crime tend, in many instances, to be one and the same thing.

There has been so much rhetoric expended on fighting crime in recent years that the public cannot be blamed if it tends to think the battle is more verbal than real.

This is perhaps the only serious handicap the President faces in winning support for the new program, that there has been so much talk about fighting crime that the public is understandably skeptical when it hears still more.

This does not mean, however, that it does not wish to end the traffic in drugs. It simply wonders whether it ever will end, or whether any federal program can make an effective dent in it.

The President, Congress and the public are at one in wishing to see drug traffic either eliminated or drastically reduced.

The trouble is that as one program succeeds the next, the differences seem more bureaucratic than substantial.

Division of the nation into 12 regions, each with its own drug-busting task force may succeed where everything else has failed, and everyone will wish the program well.

Still, what it really amounts to is a reassignment of a considerable number of Justice Department agents to this specific program rather than, as far as is known, any radically different approach to the problem.

For this reason, while the President's announcement of a new program has been well received, it will have to prove itself before the public will be convinced it will work.

The traffic in drugs is certainly one of the most dangerous aspects of the current crime wave. The only other one that causes as much concern is the spread of arson.

Anything that can reduce the drug traffic is worth trying. The President's task force program may be as effective as he thinks it will. In any case, it should have an opportunity to prove its worth.

But there is no disguising that the problem is difficult and complex, or that solving it will involve considerable expense.

It is impossible to win a war while conducting business as usual. This applies to the war on drug traffic and the war on crime.

If the President really wishes his new program to work, he should bear it in mind.

The Boston Herald American

Boston, MA, October 30, 1982

The crime problem has a national and international aspect that lies beyond the reach of state and local enforcement agencies which deal with only its most visible results. This is the traffic in illicit drugs and narcotics and the hidden network of smugglers and suppliers it supports.

We were pleased to hear President Reagan announce a new, concerted federal effort to attack the drug traffic.

The president's plan calls for a group of federal "task forces," which will see federal investigators and prosecutors mounting a comprehensive strategy against major drug dealers within their assigned regions.

Mr. Reagan will need congressional support in the way of a $200 million appropriation for staffing the drug task forces with new personnel. The effort will not have to make much of a dent in the illicit drug racket to justify that expense.

Our society pays and pays again for drug abuse and narcotic addiction — only beginning with the estimated $80 billion siphoned from the productive economy by the underworld. Add to that the losses from crimes committed by addicts to support their habits, and the welfare costs for families shattered by drug problems. We can well afford to spend a little more to go after the smugglers and wholesalers who make it all possible.

THE ATLANTA CONSTITUTION

Atlanta, GA, October 18, 1982

Drug rats in Florida, feeling the heat of a concentrated, prolonged fight against illegal drugs by a federal task force, are scampering in large numbers to other states. Now, President Reagan promises federal eradication efforts will spread nationwide.

The president announced Thursday a massive program to stop illegal drug trafficking in America with special federal task forces in 12 cities, including Atlanta, and 1,000 new crime-fighting agents. The annual cost of the program is estimated at $200 million.

The Florida action shows the approach can work. Florida officials, with their state's long coastline and proximity to Latin America sources of illegal drugs, had been fighting a major but losing battle against drug smuggling for several years. With the organization in Florida two years ago of a federal task force involving federal prosecutors and FBI, Drug Enforcement Administration and U.S. Customs agents, drug smugglers increasingly found it more convenient to take their business to other states.

Annual sales of illegal drugs in the United States approach $80 billion. With such huge funds, drug-smuggling rings often are equipped with communication equipment, planes and boats superior to those of state law officers. And, unfortunately, the smugglers also quite often find low-paid local and state law officials who can be bribed.

The federal task forces don't overcome all these problems, of course. But, with the larger resources and greater expertise available to the feds, they can fight the drug smugglers with much greater firepower and efficiency. Their help is already clearly needed in Georgia; the traffickers fleeing Florida have discovered Georgia's long stretches of semi-wilderness coastline and the state's large expanses of rural land with remote airports.

Reagan said he hopes to get funding from Congress when it returns after the Nov. 2 elections and to have the program in operation by January He deserves quick congressional support.

The Pittsburgh Press

Pittsburgh, PA, October 17, 1982

Contrary to noises some Reagan administration people were making only a few days ago, the U.S. government is not about to shift its strategy in the campaign against illegal drugs away from law enforcement and toward the "education" of drug abusers.

Instead, the president and top Justice Department officials have announced a significantly stepped-up war on drug trafficking.

Taking a cue from recent successes in Florida, the plan calls for setting up federal task forces in 12 cities, enlisting 1,000 new federal agents and prosecutors, and helping local authorities create more jail space for drug peddlers and smugglers.

The program will cost an estimated $120 million to $180 million in its first year and will have to be approved by Congress when it returns for a lame-duck session next month.

The administration also will urge Congress to stiffen penalties for drug trafficking and to pass other legislation tightening enforcement of drug laws.

It's true that without drug buyers there would be no drug traffic. So efforts to reduce the demand for illicit and dangerous drugs through education and prevention programs should continue.

But in the short term, nothing works like cutting off the supply before it reaches the streets and the high-school parking lots.

When the elections are over, the returning congressmen should give the president's anti-drug plan the urgent consideration — and approval — it warrants.

The Times-Picayune / The States-Item

New Orleans, LA, October 17, 1982

Because the illegal drug trade is one of the most serious internal threats to the nation, the Reagan administration's creation of a national narcotics task force could be one of its most important programs to date.

There probably is not a city, village or hamlet in the nation that has not had problems with illegal drugs. Illegal narcotics have become a cancer in our national society, causing countless human tragedies. Drug pushers have even invaded our schoolgrounds and playgrounds, wrecking the lives of many young people. The importation of illegal drugs has become a highly sophisticated, multi-billion-dollar business that has overwhelmed the resources and manpower of local law enforcment officials and the federal Drug Enforcement Administration. The expanded federal effort is long overdue.

The program will start with $200 million, but it probably will be necessary to increase the funding as the campaign proceeds. Initially, the program calls for the creation of 12 regional task forces staffed with 1,200 federal agents.

The enormity of the highly profitable illegal drug trade is shown by the successful crackdown in Florida. As a result of that effort, spearheaded by Vice President George Bush, drug smugglers, using planes and boats equipped with sophisticated electronic equipment, shifted their operations to the coasts of Louisiana and other states. "It's like squeezing a balloon," observed Jimmy Davis, a Georgia state investigator. "You squeeze one area and it pops out in another."

Without a major federal effort, there was no hope that the drug trade could be controlled. State and local authorities are simply outspent and outmanned by their criminal adversaries.

Not only will the increased federal effort provide desperately needed support for local authorities, it should encourage officials in foreign countries to do more to halt the production and exportation of dangerous drugs to the United States.

Houston Chronicle

Houston, TX, October 20, 1982

One of the principal complaints about the interagency war against drug trafficking in southern Florida was that the successful campaign there was driving the criminals to other states within boating and flying distance of the Gulf of Mexico.

All indicators show that the combined federal effort, and particularly the use of sophisticated military equipment and techniques, has slowed the drug traffic remarkably in Florida. Before the South Florida Task Force stepped in, more than 70 percent of the cocaine and marijuana smuggled into the United States came in through Florida and the state was beginning to experience a sharp increase in drug-related crime and violence.

After the all-out war began, there was a noticeable upswing in drug traffic in other coastal states, and even inland in such states as Tennessee, where remote airstrips were utilized for ferrying in illicit drugs.

The next move, logically, would be to expand the federal interagency fight to the rest of the nation. And that is what the administration is doing. President Reagan, in announcing the campaign against organized crime (which is what drug smuggling is all about), said he believes the effort "can mark a turning point in the battle against crime."

An additional dozen task forces, including one with headquarters in Houston, will work under the direction of the attorney general to cover the nation in this expanded version of the successful Florida campaign. The task forces will have the expertise of such federal agencies as the FBI, Drug Enforcement Administration, Customs Service, Internal Revenue Service and the military to help, and the effort, coordinated nationwide, will assure there is no refuge for the criminals.

"We've taken down the surrender flag and run up the battle flag," the president said. Most Americans will say it's about time.

Buffalo Evening News

Buffalo, NY, October 24, 1982

Everyone is against crime, and so President Reagan's announcement of a new crime crackdown so soon before the November election has been interpreted in some quarters as politically motivated. Whether it is or not, it is hard to argue against the program itself, which is national in scope and designed, in Mr. Reagan's words, "to cripple the power of the mob in America."

The drive is specifically targeted to combat the traffic in narcotics by organized crime. Early in his administration, Mr. Reagan sent a task force to fight the traffic in marijuana and cocaine in southern Florida. Since then, drug-related arrests there have risen 40 percent, and drug peddlers have tried to shift to other points of entry into the country. The new national strategy is designed to combat drug dealers in every part of the country.

Twelve new special task forces will be set up across the United States by agents of the Federal Bureau of Investigation and customs and narcotics officials. These task forces will work with state and local law-enforcement officials, but a key factor will be the additional manpower of up to 1,200 federal agents and investigators.

While geared closely to the narcotics traffic and organized crime's dominant role in it, the new federal program includes other aspects designed to fight crime in general: funds to house 1,260 more inmates in 11 federal prisons; a legislative drive to close loopholes in the law and reform criminal statutes dealing with bail and sentencing; and the formation of a federal crime commission to probe organized crime, region by region, over a three-year period.

The cost of the program is estimated at up to $200 million a year, but the administration plans to draw these funds from various federal agencies. Some concern has rightly been expressed in Congress as to whether this plan might shortchange other law-enforcement services. The additional funds needed are not great considering that crime in the nation costs us $8.8 billion a year in various financial losses, to say nothing of the loss of life or the deterioration in the quality of life.

In a speech at the Justice Department, Mr. Reagan spoke eloquently of the "invisible, lawless empire" of organized crime and of career criminals who are contemptuous of our system of justice.

"They do not believe they will be caught," he said, "and if they are caught, they are confident that once their cases enter our legal system the charges will be dropped, postponed, plea-bargained away or lost in a maze of legal technicalities."

The new drive should make life more difficult for criminals in general and drug traffickers in particular. Attorney General William French Smith cited a recent study revealing that, over an 11-year period, 243 drug addicts had committed about half a million crimes, or 2,000 each. The new anti-crime drive should help to combat such drug-related crime, both by striking at drug dealers and by keeping behind bars those who have made a career of crime.

The News and Courier

Charleston Evening Post

Charleston, SC, October 23, 1982

In a speech last week in the Great Hall of the Justice Department, President Reagan unveiled a major, new, eight-point plan to launch a bold attack on organized crime, especially drug trafficking.

He referred to the perception of a new privileged class in American society — "a class of repeat offenders and career criminals who think they have a right to victimize their fellow citizens with virtual impunity." He went on to criticize our judicial system, one that lets these hoods think that, if they are ever caught, their cases will be "dropped, postponed, plea-bargained away or lost in a maze of legal technicalities."

Regettably, the president is not just referring to a perception without base. What he's saying is a reflection of the way things are in today's other world — the world of the syndicate. Our society arrived at this monstrous point in history because we, over a period of two or three decades, somehow divorced the causal relationship that used to exist between crime and punishment and adopted the thesis that man was only the product of his material environment. If heaps of money, in the form of well-intentioned but misguided social programs, were used to better the environment, then it would follow that man would become more virtuous. If there were still a criminal element left in the society, then it is the fault of society, not the individual. With such prime fertilizer, those who would find the syndicate mentality attractive, flourish.

President Reagan's plan, therefore, is based on strengthening the forces wearing white hats so more and more of the bad guys are given the opportunity to repent — at their leisure in prison. He's returning the cause-and-effect relationship to crime.

One of his plan's highlights as it strikes out at drug traffickers, is to establish 12 additional task forces, under the attorney general, to monitor key areas in the United States active with drug smugglers. Surely the coast of South Carolina, second only to Florida with its appealing inlets and bays, will receive some of that increased surveillance. And the task forces reflect more than just officers from DEA, the FBI, INS, Customs and the Coast Guard. The team will now be augmented by the tracking and pursuit capabilities of the Defense Department. The time is right to marshall all federal forces to route out what the president referred to as "the cancers of organized crime and public corruption." The task needs the cooperation of all Americans if it is to succeed.

Supreme Court Allows Limits on "Head Shops"

"Head shops," which have sprung up across the country in recent years—there are an estimated 15,000 to 30,000— sell assorted drug paraphernalia. Their stock includes everything from rolling papers and water pipes to hypodermic syringes and cocaine spoons. They also carry publications which give advice on purchasing drugs and growing marijuana and psychedelic mushrooms. It has been suggested that the increase in drug abuse among adolescents must be due in part to the prevalence of head shops, and that their existence is a continuation of the casual public attitude toward drug abuse.

The United States Supreme Court ruled March 3, 1982 that communities had the right to limit the sales of drug-related items such as pipes, rolling papers and measuring scales. The 8-0 decision (Justice John Paul Stevens did not participate) involved Hoffman Estates, a suburb of Chicago. The village had passed a law requiring head shops to obtain licenses to operate. The stores also had to keep a record of people who purchased drug-use items and were forbidden to sell such items to minors. The law was challenged by Flipside Hoffman Estates Inc., which ran a store that sold drug-use items in addition to clothing, records and jewelry. Flipside said the law was vague and violated the constitutional guarantee of free speech.

The court upheld the town law, noting that laws limiting head shops had been enacted throughout the U.S. "We hold that such legislation is not facially overbroad or vague if it does not reach constitutionally protected conduct and is reasonably clear in its application," wrote Justice Thurgood Marshall in his controlling opinion. The claim of free speech was "exorbitant" because the law was "expressly directed at commercial activity promoting or encouraging illegal drug use. If that use or activity is deemed 'speech,' then it is speech proposing an illegal transaction, which government may regulate or ban entirely."

St. Louis Globe-Democrat

St. Louis, MO, March 6, 1982

The U.S. Supreme Court ruling upholding an Illinois community's ordinance prohibiting the sale of drug paraphernalia to minors means that local governments do have the power to stop head shops from selling these items to young people.

The high court, in an 8 to 0 decision, held that the ordinance of Hoffman Estates, a Chicago suburb, which also requires drug paraphernalia stores to get a special license and record the names of customers, is not "overbroad or vague if it does not reach constitutionally protected conduct and is reasonably clear in its application."

It should be noted that there is a difference between the Hoffman Estates ordinance and laws enacted by St Louis County and at least eight cities. The former regulates the sale of drug paraphernalia to adults only. The local laws have banned the sale of drug paraphernalia used with illegal drugs to anyone.

But, using the Hoffman Estates ordinance as a guide, it becomes clear that, as a minimum, the Supreme Court will support laws that outlaw the sale of these items to under-age persons, which is probably the most important goal of laws enacted locally.

Now that the Supreme Court has spoken on this issue, the way is open for Missouri to enact a drug paraphernalia law to curb the sale of such devices statewide. It would be an effective way to prevent stores from introducing a great many young people to the use of dangerous drugs.

THE MILWAUKEE JOURNAL

Milwaukee, WI, March 6, 1982

The US Supreme Court has handed down a reasonable but limited decision on the right of communities to regulate the sale of drug paraphernalia. The far more troublesome question — whether the sale of such materials can be *banned* — has yet to be decided.

The immediate case dealt with a village ordinance in Illinois that imposed a license requirement and record-keeping rules on businesses selling "any item, effect, paraphernalia, accessory or thing which is designed or marketed for use with illegal cannabis or drugs." If the ordinance had stopped there, we think its challengers might have been right in their contention that it was unreasonably vague, leaving the dealer no sure way of knowing what the law expected.

But that doesn't seem to be the case. The ordinace is accompanied by guidelines to help both dealers and police determine what paraphernalia is covered.

The challengers also raised a free-speech issue, contending that the ordinance was unconstitutional because one of its guidelines said certain items — such as pipes, cigaret papers and clips — would be considered drug paraphernalia if they were displayed in the proximity of "drug related" literature. The guideline had a chilling effect on the First Amendment right to publish, the challengers argued.

Although we are strong defenders of free expression — it is, after all, our stock in trade — we think the argument was far fetched. Justice Thurgood Marshall, a sturdy liberal writing for the court's 8-0 majority, called the contention exorbitant.

The court undoubtedly will have to refine the decision further as other drug paraphernalia cases are appealed, but it has made a reasonable start.

TULSA WORLD

Tulsa, OK, March 5, 1982

THE U.S. Supreme Court has upheld an Illinois ordinance regulating the sale of drug paraphernalia in so-called "head shops."

The unanimous — and welcome — decision leaves some questions unanswered. But it makes one thing clear: society has a right to reasonably defend itself against the sale and promotion of drug accessories.

The arguments against the Illinois regulation were familiar. The law was vague and might violate the rights of vendors and buyers of drug items.

Not so, said the Court. In an opinion written by the tribunal's most liberal member, Thurgood Marshall, the justices overruled a lower-court opinion which held the Illinois law to be unconstitutionally vague.

"Many American communities," Marshall wrote, "have recently enacted laws regulating or prohibiting the sale of drug paraphernalia . . . We hold only that such legislation is not facially overbroad or vague if it does not reach constitutionally protected conduct and is reasonably clear in its application."

That makes sense. And it also hedges against a truly abusive application of the law that might threaten free speech, the protection against illegal search or other individual rights.

Lawmakers will have to be specific in defining the outlawed material. They will have to be careful not to trample on recognized legal concepts. But the Court leaves little doubt that communities can protect themselves against the "head shop" nuisance and they can do it without violating the Constitution.

The opinion is good news, and not only because it is a sharp blow against a growing public pain in the neck. It also suggests the Court is mellowing on law enforcement issues — giving the general public a little break at the expense of would-be lawbreakers.

Score one point for John Q. Public, zero for drug promoters.

The Cincinnati Post
Cincinnati, OH, March 10, 1982

Two Supreme Court decisions have given the nation a welcome opening to combat the sleazy fringe of the drug business.

By a vote of 8-0, the court upheld an ordinance in the village of Hoffman Estates, Ill., regulating the sale of drug paraphernalia.

The ordinance requires the licensing of shops that sell "roach clips," bongs, rolling paper and similar items designed for use with marijuana and other drugs; requires adult purchasers to sign a roster available for police inspection; and, most importantly, bans entirely the sale of the stuff to minors.

The court rejected arguments that the law was unconstitutionally vague and an infringement on "free speech."

This is good news for Cincinnati and the suburban communities of Reading and Forest Park, as well as communities around the nation which have been trying to rid themselves of "head shops." It's a real "downer" for the $3-billion-a-year drug paraphernalia business.

A second Supreme Court decision this week upheld a law in New York's Westchester County which flatly prohibits the sale of drug paraphernalia.

American parents now have won two significant victories. The court has made clear they need not stand helplessly by and permit the seduction of their children. In upholding the Hoffman Estates and Westchester County ordinances, the court has given them model laws that can confidently be adopted everywhere.

DESERET NEWS
Salt Lake City, UT, March 5, 1982

Utah's new drug paraphernalia law is on more solid ground now that the U.S. Supreme Court has ruled 8-0 in an Illinois case that local governments have the authority to ban sale of drug-related accessories to juveniles. At least 10 states have passed anti-paraphernalia laws that generally seek to put what are called "head shops" out of business.

When the Utah anti-paraphernalia law was proposed in the 1981 Legislature, some head shop owners argued that it would scarcely deter persons who want to use drugs. They pointed out that pipes and other items adaptable to drug use can be readily obtained at standard stores, even though they're illegal at stores dealing in drug use articles.

As the Supreme Court decision acknowledged, such laws do encounter enforcement problems. As Justice Thurgood Marshall noted: "We do not suggest that the risk of discriminatory enforcement is insignificant here. (But) we are not prepared to hold that this risk jeopardizes the entire ordinance."

Those risks are insignificant compared to the need to stamp out drug use, especially among high school and junior high students. As Sen. Fred W. Finlinson noted in proposing the drug paraphernalia law:

"If certain drugs are outlawed, why should people be able to buy the paraphernalia directly associated with drug use?"

This law also gives prosecutors an extra weapon in fighting drug abuse. In plea bargaining, for example, a paraphernalia charge might be dropped if the suspect pleads guilty to drug possession.

The war on drug use is too important not to use every reasonable weapon.

THE INDIANAPOLIS STAR
Indianapolis, IN, March 5, 1982

Crocodile tears are flowing again for the sellers of alligator clips and the like — those poor, unwitting "head shop" operators who shouldn't be held accountable for the proclivities of their wayward patrons.

It is enough to make a strong man cry, civil liberties groups contend, the way "gift shop" operators are hassled for selling cute little spoons, unique electrical connectors and water pipes for emphysema sufferers. It's not their fault if the items are misused by cocaine and pot fanciers.

Still the hard-hearted Supreme Court this week ruled that local governments may restrict the sale of drug-related accessories. The court upheld an ordinance in a Chicago suburb which prohibits head shops from selling to minors. In addition, the ordinance requires stores to keep a record of the name and address of each purchaser.

The decision, limited as it is, may help reinforce local and state laws that seek to reduce drug traffic by targeting those who sell drug-related paraphernalia. So here's a cheer for a small, but perhaps significant, victory.

In 1979, the Indiana General Assembly passed a law making it illegal to manufacture, sell or own a device for consuming illicit drugs. Two previous paraphernalia laws, passed in 1975 and 1977, were overturned but the 1979 law was upheld by a federal court in December 1980.

The Indiana law is modeled after legislation drafted by the U.S. Drug Enforcement Administration. Both critics and supporters say its vulnerability hinges on intent. Drug accessories are outlawed only when the user or seller has an illegal intent.

Paraphernalia laws have become a cause celebre with the American Civil Liberties Union and the organization argued against the Illinois town ordinance. That defeat, however, is not about to dissuade the organization from its crusade. Nor is the high court ruling going to still the controversy over the Indiana law and similar statutes enacted in other states.

But the ruling does give a measure of assurance that courts, at long last, are beginning to see through the sham rhetoric about the rights of "victimized" head shop owners. Perhaps the minor victory can be turned into a major one.

THE COMMERCIAL APPEAL
Memphis, TN, March 7, 1982

THE CLOSING or regulation of "head shops" won't solve the drug problem, but a Supreme Court decision that permits regulation at least will give those who are concerned about drug abuse another chance to say they don't intend to look the other way.

The court decision involved a Chicago suburb's law that requires a $150 license to sell items "designed or marketed for use with" illegal substances, including marijuana and cocaine. It bars sales to minors, requires stores to keep logs of purchasers' names and addresses, and provides for fines of up to $500.

Opponents of this kind of legislation may argue that regulation or prohibition won't work any more than the former constitutional amendment against the drinking of alcohol did. But the drug problem has to be combatted in many ways. A "head shop" law is just one of them.

To ignore the trafficking in drug paraphernalia is, in a sense, to accept it, and to tell users, especially young ones, that what they're doing is all right as long as they can handle it. And that attitude, along with denial that the problem exists, has helped contribute to what some authorities consider an epidemic of drug abuse among American teenagers.

Like the teacher in the CBS movie "Desperate Lives," which was shown Wednesday night, parents and persons in positions of authority have to care and be willing to take any reasonable actions to prevent drug use by young people. Otherwise, the use will grow, as it has been doing.

The Supreme Court didn't speak to the issue of whether the sale of drug paraphernalia can be banned. So the constitutionality of a Tennessee bill sponsored by Sen. Tommy Burks (D-Monterey) is perhaps uncertain. That bill would prohibit sales to buyers of any age specific items that Burks contends are clearly for drug use. Use or possession of the banned items would be a misdemeanor. Selling them would be a felony.

Tennessee's experience with the Larry Parrish antipornography law should still be fresh enough in the memory of legislators and others that they'll be careful about trying to ram through any bill that might violate constitutional rights.

BUT, WHETHER IT'S prohibitory or just regulatory, a "head shop" law is needed to help reflect a change of attitude about drug problems, as well as to provide another specific, if limited, legal attack on them. These shops aren't innocent ventures in free enterprise. Nothing involved in the drug scene is.

Drug abuse won't go away if factors that contribute to it are ignored, because it's a sickness of the mind and body. If drug usage by teenagers was reduced even 5 per cent by a law that cut off the enabling paraphernalia, the law would be worthwhile.

The News and Courier

Charleston, SC, March 9, 1982

Recently, the Supreme Court upheld the right of a community to curb illegal drug use through regulating the sale of drug paraphernalia at so-called "head shops." While not banning the businesses all together, the justices okayed an ordinance of an Illinois town that requires such shops to obtain licenses for selling items "designed or marketed for use with" illegal drugs such as marijuana or cocaine.

That's a step in the right direction, although it would be preferable to see the sale of such equipment banned entirely. Much, if not all of it, can be used only in conjunction with breaking the law.

The local reaction to the Supreme Court decision was self-damning. One shop owner, crediting paraphernalia with helping build his business, commented "mark-ups are high."

Another local merchant, ticking off some respectable occupations of people ("businessmen, officers and detectives") who trade with him, said "It's going to infringe on their rights (for us) not to be able to sell."

A third head shop manager said such ordinances are "attacking the problem from the wrong end." It's not the wrong end of the (self-admitted) problem, it's another facet of it. We have consistently supported law enforcement agencies in their continuing uphill struggle with drug smugglers. We have called for higher bail bonds for those caught and tougher sentences for those convicted. If outlawing the sale of paraphernalia drives the business underground and makes it just a little more expensive and harder to obtain, then society will be better served. The bill, introduced last week in the General Assembly, that would ban head shop sales, merits approval.

THE DAILY HERALD

Biloxi, MS, March 5, 1982

The Supreme Court's ruling this week legalizing laws that restrict drug paraphernalia sales may do more good for American society than the justices will ever know. The court upheld the drug paraphernalia restriction law adopted by Hoffman Estates, Ill.

Until that ruling, state and local officials had wrestled with the question of what to do about head shops, those businesses which hawked, among other goods, items obviously intended only for use in partaking of illegal drugs.

Mississippi and the Gulf Coast are included in those localities whose officials and leaders have been concerned about the presence of head shops, but had been stymied in efforts to arrive at a consensus of what could be done, legally, to ban or regulate them.

In a two-part series last March, Ron Grove explained for *The Daily Herald* readers the worrisome problem and the positions Coast leaders held. Educators, law enforcement officials and legislators interviewed for those reports favored some type ban on the sale of drug paraphernalia and drug-oriented publications. Their general agreement dissolved, however, when the question of implementing their desires was posed.

Capt. Ed Dickey of the Mississippi Bureau of Narcotics, Gulfport assistant Police Chief H. T. Hargrove and Biloxi Police Chief Ed Ryan agreed there should be some restrictions on paraphernalia. School Superintendents Dr. Olan Ray of Biloxi and Dr. Mercer Miller of Gulfport and Sen. George Smith and Rep. Dennis Dollar expressed concern that paraphernalia and drug publications are readily accessible to minors.

They believe, and with good reason, that young people are influenced by seeing head shops in Coast shopping centers and alongside other businesses. They are influenced when they see their peers purchasing and displaying hash pipes and roach clips and reading *High Times* or *Marijuana Grower's Guide* and other such publications.

These influences could, and probably do, make young people more receptive if and when they are approached by drug pushers, adding to the drug problems that already exist in our communities.

This week's Supreme Court ruling may have adverse effects on the 23 states and hundreds of localities that have adopted the model ordinance drafted by the U. S. Drug Enforcement Administration three years ago. It prohibits the sale of items "intended for use or designed for use" with illicit drugs. The model ordinance obviously leaves wide areas open to reasonable disagreement in applying this vague test to, let us say, a small spoon or a small pipe.

Given the guidance of this week's ruling, those communities like the ones along the Coast which have been delaying adoption of any restrictions on head shops can now move ahead, secure in the knowledge that the court condones barring sales of regulated items to minors and making records of all sales, including the names and addresses of customers, available to police. These two conditions are part of the Hoffman Estates law. It is reasonable to assume that the court would also look kindly upon other restrictions a community might want to adopt, providing the restrictions did not tread upon Constitutional proscriptions.

Still questionable is the Constitutionality of a law that would ban all sales of drug paraphernalia. Such a law, we believe, would not survive Supreme Court scrutiny, nor would a law banning publications of the *High Times* variety.

Gulf Coast communities, and the state, now have the responsibility of adopting laws and ordinances to regulate drug paraphernalia sales. There is no longer an excuse for inaction.

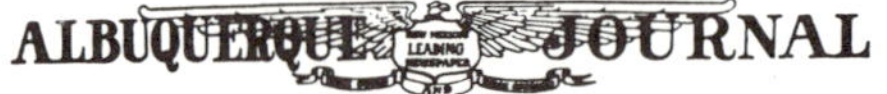

ALBUQUERQUE JOURNAL

Albuquerque, NM, March 7, 1982

The U.S. Supreme Court may have made the correct decision in opening the legal door to local laws regulating or banning sale of drug paraphernalia, but it almost certainly has opened the door to continuing expensive and time-consuming litigation on the subject all over the country.

We generally oppose the regulation or proscribing of otherwise innocuous items, because of their potential for illegal application.

But there are some items sold in "head shops" that have no discernible legitimate application. Such things might include "bong" pipes, used solely for the smoking of marijuana, and kits for testing for cocaine.

The danger is that zealots will take the Supreme Court paraphernalia ruling and cut too broad a swath. Writings of all sorts—including those that advocate or explain drug abuse — should be constitutionally protected.

Drug paraphernalia which has legal applications should remain legal—and more important, free from harassment. In this category we would place everything from cigarette papers and soda straws, to spoons of all kinds.

But we will almost certainly face the problem of selective enforcements which would find cigarette papers in a "head shop" deemed paraphernalia, while the same item in the posh tobacconist's shop would remain inviolate.

The Supreme Court has opened the door to the regulation or banning of sale of drug paraphernalia. Unfortunately, untold numbers of unorthodox entrepreneurs across the country will face arrest and legal costs before the court finally defines the limits of the doorway.

The Providence Journal

Providence, RI, March 13, 1982

"Head shops" feed on illegal drug abuse. They market the utensils and other paraphernalia that are part of the drug culture and in so doing promote an activity that is prohibited by law. It is time to put such places out of business.

Two bills that would ban the manufacture and sale of these materials are under consideration by the General Assembly. The House and Senate measures are similar but the House version would also prohibit the possession of specific articles.

Said Sen. Lowell W. Kinch, D-Pawtucket, a sponsor, "I feel that this blatant exploitation of the so-called 'drug culture' of this nation makes inexperienced young people think that fooling around with drugs and other controlled substances is the smart and fashionable thing to do. Actually, drug addiction usually leads to a life of crime, horror and degradation."

Making it difficult to purchase the accoutrements of drug use would not, of course, stop the users. But it would remove from the legal marketplace products that carry a message of approval, an implication that there is nothing wrong with buying illegal substances and using them illegally as a source of entertainment.

In today's letters column, Mark A. Refowitz, director of development for Marathon House, the drug rehabilitation program, writes from the perspective of one who has seen the consequences of drug abuse firsthand. He calls on the community, as do these newspapers, to take a stand against this kind of commerce and to stop sending mixed messages.

There was a time when the constitutionality of legislating against drug paraphernalia and those who make and sell the stuff could be called into question. No longer is that true. The U.S. Supreme Court has upheld the constitutionality of an ordinance adopted by Hoffman Estates, Ill. that regulates the sale of these materials. And subsequently it refused to hear a challenge to a Westchester County, N.Y. law that bans the sale of drug use items. At least by implication, it has approved the wording of the model law endorsed by the federal Drug Enforcement Administration.

Whether banning possession, as proposed in the Rhode Island House bill, would pass constitutional muster is in question.

Some 30 states and several hundred municipalities have already enacted laws regulating or banning drug paraphernalia. Rhode Island should do likewise by approving the Senate bill, S-2388, as a message to the drug culture that not only does the state refuse to cooperate in this ugly business but also that it will severely punish those who do.

The Wichita
Eagle-Beacon

Wichita, KS, March 8, 1982

The U.S. Supreme Court unanimously has upheld a Chicago suburb's ordinance banning the sale of drug-related paraphernalia to minors and putting tighter controls on the sale of such items generally. Thus, the high court seems to have given its blessing to similar laws in hundreds of other communities and about 30 states, including Kansas.

By ruling no constitutional rights are violated by the Hoffman Estates, Ill., restrictions on sales of goods "designed or marketed for use" with illegal drugs, Justice Thurgood Marshall, who wrote the court's opinion, seems to have taken care of arguments by lawyers for the $1.5-billion-a-year drug culture industry that such laws tend to be ambiguous and discriminatory.

Justice Marshall found the wording clear enough both to make obvious the intent of the Illinois law and to protect sellers' rights in cases where it can be demonstrated items were sold for other than illegal purposes.

Kansas' law, whose constitutionality — except for a section dealing with advertising — was upheld last fall by U.S. District Judge Patrick Kelly, is much more specific. It even identifies many prohibited items by their common street or drug-culture names — roach clips (used for holding marijuana cigarettes that have burned down too much to be held otherwise), bongs (small pipes), and so on.

Concerned parents and others around the country will welcome the high court's ruling. At congressional hearings in 1980, proponents of tighter drug-control legislation displayed such youth-appeal "head shop" items as "grass, stash and practice kit" containing a bag of alfalfa and a 20-page booklet telling how to roll practice "joints" and what to wear to real pot parties. In Wichita, last year, authorities closed down a store dealing in "legal" simulations of street drugs intended, they suspected, for distribution to school children.

The new ruling should help keep such nefarious activities under control.

Post-Tribune

Gary, IN, March 15, 1982

The U.S. Supreme Court isn't offering much sympathy to "head shop" operators who peddle drug paraphernalia. That's good, because the sympathy would be misplaced.

Twice in the last several days the high court has said that state or local officials can regulate the sale of such items. First, it upheld an Illinois village ordinance that requires shop owners to get a license to sell the items. Then, it refused to hear a challenge to a New York law that banned the sale of "drug paraphernalia." That law applied to Westchester County.

Obviously those rulings will encourage tighter restrictions. How they will affect Indiana's state law depends upon some rulings from the State Supreme Court, but local "head shops" could be in jeopardy.

Drug accessories are outlawed only when the user or seller has an illegal intent, which does raise a delicate point about rights. But let us not weep for shop operators who protest that they should not be held accountable for what their customers do with the equipment they buy. The most common are clips for smoking marijuana, but some shops also sell funny little spoons, which obviously are not for the sugarbowl, and various other items.

Free enterprise is one thing. Encouraging drug abuse is another. Quite another. The message from the courts seems to be that the freedom to do business is no more absolute than any other freedom. Enforcing the "head shop" laws must be done carefully, not arbitrarily, but it should be done.

Syndicated Columnist Carl Rowan says that once when he and a camera crew went into a "head shop" in Washington, a man buying a bowl used in taking cocaine said, "You could save me if you could get me off cocaine." The columnist says what he remembers most vividly about that is that the shop owner's business was to make money off people hooked on drugs — even to drag more people into it.

Those clips, bowls, spoons, etc., aren't just collectors' items.

Herbacide Paraquat Sprayed on Georgia Marijuana Fields

The United States Drug Enforcement Administration (DEA) August 12, 1983 used helicopters to spray the herbicide paraquat on several patches of marijuana fields in White County, Ga. The widely publicized federal action drew numerous protests. A federal district judge Aug. 12 issued a temporary restraining order against further spraying in the north Georgia area. Most of the criticisms leveled against the spraying concerned risks to the area's residents, who were warned of the spraying only 15 minutes before it began.

The DEA spraying was the first of its kind undertaken by federal officials, although Florida authorities had used paraquat against marijuana in 1982. The DEA indicated, however, that other U.S. areas had recently been targeted as sites for possible spraying. Paraquat is a widely used but toxic herbicide that is usually sprayed from ground level. According to a spokesman for the Centers for Disease for Disease Control in Atlanta, over 1,000 persons had died from paraquat poisoning since the herbacide had come into wide use in the 1960's. The federal action in Georgia reportedly destroyed 50 to 70 marijuana plants. To protect against the possibility that sprayed plants would reach marijuana smokers, the plants were pulled up after they were sprayed. A DEA spokesman called the Georgia operation successful and said it would send a "symbolic message to marijuana growers." The federal government said it was going to use films made of the spraying operation to try to convince authorities in Colombia to use paraquat to destroy marijuana crops in that country, the source of much of the marijuana used in the U.S.

The Miami Herald
Miami, FL, August 20, 1983

BEFORE the Government begins to spray the herbicide paraquat on marijuana fields in 40 states, it ought to take a cue from the Florida experience. Florida tried it and found that paraquat spraying doesn't work. State officials quietly abandoned the program.

Now the Federal Government wants to have a go at it. White House and Drug Enforcement Administration spokesman said the other day that the Administration plans to spray paraquat on Federal lands in 40 states.

A "trial run" was conducted in the Chattahoochee National Forest in northern Georgia. Federal officials called it a success. But a U.S. District Court judge issued a temporary restraining order to bar the Government, for the moment, from further spraying.

Florida used paraquat to encourage Colombia, where much of the U.S. marijuana supply originates, to do likewise. Gov. Bob Graham pushed paraquat in his 1982 re-election bid.

But the herbicide is a powerful killer. Mere drops can kill a human. Further, the chemical endangers food and water sources. The area to be sprayed must be strictly controlled and the weather cooperative. Florida was sued twice and feared becoming enmeshed in even more lawsuits.

The Reagan Administration would be wise to learn from Florida's mistake. It can better influence foreign countries to control marijuana through direct negotiations. It can better control domestic marijuana by other measures.

Paraquat is a trap. Don't fall for it, Mr. President.

ST. LOUIS POST-DISPATCH
St. Louis, MO, August 24, 1983

Federal drug enforcement officials have been temporarily halted by a court order from spraying marijuana patches in Georgia with the poisonous herbicide paraquat. But they are not taking the order sitting down. Late last week they took to the air over Kentucky and sprayed patches of pot in the Daniel Boone National Forest, despite objections of state officials and others about the threat that the spraying poses to health and environment.

In one sense, the federal government's insistence on the paraquat approach to pot can be seen as evidence of its determination to assert its authority over federal forests — without regard to anything state officials might say. On another level, it is proof that the U.S. government will practice at home what it has preached abroad.

But what is perhaps most striking about the operation is the extent to which it is characterized by technological overkill.

When federal agents took to the air over Kentucky, they used, according to an Associated Press report, no less than three helicopters for the task. When they returned, mission accomplished, three tiny plots of pot, each about 20 feet by 40 feet, had been sprayed. In other words, the federal government's display of air-and paraquat-power rid the world of three pathetic patches of pot that together took up less space than a small back yard in the suburbs — less than 6 percent of an acre.

We have no idea how many thousands of dollars the operation cost, nor would we venture a guess at what it will cost all concerned before the lawyers on all sides are done with it. But of this much we are sure: A small crew armed with a scythe — or even one of those newfangled gas-powered weed cutters — and a few plastic bags could have put those illicit fields out of commission for a whole lot less.

The Chattanooga Times
Chattanooga, TN, August 16, 1983

The federal Drug Enforcement Administration's decision to use paraquat to destory marijuana fields in this country is unwise. It will make no substantial contribution to curbing the serious drug problem in the United States and presents a disproportionate danger to the environment, wildlife and human health. We applaud Gov. Lamar Alexander's refusal of the DEA offer to spray the toxic herbicide in Tennessee.

Last Friday DEA agents sprayed several small plots of marijuana on the outskirts of the Chattahoochee National Forest in Georgia. Although the state of Florida used paraquat last year, this was the first time federal agents have employed the herbicide. Georgia Gov. Joe Frank Harris welcomed the initiative, saying, "We're sick and tired of drug problems and we're going to do something about it."

There is no argument the nation is sick and tired of drug problems. Untold thousands of lives have been damaged if not destroyed by drug abuse. A large proportion of property and violent crimes are associated with the lucrative drug trafficking industry, and it is the business of the government to combat those crimes and the flow of dangerous drugs. But it is the responsibility of the government to target drug enforcement activities at the source of the problem and to avoid losing perspective on the problem in their zeal to demonstrate that they are doing something about it.

Drug enforcement officials complain they haven't enough money to wage their war on drugs, which would indicate they should set priorities for their operations. Enforcement should be aimed at the most dangerous drugs and large smuggling operations which carry the marks of organized crime and involve the potential for corruption of law enforcement officers. Wiping out a few, small domestic marijuana crops provides publicity for the DEA, and, in this case, Gov. Harris, but it hardly advances efforts to combat the serious drug problem.

Paraquat is a highly toxic herbicide which can cause severe respiratory problems and death if ingested by humans. Residents of White County are justifiably alarmed about the dangers of the spraying; one citizen said it brings to mind the use of Agent Orange in Vietnam. U.S. Rep. Ed Jenkins properly stated, "The use of paraquat-armed aircraft to spray minute patches of 10 to 20 plants of marijuana when these plants can be easily and safely destroyed by hand defies common sense and economics."

But Gov. Harris is apparently unconcerned about potential contamination of the environment, wildlife and innocent by-standers. And he has callously dismissed the health risk to marijuana smokers: "We don't have any responsibility to those people," he said. "They do that at their own risk." But the fact is that "those people" are, by and large, not hardened criminals but otherwise law abiding people who make up a substantial proportion of the population and reject the laws against smoking marijuana the same way the laws against alcoholic beverages were flaunted during Prohibition.

Raining poison from the skies is, at best, overkill when it comes to combatting marijuana use. The misguided paraquat offensive represents a considerable expenditure of public funds which would be better used to combat the real problem of dangerous drugs. It should be quickly abandoned.

THE LOUISVILLE TIMES

Louisville, KY, August 18, 1983

The recent activity of the powerful U.S. Drug Enforcement Administration gives the strong impression of a government agency under confused and not altogether rational leadership.

Last week, the DEA lurched into Georgia to spray marijuana plants found near the edge of Chattahoochee National Forest with Paraquat, a potent plant killer. There was no sensible explanation for this plan to destroy small, scattered patches of pot plants with a chemical that is deadly to wildlife and human beings and can poison water supplies.

Kentucky, considered a major center of illegal marijuana cultivation, was supposed to be the next stop for the Paraquat sprayers. Pot grown in Daniel Boone National Forest is the target. But a public outcry, congressional protests and a federal court order temporarily restraining use of the herbicide in Georgia have thrown the program into confusion and disorder.

If a reasonable case can be made for aerial spraying on or near federal lands, then residents of the areas involved should have been carefully prepared in advance. Many Kentuckians, however, would not be impressed by the weak official explanation. The use of Paraquat here, say the feds, will persuade authorities in Colombia and Mexico to spray pot grown in their countries for American consumption.

There's no assurance that the Latin Americans will follow our example, of course. But even if a herbicidal attack on marijuana were desirable from the standpoint of law enforcement and foreign relations, the DEA is going about it the wrong way.

Helicopter spraying is notoriously inaccurate. A slight wind can carry toxic mist into adjoining woods and farms. The danger is all the greater because the targets are for the most part small patches of the weed. Ground-level spraying is far preferable.

The increasing efficiency of state police efforts to find and destroy marijuana in Kentucky, Indiana and other states makes it difficult, however, to justify any use of dangerous chemicals.

As staff writer Al Cross reports in two recent *Courier-Journal* articles, detection becomes more sophisticated every year. Kentucky leads the nation in the number of plants confiscated so far this summer, and arrests are four times greater than at this time in 1982. Indiana troopers believe they may nab 80 per cent of the Hoosier crop.

Domestic cultivation of pot, especially on public lands, is a legitimate federal concern. But the Paraquat attack is superfluous in light of state police successes.

Moreover, spraying a deadly chemical in Kentucky woodlands may be more damaging than the problem it is intended to address. Sen. Wendell Ford, U. S. Rep. Hal Rogers and other congressmen should continue their efforts to bring DEA to its senses.

THE ATLANTA CONSTITUTION

Atlanta, GA, August 16, 1983

In his first public difference with Gov. Joe Frank Harris, Lt. Gov. Zell Miller had some harsh words Monday for the governor's decison to allow paraquat spraying on plots of marijuana in the north Georgia mountains.

It does not matter that the spraying, carried out on a limited basis, has now ended. What does matter is that the small-scale "symbolic" nature of the spraying was not advertised very well in Georgia's mountain communities.

As a result, unnecessary fears and anger were generated about a decision to use north Georgia as the federal government's first guinea pig for domestic paraquat spraying.

The Drug Enforcement Administration also demonstrated a carelessness and insensitivity to the region by choosing the peak tourist season in the mountains to announce plans to spray areas in national forests.

Making the timing and hype even more gratuitous, the exercise was not even conducted mainly to reduce marijuana cultivation, but to persuade Colombia to follow suit on its own, much more extensive cultivation of illegal drugs.

Said Lt. Gov. Miller:

"The point of this excercise was called sending a 'symbolic message' to Colombia. 'Sending a message' cuts two ways. We have never had the economic benefits in those mountains that other sections of the state have — no industry, just a little tourism that's finally beginning to come along. I wonder how many potential tourists in north Georgia saw the evening news and got the message 'spraying near Helen and 'Unicoi Lodge' and decided to stay home.''

Gov. Joe Frank Harris' commitment to cooperating with the DEA in an all-out war on drugs is commendable. But Georgia is too densely populated and marijuana cultivation too limited to use this state for extensive paraquat spraying.

Fortunately, the spraying has ended. Gov. Harris, having listened to the public outcry about use of the highly toxic herbicide, undoubtedly will decide that digging and burning are less costly, both politically and otherwise, methods of destroying home grown dope.

DAYTON DAILY NEWS

Dayton, OH, August 16, 1983

More poison for the masses:

Georgians have a right to be unhappy with the United States government for its spraying of the herbicide paraquat on federal lands in their state.

The spraying was part of the Drug Enforcement Agency's all-out attack on pot being grown on federal lands. There's nothing wrong with the feds wanting to curb these illegal operations. But spraying paraquat, a toxic herbicide known to cause respiratory problems if inhaled and death if ingested, is asking for hostile public reaction. Not only is paraquat a danger to humans, it also affects birds and wildlife.

DEA officials insist that the spraying was done in controlled "beams" so only small areas were involved. And authorities will go in and remove the plants when they're dead.

So why not cut the plants out instead of going first to the expense of spraying? The psychological side effects of the word "paraquat" is one reason. People, fearing lung damage from smoking paraquat-sprayed marijuana, will be reluctant to buy any pot grown in areas being sprayed. National Organization for the Reform of Marijuana Laws says that the Reagan Administration hasn't been able to sell Latin American countries on paraquat spraying of their crops if the United States won't use it on its home grown stuff. Now it's being used in this country.

The outrage of Georgia officials and citizens, which included a $15 million lawsuit against numerous federal officials, forced the U.S. government to back off in Georgia.

The feds, however, continue to map marijuana plots in other areas, such as the Daniel Boone National Forest, because the government hopes Kentucky will go along with the spraying program. Kentucky should decline the offer. The amount of marijuana being grown on U.S. park land can't be so overwhelming that it justifies exposing the general population to the dangers of paraquat.

The Oregonian

Portland, OR, August 20, 1983

The possibility that the federal Drug Enforcement Administration will extend its marijuana eradication program to Oregon, using the herbicide paraquat, is reason for concern, not entirely because of the risk of spraying a lethal poison but also because it would be another waste of tax dollars.

The government does not need to rent expensive helicopters and buy thousands of gallons of a highly toxic herbicide just to eradicate small plots of marijuana, which in some cases agents have observed for weeks. A couple of officers can uproot by hand half an acre of marijuana in a couple of hours, haul it off in a pickup truck and burn it. That is the way any sensible taxpayer would do it.

The national marijuana-cum-paraquat war, now concentrated in Southern states where it has caused a public outcry, is an expensive show-and-tell project. It is designed to calm the fears of Latin American countries by showing that paraquat spraying in remote areas is both safe and effective, that it is good enough for Americans, even if it costs a bundle to prove it.

Recently money was wasted in spraying paraquat by helicopter in five plots in Georgia, each hardly bigger than a king-size waterbed. Each plot could have been pulled up in minutes by one agent.

Farmers in Oregon and all other states have been using paraquat, a quick-acting weed and grass killer, to "burn down" vegetation for many years. But they usually do not use aircraft to spray paraquat, which, like countless other substances, will kill anyone who drinks it. At least two persons have died that way in Oregon.

Another risk with using paraquat on marijuana is that, while it will quickly kill the plant in several days, the crop may be harvested and sold after being sprayed, if done promptly, exposing smokers to serious lung damage from the paraquat residue. This concern has caused the federal program in some cases to set up manpower-wasting ground watches to see that sprayed plants are not immediately harvested.

In any toxic spray program there are certain environmental risks. Materials miss targets and kill other vegetation or animal life. Helicopters crash and chemical delivery trucks run off the road and burst their tanks in streams, as Oregon has seen this summer in accidents in the Sevin forest spray program.

So far, despite the national paraquat demonstration effort, marijuana remains plentiful on the street. And there is little evidence Latin Americans are getting out of the lucrative drug business, which is astronomically more profitable than raising coffee, or growing sugar cane.

The Saturday OKLAHOMAN & TIMES

Oklahoma City, OK, August 27, 1983

MORE than 70 arrests resulting from a 10-month undercover investigation aimed at halting drug trafficking at schools in several cities in eastern Oklahoma County point up the ludicrous position of those who oppose the federal government's use of the herbicide paraquat to kill marijuana plants on public land.

The size and scope of trafficking in marijuana are indicated in the number of arrest warrants issued for suspects in Midwest City, Del City, Choctaw, Nicoma Park and Oklahoma City.

The warrants were issued following an expansion of undercover operations last fall when officers posing as high school students infiltrated the schools and gathered information on illegal drug sales.

Police said most of the suspects being rounded up in the latest raids are being charged on marijuana complaints. A police spokesman said many of those being arrested were selling drugs to minors and one suspect was selling an estimated $4,000 worth of marijuana per week.

A major reason for the proliferation of marijuana trafficking is the accessibility of the drug. It can be grown practically anywhere. That is the reason the motives of many of those opposing the government's use of paraquat are questionable.

The federal Drug Enforcement Administration said the use of the herbicide sprayed from a helicoptor would not endanger human health or environment. The DEA has sprayed small marijuana patches on federal lands in Georgia and Kentucky and said its use is being considered in as many as 40 states.

This has prompted a lawsuit and stated opposition from some politicians. Certainly there would be health risks for anyone who smokes pot sprayed with paraquat. The governor of Georgia had an answer for that complaint — pot smokers light up at their own risk.

St. Louis Globe-Democrat

St. Louis, MO, August 18, 1983

State officials in Missouri and Illinois are reported to have decided to oppose the Federal Drug Administration's possible spraying of marijuana plants on federal land with paraquat.

The fear by critics of the paraquat spraying program is that some of the marijuana sprayed with paraquat might find its way to drug users and injure their lungs. However, federal drug officials say the health hazards of paraquat have been exaggerated. They say that paraquat turns plants to dust within 72 hours, and that they watch the plants during that time to see that they aren't harvested.

In any event, the FDA should go ahead with spraying paraquat in Missouri and Illinois, and other states where there are large growths of marijuana on federal land, and let the drug abusers beware.

Why should Missouri and Illinois officials be so solicitous of drug abusers anyway? If paraquat is the best way to eradicate these enormous growths of marijuana, they should be encouraging the federal government to get rid of these large plots of marijuana that now cover large tracts of federal land. There also should be no sympathy for those who are growing pot illegally so they can get rich selling the drug to addicts. Their "business" should be wiped out rather than be protected.

In Missouri's case, it would seem that the Bond administration would be anxious to have federal assistance in eliminating the enormous amount of marijuana grown in Missouri. The state marijuana crop is said to be one of the three largest in the country.

This country has urged other nations to use paraquat to destroy their marijuana crops. If states act to stop the federal government from using paraquat on these plants in the United States, it might cause other nations to decide our government isn't really serious about curbing drug abuse, and they might relax their drive against drugs as well.

The News and Courier

Charleston, SC, August 27, 1983

In the controversy over the U.S. Drug Enforcement Administration's plan to spray paraquat on marijuana fields in 40 odd states of the union — but thwarted, so far, in the Carolinas — the real issue has been lost.

The fact is that the DEA is going about what is quaintly called "the domestic cannibis erradication program" in the wrong way. The DEA is merely playing at wiping out home supplies of pot. But, in the process, the DEA is playing with poison.

The boys and girls in the DEA are obvously in love with their program. It's so dashing. They come humming in over the trees in their helicopters. Then it's "sprays away" — or whatever the expression is. Then off to the next field of pot.

Not that we have any overwhelming concern for the health of pot smokers, but forgive us for spoiling the fun if we ask why the DEA agents cannot cut the plants and burn them? It would save on costly chemicals, for a start. But the major economy would lie in averting the danger of causing massive damage to other crops, to wildlife and to humans not connected with the growing, distribution or consumption of marijuana.

Paraquat is an extremely useful agent in no-till farming. As long as it is used strictly in accordance with precise instructions, it will cause no harm. But paraquat was not meant to be sprayed from helicopters. Indeed, its scary reputation has been partly caused by its improper use in some Third World countries. Improperly used, paraquat can be highly toxic. This has been firmly emphasized by the state Commissioner for Agriculture D. Leslie Tindal, who is on record as saying: "I am not at all satisfied...that aerial application of this chemical in large areas is safe. Paraquat, even in water-diluted form, is potentially hazardous to humans, animals and other wildlife. Not only could it destroy wildlife, but it could also destroy human life."

There is no recorded instance of the improper use of paraquat in South Carolina. But there are plenty of incidents of aerial spraying, although not of paraquat, which are remembered because of the toll they took on nature and wild life.

Chemicals are very tempting to use because they are often a substitute for hard physical work. But the price you pay for not resisting the lazy option could be incalculably high. It's time to call off the cannibis caper. The DEA should be busy stopping supplies of pot and other drugs from coming into the country from abroad and breaking up the distribution network. Or is that also too much like hard work?

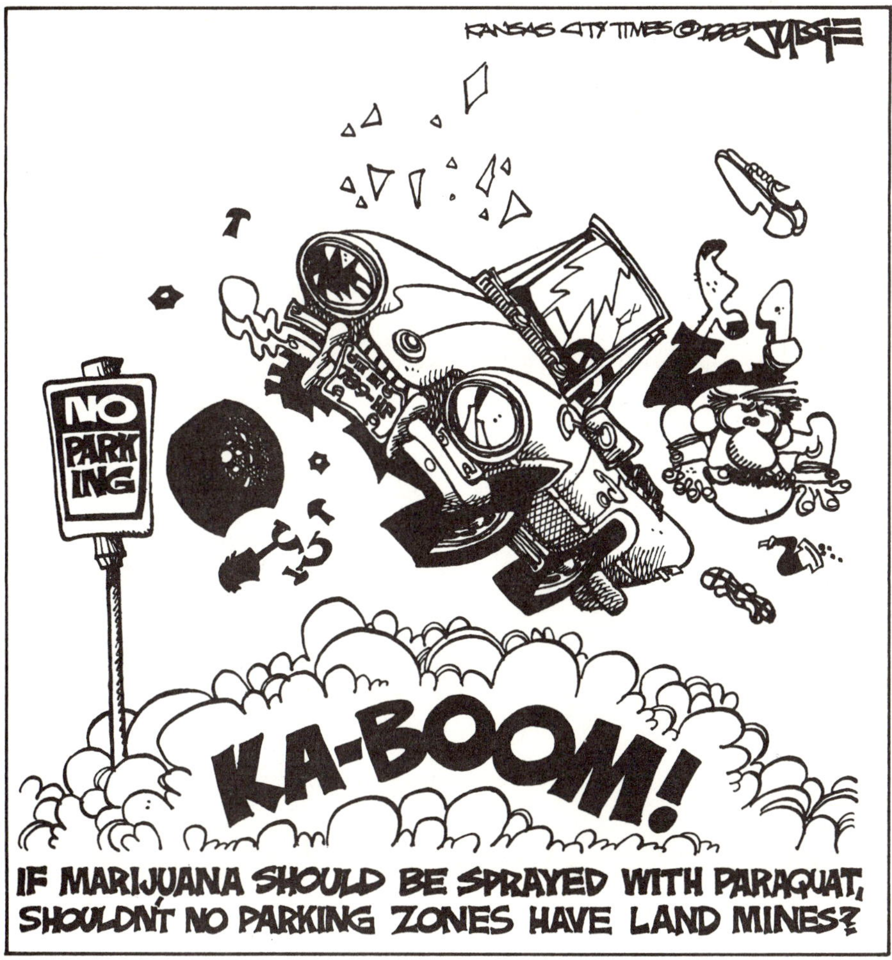

St. Petersburg Times

St. Petersburg, FL, August 20, 1983

The U.S. Drug Enforcement Administration (DEA) is so high on aerial paraquat spraying as a deterrent to marijuana smoking that it has lost sight of the threat to public health — if, indeed, it considers millions of American pot smokers worthy of protection.

The federal enforcers intend to spray the deadly herbicide in up to 40 states, including Florida. DEA planes sprayed the Chattahoochee National Forest in northern Georgia last week until they were halted by a federal judge in Atlanta. Then they headed for the Cherokee National Forest in eastern Tennessee, but were unable to find suitable marijuana patches.

TENNESSEE Gov. Lamar Alexander, saying the state does an adequate job of pulling up and burning marijuana, has denied permission for paraquat spraying on state and private land.

The superintendent of the Great Smoky Mountains National Park, surrounded by national forest, says he will not permit spraying there.

Florida Gov. Bob Graham should stop the DEA's deadly squadron before it crosses our borders.

State Department of Law Enforcement Director Robert Dempsey is prudent enough to realize that aerial paraquat spraying creates environmental and health hazards. Before any spraying in Florida, Dempsey says the DEA should seek state approval and follow state guidelines.

BUT DEMPSEY'S concern is not enough protection from the DEA's dangerous expedition. Paraquat is poison for people, as well as plants. It kills marijuana in a few days, but if the contaminated plants are quickly harvested, they can pass for normal. Inhaling paraquat can cause irreversible lung damage.

Granted, the commercial trafficking in, and possession of, marijuana are illegal. People should not smoke it, but government surveys show that about two-thirds of all young adults have tried pot and millions of Americans use it regularly as a recreational drug.

If paraquat simply destroyed the marijuana crop, aerial spraying might be defended. But it does much more that. It is a needless risk to persons who happen to be in the forest or park being sprayed.

The DEA's poison planes are a terror tactic. Although pot smokers are breaking the law, they don't deserve the death penalty.

Pittsburgh Post-Gazette

Pittsburgh, PA, August 24, 1983

You have to wonder what they were smoking at the U.S. Drug Enforcement Agency in Washington when they ordered plots of marijuana in the Chattahoochee National Forest in Georgia to be sprayed with the herbicide Paraquat, a federally licensed weedkiller that can cause severe respiratory ailments and death if ingested.

Last week, a U.S. district judge issued a temporary restraining order preventing the DEA from continuing spraying the forests, which make up two-thirds of northern Georgia. But that has not necessarily put an end to it. The DEA has plans to spray federal lands in 40 states and the restraining order only restricts sprayings at the Chattahoochee National Forest — and even that order is only temporary.

The debate over the use of Paraquat started back in the late '70s when it was learned that the government had provided funds for spraying the herbicide on marijuana fields in Mexico in an attempt to wipe out plants exported to the United States. A government report issued in 1979 said that smoking marijuana contaminated by Paraquat can cause serious, sometimes irreversible lung damage when inhaled in large amounts.

The DEA's recent actions were challenged in court by Citizens Opposed to Paraquat Spraying (COPS), an ad hoc citizens' group of about 300 who became alarmed when they learned of the sprayings. The group contends that the government gave no warning before the plots were sprayed and believes the herbicide, which they said was sprayed on a windy day, presented a danger to campers and hikers in the area.

Even Chevron, the manufacturer of Paraquat, recommends that the herbicide not be sprayed by air because it is too difficult to control. Spurning this advice, the government sprayed by helicopter in Georgia and, according to an opponent of the spraying, "spilled a lot on a public highway and just let it evaporate." The suit charged that campers in the area "reported nausea, headaches, and other symptoms associated with paraquat poisoning."

Finally, there's an irony to this dangerous federal spraying. The government was concerned about marijuana plants found on six or seven patches, or a total area of about 700 square feet. According to a DEA spokesman, there were only about 70 marijuana plants on those plots. Rather than court the risks of spraying poisons over the countryside, the government could have dealt with those weeds by using a couple of machetes.

Federal Task Force Established; Military to Fight Smuggglers

Attorney General William French Smith January 20, 1983 announced that the first staff members had been assigned to 12 new regional task forces that would investigate drug trafficking by organized crime. The task forces, modeled on a federal group operating in South Florida, were to take the lead in the Reagan Administration's battle against illegal drugs. Smith said that each group would initially be staffed by four federal prosecutors and 18 agents. The agents would come from the Federal Bureau of Investigation (FBI), the Drug Enforcement Agency (DEA), the Internal Revenue Service (IRS), the Customs Service and the Bureau of Alcohol, Tobacco and Firearms. In all, 1,600 agents and prosecutors were to be assigned to the groups. Smith said each task force would concentrate initially on two "high quality cases—those involving major trafficking by major organized crime groups."

Presidential counselor Edwin Meese 3rd March 23, 1983 announced the stepped-up use of the Navy and Air Force in the nation's battle against drug smugglers. Participation by the military in regular law enforcement activities had been allowed by federal legislation passed in 1982. Meese said the use of the military would be coordinated by Vice President George Bush. Meese cautioned that it would "take a long time to implement this program and a long time to see the results." Navy ships would be used to intercept vessels suspected of carrying drugs. Air Force planes and radar units would search for small planes loaded with drugs.

The Times-Picayune
The States-Item

New Orleans, LA, October 22, 1983

A subcommittee of the U.S. House of Representatives paints a grim picture of the effort of local and federal authorities to combat illegal drugs. In a preliminary report, the government operations subcommittee concludes that the authorities are losing the drug war despite the stepped-up efforts of the Reagan administration.

The illegal production of marijuana in the United States has grown so rapidly in recent years that it is "overwhelming the abilities of most local jurisdictions," said the panel. In addition, "We find that smugglers are currently beating even the best of our efforts," said subcommittee chairman Glenn English of Oklahoma. "In fact, according to the Food and Drug Administration, the streets of our major cities are literally awash in cocaine that is purer and cheaper than it was before the inauguration of the vice president's South Florida Task Force."

The Reagan administration has been innovative in its effort to combat the smuggling and distribution of illegal drugs. In some instances, military aircraft, ships and boats have been committed to a widespread effort to apprehend smugglers, particularly in coastal states.

Support for local authorities has also been increased. Additional federal manpower has been committed to the campaign.

But it is obvious that much more needs to be done to have a major impact on the illegal drug trade.

The subcommittee offers some worthwhile recommendations:

—The Justice Department and the Food and Drug Administration should provide more leadership to local authorities and improve information collection systems.

—The government should be more vigorous about eradicating marijuana crops on federal lands.

—Local jurisdictions should have more access to federal resources and equipment, particularly those of the Defense Department and the National Guard.

It has long been apparent that local authorites are far outspent, outmanned and outgunned when it comes to combatting wealthy drug smugglers and distributors. Only a determined and prolonged effort by the federal government will suffice to cope with the spreading tide of illegal drugs.

The San Diego Union

San Diego, CA, May 23, 1983

The use of military ships and planes to help stop drug smuggling into South Florida has worked so well that the 12,000 pounds of cocaine and 3 million pounds of marijuana seized under the program last year equaled the quantities confiscated on land by the Drug Enforcement Administration.

But the success of the Reagan administration's South Florida Drug Task Force has bred new problems. Drug traffickers driven out of Florida are beginning to concentrate around other locations in the United States, including Southern California.

We welcome, therefore, the announcement that a new National Narcotics Border Interdiction System under Vice President George Bush will use the ships, planes, and intelligence resources of San Diego area military installations to apprehend drug smugglers off our coast.

Utilizing Navy ships and planes on regular patrol from San Diego to track suspicious craft until the Coast Guard arrives to investigate makes a lot of sense. Eventually, Coast Guard personnel may be stationed aboard Navy vessels for quicker action against the smugglers. Authorities believe that so-called mother ships carrying thousands of tons of marijuana travel several hundred miles off San Diego as they move north to unload their cargoes.

The involvement of the military should strengthen an expanded drug enforcement program already being implemented. The administration previously had announced creation of 12 regional drug task forces, including one headquartered in San Diego, to coordinate the battle against this illicit trade within the country.

The beefed-up interdiction system and the new regional task forces can't be expected to stop the narcotics traffic altogether. But such wise use of available resources ought to put a significant dent in what has become both a national peril and a national disgrace.

The Kansas City Times
Kansas City, MO, March 1, 1983

The administration's assault on illegal drugs has been judged a standoff between government agents and traffickers. That is not necessarily good news, but even a stalemate in this instance must be considered progress.

Seizures of cocaine nearly tripled and those of heroin were about double over the previous year. Destruction of domestic marijuana reached an all-time high. Government officials acknowledge, however, that street supplies of heroin and cocaine became more plentiful. Both sold for less and were purer. The price of marijuana remained about the same.

Whatever anti-drug gains occurred came with a minimum of financial assistance. In the early going the administration seemed more concerned about denouncing crime than taking decisive action. Officials stressed economies, including key personnel cuts. That left fewer agents to try to keep pressure on the traffickers. Much of the serious activity centered in South Florida, where a special task force headed by Vice President George Bush was set up in an attempt to curb the flow of illegal drugs into this country.

Last fall the administration called for the hiring of up to 1,200 more agents and investigators, as well as establishment of task forces around the country, as a means of fighting organized crime, including drug trafficking. There seemed to be a recognition at that time the anti-crime fight would require additional money. The cost of the president's new program was set at $200 million.

As law enforcement authorities know all too well, drug abuse is only one part of the problem. Addicts must steal or rob, perhaps both, to support their habit.

So cracking down on drug traffickers not only helps dry up narcotics supplies, it has a direct impact on other crime. The administration should keep up the good fight and not fear spending money in the process.

FORT WORTH STAR-TELEGRAM
Fort Worth, TX, February 6, 1983

We are in a war in this country.
A war on drugs.

It sometimes seems to be poorly fought, and poorly funded, when compared to the enormity of the drug traffic against which the war is waged. But the effort is growing.

Increased attention on the federal level has at least enabled the Drug Enforcement Administration, U.S. Customs officers, the FBI and the Coast Guard to hold the line against importation of drugs. While the drug traffic has grown, federal agencies have continued to seize more than 10 percent of the contraband.

We're in that same war here in Texas, with the combat targeted on distributors and street dealers.

And Department of Public Safety Director Jim Adams cites increased success on the state level since the Legislature, at the urging of Gov. Bill Clements, passed in 1981 a body of laws incorporating stiffer penalties, wiretap authority and other aids to increased vigilance, particularly against dealers who prey on school students.

Clements has left the governor's office to Gov. Mark White, amid a certain amount of acrimony, but both men earn the plaudits of the people because the state's war on drugs — begun under Clements — continues, and may even be expanded, under White.

White has said he will ask for more narcotics agents and still tougher penalties for drug dealers.

It's one war we all support.

THE ☁ SUN
Baltimore, MD, September 20, 1983

In "War on Drugs," an investigative series by reporter Ann LoLordo that concludes in *The Sun* today, several points were made that every citizen ought to know:
• City police under Commissioner Frank J. Battaglia and Capt. Joseph P. Newman, chief of the Narcotics Task Force, are waging an inspired battle against drug criminals, employing more than triple the resources of just two years ago.
• State's Attorney Kurt L. Schmoke and his assistant for narcotics, John N. Prevas, have increased prosecutions in serious narcotics cases by 50 percent in just one year — and are winning twice as many prison sentences as a year ago.
• The Federal Bureau of Investigation, the Drug Enforcement Administration and the U.S. Attorney for Maryland have increased their efforts, with a special task force set up for this region.
• Police, health and social workers are putting in more time and spending more money to prevent youths from getting hooked on drugs and help addicts end their dependency.

Yet, despite all this, the war is not being won here. Drug traffic is being "contained," in the words of U.S. Attorney J. Frederick Motz, but "You're never going to get rid of it," in the words of Kurt Schmoke. It is a war that never ends.

This is hardly a criticism of the people in the front lines of the war. People can only do so much, no matter how dedicated and professional. The fact that the drug traffic continues means even more resources must be found for law enforcement, prevention and treatment. Targets all along the network that make drug trafficking profitable must be attacked.

Local and regional efforts are not enough. Overseas opium poppy fields and heroin processing plants, and all distribution facilities, must be dealt with. Congress should think strongly about amending foreign aid laws to penalize countries responsible for the flow of drugs into the U.S., and the president perhaps ought to reconsider his opposition to legislation creating a cabinet-level drugs "czar" — or to come up with his own initiative to elevate and coordinate federal drug efforts.

Drug addiction flourishes in the slum-ghetto environment of joblessness and despair. The addict pays for his habit with crime, and his victims are all of us. The profile of the typical addict is known to social scientists. But as Dr. David Nurco of the University of Maryland Medical School has pointed out, what we don't know is the profile of the typical "invulnerable." What is different about the youth who lives in the same hopeless environment as the criminal addict but never turns to drugs? Can that difference be learned and taught? This is worth pursuing.

So is the goal of eradicating the slum-ghetto culture by creating jobs and other avenues out. Meanwhile, the war goes on, and those in the trenches on society's side deserve commendation and support.

The Boston Herald
Boston, MA, September 14, 1983

FROM NEWS accounts this summer of some record-breaking drug seizures, one would think the waters off Massachusetts were packed with the sleek sloops of drug traffickers. Well, it must have seemed that way to the state's top law enforcement officials and to Gov. Michael S. Dukakis too, because the governor and Attorney General Frank Bellotti have agreed to what they call a "scorched earth" policy toward drug traffickers.

The new policy will mean nothing is sacred any more — not the drug dealer's home or boat or car or liquor license or anything that can be attached and carted off by police or Revenue Department officials. The new get tough policy is more than just an attitude, it represents a new type of extensive cooperation between law enforcement and the executive agencies of government.

Now part of the policy will need legislation. One proposal would allow money from the sale of seized vessels and vehicles to go directly to the offices of the district attorneys that helped in the capture, rather than to the state's general fund. That would provide not only added incentive in the war against drugs, but added resources as well to the front line troops.

One of the prime beneficiaries would be Bristol County District Attorney Ronald Pina, whose territory includes the ports of New Bedford and Fall River, where a number of large drug seizures have been made recently. Pina's office would also be granted special state police powers to make pursuit of the drug traffickers easier.

The policy is great news for those who don't want to see us become the Fort Lauderdale of the Northeast, and it sure will be bad news for the drug trade.

Rocky Mountain News

Denver, CO, October 4, 1983

DESPITE the Reagan administration's highly publicized crackdown on drug smuggling, there doesn't seem to be any shortage of the stuff in the United States.

A South Florida law enforcement officer told a congressional task force on international narcotics control recently that an unprecedented flood of cocaine and marijuana is coming in from the Bahamas.

Heavy narcotics shipments from Latin America also are reported crossing the borders in the Southwest and West.

Sen. Dennis DeConcini, D-Ariz., complained that the United States lacks a "war plan to attack drug smugglers," and suggested establishing a Cabinet-level "drug czar."

Whether there is need for such an office is arguable. In fact, President Reagan last year vetoed a bill that would have established one. But it's pretty obvious that better coordination of the fight against drug smuggling is required.

One thing that would help is prompt confirmation of a permanent director for the federal Drug Enforcement Administration.

Francis M. Mullen Jr., former executive assistant director of the FBI, has been acting head of the drug agency for more than two years. His confirmation as permanent DEA director was held up in the Senate Judiciary Committee largely because of opposition from Sen. Orrin Hatch, R-Utah.

Hatch dragged his feet for so long, for so many reasons, that his opposition almost took on the nature of harassment.

Mullen was handpicked by FBI Director William Webster to head DEA. Lack of confirmation is said to have created morale problems at the agency. And that can't help but hamper its work.

The Judiciary Committee has finally approved the nomination and the Senate is expected to act on it shortly. Maybe then we'll see action in the fight against drug smuggling.

The State

Columbia, SC, December 4, 1983

THE CANCER of illicit drugs continues to plague South Carolina but obviously action and, more importantly, results have begun to replace words in the battle against the smuggling.

The success in convicting the two dozen law-breakers netted in Operation Jackpot, code name for a federal investigation of an illegal operation dating from the early 1970s, serves to warn those who ply their nefarious trade in the Palmetto State.

The latest convictions in November involved four members of the so-called Riley ring. The third trial of Jackpot defendants just got under way.

The Jackpot prosecutions are a welcome culmination of President Reagan's push, launched Oct. 2, 1982, to target the fat cats of the drug trade. The drive wisely focused on the overlords' distribution networks rather than on local pushers. The object was to nab those who prey on the vulnerable before the sellers take to the school playgrounds and the streets.

U.S. Atty. Gen. William French Smith then noted that illicit retail drug sales in 1980 topped $79 billion — an amount he said roughly equaled "the combined profits of America's 500 largest industrial corporations."

The anti-smuggling war is vital, and not merely because drugs are illegal. The drug epidemic is at the heart of crime in America. Aside from the human misery, the economic and personal losses drugs inflict on the nation are enormous. While the vice merchants amass wealth, society pays the toll in crimes committed by addicts to support their habits, welfare costs for families wrecked by drugs and in countless other ways.

Smashing the drug network would have a major effect on crime because the battle against the drug overlords is in part one against organized crime, which is deeply involved in the racket.

But the war is far from being won. In November, three major seizures of drugs were made off the coast of South Carolina, whose inviting inlets, coves and bays have proved attractive to smugglers after successful crackdowns in and off Florida.

Nor will the day be carried with wholesale convictions. Still needed is a greater emphasis on anti-drug education for young people. For users create the demand that makes the business so lucrative that the misery peddlers are willing to risk jail for big bucks.

The problem is difficult, complex and costly. But determined efforts like Operation Jackpot finally are showing concrete results where rhetoric once prevailed.

DESERET NEWS

Salt Lake City, UT, March 23-24, 1983

For years, presidents' wives have busied themselves with worthwhile projects while their husbands were in office. Lady Bird Johnson urged beautifying America; Jacqueline Kennedy undertook a historic restoration of the White House; Pat Nixon devoted herself to several causes, including educational programs, community self-help undertakings, and volunteer work.

Rosalynn Carter, said an Associated Press biographer, shared "a political partnership" with her husband Jimmy "unequaled in the White House since the days of Franklin and Eleanor Roosevelt."

Of all these worthwhile projects, perhaps none is as important to America's long-range well-being as First Lady Nancy Reagan's efforts to combat drug and alcohol abuse by school-age children. As part of that program, it was announced this week, she plans to host two prime-time public TV specials next November aimed at grass-roots attempts to stamp out abuses among young people.

"We are in danger of losing an entire generation," says Mrs. Reagan, "unless we act now to educate ourselves and our children."

Certainly that's a commendable aim. National figures show:

— Two-thirds of all children experiment with an illicit drug before they finish high school.

— One in 16 high school seniors smoke marijuana regularly. The same number use alcohol daily.

— Drunk driving is the leading cause of death among 15- to 24-year-olds.

The drug program's aims are ambitious and well-funded. The $2 million project seeks to establish at least one drug abuse task force in each school district in the nation. It will be up to these task forces to develop educational, informational, and treatment programs in their areas.

Can there be any more worthy cause for the nation's first lady to be associated with than to get kids off drugs and alcohol? Mrs. Reagan deserves strong national support for this most vital cause.

The Seattle Times
Seattle, WA, October 26, 1983

FEDERAL agents in the Pacific Northwest rate public commendation for some first-rate police work leading to the largest seizures of cocaine and heroin in this state's history.

But news of the arrests of four persons and confiscation of large amounts of the drugs also serves as a worrisome reminder that illegal trafficking in dangerous drugs — especially cocaine — continues to be a large piece of unfinished business on the law-enforcement agenda. It also represents a major issue for law-abiding citizens in general, since drugs still figure importantly in the overall picture of crime in American society.

The sheer magnitude of the most recent seizures — 10 pounds of cocaine with a wholesale value of $400,000, intended for delivery to Vashon Island, and 1.7 pounds of heroin, worth perhaps $800,000, confiscated at the Blaine border crossing — provides insight into dimensions of the larger problem. That is because vastly more contraband continues to exist in the marketplace than is taken out of circulation.

The dangers of heroin long have been clearly understood. But there is far less appreciation of cocaine's detrimental side effects. A widely prevailing but incorrect belief that cocaine is not a dangerous drug explains its widespread popularity, an acceptance that complicates the task of enforcement agencies.

Even with intensified efforts to curb cocaine trafficking, agents estimate they're able to seize only about 10 percent of the 100,000 pounds of cocaine smuggled into the U.S. each year, almost all of it from Bolivia, Colombia and Peru.

Lacking assistance from the governments of those countries, U.S. authorities must fight largely a single-handed battle. To their credit, they continue the effort against very tough odds.

THE DAILY HERALD
Biloxi, MS, June 15, 1983

Despite the rhetoric of elected officials at all levels of government, the United States continues losing in its war on drugs and eventually, words of condemnation will need to be replaced by action. This week's General Accounting Office report gives additional documentation to the losses and adds to the sense of urgency for changing federal strategy and tactics.

GAO, an arm of Congress, recommended creation of a drug "czar," a Cabinet-level official who would be in charge of coordinating the efforts to halt the deluge of illegal drugs flowing into the country. Congress last year passed legislation similar to GAO's current recommendations, but President Ronald Reagan vetoed it. He since has announced plans to create a series of task forces, similar to the one that obtained some success in South Florida.

Vice President George Bush, who headed the Florida task force, is expected to announce six more such task forces on Friday. The task forces ought to be given the opportunity to stop the incoming flow of drugs.

Despite an increase in federal resources devoted to drug interception from $83 million in 1977 to $278 million last year, the government's record is pathetic. It seized only 16 percent of incoming marijuana and less than 10 percent of the heroin, cocaine and other hard drugs. The record is too weak to dis-courge smugglers, much less deter them.

Another indication of the failure of the federal efforts is a Drug Enforcement Administration report issued this week. DEA reports an increase in the heroin supply, a reduction in price and a rise in drug purity, accompanied by an increase in deaths and emergency room admissions for heroin overdoses.

Estimates are that the illegal drug business has grown to sales of $100 billion annually in the U. S. A national survey in 1981 found 23 million marijuana users and five million regular users of cocaine.

Both the GAO study and a Gannet News Service 14-month investigation into the war on drug found that federal agencies involved in the struggle squabble with each other, are disorganized, communicate poorly with one another and suffer inefficiency when called upon for joint efforts.

In contrast, drug smugglers have increased their organization and efficiency, applying substantial protions of their outlandishly high profits to obtaining expert assistance and sophisticated equipment to avoid interception and arrest.

There must be a turnaround. If the new task forces fail to produce substantial gains in a reasonable period, the president and the Congress must then implement the GAO concept.

OKLAHOMA CITY TIMES
Oklahoma City, OK, December 20, 1983

IT'S going to take more than the expertise of the cloak-and-dagger boys of the CIA to make a dent into massive airborne smuggling of marijuana and narcotics through U.S. southern borders.

That becomes obvious with knowledgeable figures of illegal drug smuggling operations cited by Oklahoma's Rep. Glenn English, who has become recognized in Congress as an expert in that field.

English's war on drugs has spurred the Reagan administration to increase its efforts to combat the flow of narcotics into this country. The administration last summer established the National Narcotics Border Interdiction System (NNBIS). It is comprised of eight regions around the perimeter of the United States and is headed by Vice President George Bush.

When he took over the NNBIS, Bush ordered the CIA to get involved in drug smuggling intelligence to be a part of the war on drugs.

But English last week said airborne drug smugglers still are operating with impunity, flying their illicit and deadly cargoes into the United States through Puerto Rico. He said the smugglers are hauling in cocaine from Colombia, 400 miles from the island of Puerto Rico, in private aircraft that land on "30 or 40" air strips, some of which are guarded and fenced off from law enforcement officers.

English said the drug smugglers can file a flight plan from any commercial airport in Puerto Rico and "enter any U.S. cities without clearing customs or undergoing any inspection. They are subject to no more checks than you would receive flying from Dallas to Oklahoma City."

He contends there is little or no hindrance to drug trafficking, mainly because of lack or severe shortage of federal drug enforcement officers and lack of authority to intercept smugglers.

He said he will seek new regulations, or possibly legislation, for the U.S. Customs Service to fence off the contraband drugs from the mainland United States.

Certainly, air cargo coming into the United States from Puerto Rico should be subject to customs inspection.

Houston Chronicle
Houston, TX, October 17, 1983

There has been some debate of late, especially in hearings before the House Select Committee on Narcotics Abuse and Control, about the effectiveness of the federal drug task force that has been fighting the flow of drugs into the United States.

The usual complaints center around the cost, the fragmented nature of the federal effort and the ability of drug traffickers to merely change their operations to other locations. One congressman at the hearings said the program was netting the little people, not the "big guys."

The debate serves a useful purpose in that the legitimate problems and possible flaws in the program are being discussed; however, the obvious success of the task force in zeroing in on the trouble spots should not be overlooked.

Before the task force went into operation, the drug traffickers were conducting virtually open warfare in southern Florida. With several government agencies cooperating, including the military, the traffickers found the going tougher and justice a little swifter. The task force definitely made a difference in Florida.

The statistics indicate the drug flow is still high, but who can say what the figures would have been had the task force not been operating? Yes, some of the dealers moved their operations into rural Georgia and Tennessee, even into coastal Texas. But the federal program, again with the cooperation of several federal agencies, has been expanded to cover the entire nation.

One thing is certain: The fight cannot stop. There are governments in Latin America that cannot or will not control the cultivation of drug-producing plants and the processing of drugs explicitly for smuggling to the United States, where there unfortunately is still a ready market. The best way to cut down on the human toll these illegal drugs exact is to meet the challenge. Right now the task force seems to be doing that.

Reagan Vetoes Crime Bill; Opposes 'Drug Czar' Provision

President Ronald Reagan January 14, 1983 vetoed a comprehensive anticrime bill approved by the 97th Congress, saying the bill would have "an adverse impact on our efforts to combat drug abuse." Although he approved of several of the bill's seven provisions, the president strongly opposed a section of the bill that would have established a cabinet-level position for an official, popularly known as a "drug czar," to oversee federal antinarcotics efforts. The President said the "so-called drug czar provision was enacted hastily without thoughtful debate and without benefit of any hearings." In refusing to sign the bill, Reagan continued: "The war on crime and drugs does not need more bureaucracy in Washington. It does need more action in the field, and that is where my administration will focus its efforts."

Reagan also opposed provisions of the bill that would have imposed mandatory sentences on persons who were repeatedly convicted of committing crimes with handguns, and that would have given local prosecutors veto power over federal indictments. He called the latter provision "an unworkable and possibly unconstitutional restraint on federal prosecutions."

Sen. Joseph R. Biden (D, Del.), a sponsor of the crime bill, said Reagan had rejected a compromise that he and several other senators had offered. Under the compromise proposal, the attorney general, rather than a new appointee would be named the drug czar until Congress could act to weaken the powers of the new position. "This administration has always been strong on rhetoric about crime but weak on substantive action," Biden said. He called working with Reagan on crime issues "an uphill battle."

The Arizona Republic

Phoenix, AZ, January 16, 1983

THE good went down the drain with the bad when President Reagan's pocket veto killed anti-crime legislation fashioned hastily by the lame duck session of Congress.

The bill's worst feature was the creation of a Cabinet-level "czar" to take control of disparate federal anti-drug programs and direct enforcement from a single office.

The president was wise in killing the measure, although attractive features the administration had requested also were lost.

Drug trafficking, indeed, is a menace of terrifying proportions. Illicit and illegal drugs succor the greed of vice lords, and work destructively on addicts.

But the notion that a "drug czar" is the solution is plain silly.

The administration has made workable strides in exacting more cooperation and coordination among agencies whose statutory authority gives them differing forms of reach into the world of drugs.

Little more could be done with a "drug czar" — unless, of course, the very Democrats in Congress who complain of Interior Secretary James Watt's heavy-handed methods want a "czar" who would run roughshod over established lines of authority and thumb his nose at even the wishes of Congress.

Turning to the "czar" approach to solve the drug problem would merely invite creation of more "czars." Congressmen no doubt could justify czars to provide crash solutions to unemployment, farm foreclosures, worker productivity, industrial automation.

The peevish reaction of Sen. Dennis DeConcini, D-Ariz., to the veto was especially childish.

On hearing of the veto, DeConcini petulantly took a swipe at U.S. Attorney General William French Smith — "I hope [he] is enjoying playing tennis at John Gardiner's [Tennis Ranch] while crime continues to go unchecked."

It was left to *Republic* reporter Don Harris to point out that DeConcini failed to mention that he also was scheduled to be at the Gardiner resort in Paradise Valley with the attorney general and other senators for a tennis match benefitting Hospice.

Should the attorney general have asked Sen. DeConcini if he is ignoring his senatorial duties, and allowing national problems to go unchecked, by being here to play tennis?

Sen. DeConcini should be cautioned about pretending to be an expert on drug wars.

His vaunted venture into drug enforcement — creation of the Border County Drug Strike Force while he was Pima County attorney — was a failure.

Not only did the strike force not live up to then-county attorney DeConcini's hopes, it became a multi-million dollar bureaucratic fat cat whose director resigned in the face of allegations of mismanagement of funds and equipment, and which now has been disbanded by the Legislature.

DESERET NEWS

Salt Lake City, UT, June 16-17, 1983

While the flow of illegal drugs into the U.S. is rising, federal efforts to stem the tide are fragmented and largely ineffective. Maybe the time has come to knock down the bureaucratic walls and put a "drug czar" in charge.

That is the recommendation in a report issued this week by the General Accounting Office, an investigative arm of Congress. It deserves serious consideration for the following reasons:

— Only 16% of the marijuana being smuggled into the country is seized by federal agents and less than 10% of the hard drugs such as cocaine and heroin. Most of the arrests are of low-level violators who average less than a year in jail. The big dealers and smugglers usually avoid capture.

— Authority and reponsibility to intercept the drug flow are divided among three agencies in three different departments, all with different goals, programs and priorities. The three agencies are Customs, Coast Guard, and the Drug Enforcement Administration.

What is needed is a single drug enforcement strategy with one office responsible for getting the job done.

Such a recommendation was contained in a crime package passed by Congress last December. But it was vetoed by President Reagan, who said it would just add another layer to the bureaucracy.

However, the aim is to reduce the conflicts caused by bureaucracy. And obviously, the present system is not effective.

Spending more money on the problem doesn't work. For example, from 1977 to last year, the funding for interception of drug smuggling more than tripled — from $83 million to $278 million. Yet the percentage of drugs seized has not increased significantly.

Illegal drugs are a cancer eating away at the body of the nation, but too many doctors are trying to operate from different angles. Let's put the knife in the hands of one chief surgeon.

The Dispatch

Columbus, OH, January 21, 1983

THE BILL that would have created a "drug czar" to coordinate the federal efforts to fight illegal drug trafficking deserved to die and President Reagan was right in vetoing it. Anti-drug efforts and good government are better served without the bill.

The bill would have allowed the president to appoint a high-level official to coordinate the investigation and prosecution of drug traffickers. This official would have had the authority to tell Cabinet secretaries how to use the resources of their departments in the fight against drug abuse. Such authority would substantially redefine the roles of the Cabinet members and would set a precedent that could lead to an entire new structure for the executive branch. Such a change could not be tolerated.

This grievous flaw was compounded by the fact that the bill failed to recognize the considerable inter-agency cooperation already taking place within the Reagan administration to fight the drug problem. It is significant to note that each agency that is now part of Vice President George Bush's anti-drug program opposed the drug czar legislation.

And the bill, coming as it did at a time when 12 regional narcotics task forces are being formed to crack down on drug abuse, failed to recognize that substantial gains were possible within the existing structure of the federal 'government. The bill was simply a throwback to former days when the prevailing wisdom was that more government, bigger government could solve any problem that arose. The truth is that the czar-type approach to problems is often inefficient and counterproductive since it simply makes for more paperwork and vastly complicates the solution-finding process.

Reagan is committed to curbing drug abuse in this country, and his commitment is enhanced by his decision to veto the drug czar bill.

The Register

Santa Ana, CA, January 14, 1983

President Reagan has before him a product of the lame-duck Congress that purports to be anti-crime or anti-drug legislation. If he fails to sign it by midnight, the bill would not become a law. That's what his Justice Department brass want him to do, and for once we're inclined to agree with them.

HR 3963 is a potpourri cooked up by congressional staff members, consisting of measures that had won favor in either the House or Senate. Justice officials are most troubled by a provision creating a "drug czar," a Cabinet-level official who would be responsible for coordinating narcotics-law enforcement among various departments (Justice, Treasury, and Transportation all have a piece of the action now). What troubles the prosecutors is that as the legislation is written, this new official would have the authority to order such titans as the attorney general to follow his priorities.

It's probably not in the cards for the federal government to start decriminalizing drug use; that would be too sensible a concession to reality. Even those who defend existing drug laws, however, would do well to be wary of yet another crusade, to be waged by this new Cabinet officer (and a huge department soon enough, you may be sure). The federal government's record in waging crusades designed to reform personal behavior was exemplified in *Califano v. Cigarette Smoking*. A period of fiscal crisis, when federal deficits of $200 billion per year are possible, is hardly the time to be launching another one.

Other provisions of HR 3963 are questionable as well. One section would create an Office of Justice Assistance funded with $130 million for grants to local and state law enforcement agencies, a successor to the Law Enforcement Assistance Administration of bitter memory. Another would let state and local prosecutors decide whether "career criminals" would be handed over to the federal court system. The Justice Department doubts the constitutionality of that one. We'd like to see bankruptcy handled adequately first.

Perhaps the most astounding piece of advice Reagan got regarding this bill came from Sen. Strom Thurmond, R-S.C. Acknowledging that as written it had some problems, he urged Reagan to sign it anyway and let Congress pass additional legislation to smooth out the troublesome wording. This is not a tailor we'd trust with our alterations.

Sen. Joseph Biden had a double-edged observation. Noting that it took a long time to get a consensus for HR 3963, he predicted: "If this falls apart...there will be no anti-crime legislation in the Reagan administration."

A cost-benefit test of past "anti-crime" efforts, paired with Biden's assessment, would only add to the hope that the president leaves the Oval Office tonight with this latest measure still on his desk.

San Francisco Chronicle

San Francisco, CA, January 6, 1983

THERE IS A backstairs fight on in the White House these days attempting to persuade President Reagan to veto a package of anti-crime measures lumped into one bill passed by the lame-duck Congress before its members scampered home for Christmas. We join some so-far anonymous officials in the Justice Department in urging that the measure be vetoed before it becomes law January 14.

There are a number of worthy, undoubtedly useful sections in the law, which seems to have acquired new appendages at every stop in the committee and House and Senate conference process. They deal with guns, attempting to halt a growing national flood of fraudulent identification cards and new and tougher narcotics penalties. There is even a provision responding to the Tylenol case by making it a federal crime to adulterate packaged food and drug products.

But the bill would also create a new cabinet-level "drug czar." The new director of National and International Drug Operations and Policy would be appointed by the president and confirmed by the Senate. He would have authority over other cabinet officers, including the attorney general, the nation's highest law enforcement officer, in developing and carrying drug law enforcement programs.

THE IDEA IS that of Senator Joseph R. Biden Jr., D-Delaware, the ranking minority member of the Senate Judiciary Committee. He believes that creation of the new position is necessary to "get some results" in halting the drug trade.

There is almost unanimous public agreement that the nation has a serious drug problem. There should be agreement that many agencies of government are involved in efforts to abate the huge flow of illegal substances and that their efforts should be coordinated. But creating a new office with such sweeping power seems overreaction by far. It is a response of political panic. Placing one cabinet member between other members of the cabinet and the president simply to handle an aspect of the national crime problem does not make administrative or legal sense.

It is charitable to attribute this legislation to the turmoil in which Congress found itself in the last few days of the last session. It is necessary, however, to urge President Reagan to correct a serious mistake.

The Orlando Sentinel

Orlando, FL, January 7, 1983

A new crime bill will become law if the president signs it by Jan. 14. It will make tampering with drugs and food a federal felony, toughen fines for trafficking in illegal drugs, and give government new power to seize assets tied to drug-trafficking.

Despite such worthy provisions, the president should veto the bill because of one overriding flaw: It will create a new Cabinet-level office to oversee the federal fight against illegal drugs.

Better coordination and a higher priority are needed for drug enforcement; a director of National and International Drug Operations and Policy is not.

The current Balkanization of drug-fight duties is inefficient. Few would argue otherwise. The job is divvied among 10 federal agencies, including the IRS, the CIA, the Customs Service and the Bureau of International Narcotics Matters. This means turf fights and poor coordination. For example, the Bureau of International Narcotics Matters was isolated from planning for the drug-enforcement initiatives President Reagan announced in October.

But this issue belongs at the Justice Department, squarely under the direction of Attorney General William French Smith. The attorney general should be able to get whatever interagency cooperation and office-shuffling he needs. The importance of the drug issue argues for its consolidation at Justice rather than in a Cabinet-level office distinct from any department.

Other than this bureaucratic foolishness, the bill's crime provisions are positive and non-controversial. After a veto, they quickly can be passed again.

The Seattle Times

Seattle, WA, January 20, 1983

PRESIDENT REAGAN showed good judgment in vetoing legislation that would have created a "drug czar" to run the government's drug-law enforcement.

To appoint a "czar" with sweeping powers would have been politically popular. Some even would have looked upon it as a cure-all to the drug problem.

Reagan rightly said the war on crime and drugs doesn't need any more bureaucracy but, rather, "more action in the field." This was an example of putting emphasis on real effort rather on a simplistic, politically appealing solution.

FORT WORTH STAR-TELEGRAM

Fort Worth, TX, July 12, 1983

A congressional panel was on target last week when it called for greater coordination and more cooperation between the agencies that have been charged with the task of waging the federal government's war on drugs.

It is a war that has had a promising beginning. The South Florida Task Force is a good example of that. Formed at the urging of the Reagan administration and headed by Vice President George Bush, the task force has registered a number of successes in a campaign aimed at stemming the flow of drugs into this country from Latin America and the Caribbean area.

But those successes have spawned other problems. A number of drug smugglers were trapped in the task force's net, but many others merely moved their areas of operation. Authorities report now that drug traffic has increased along the hard-to-patrol U.S.-Mexican border.

As the drug war has intensified, however, so have interagency problems. No one bureau or governmental department currently has the authority to control the total anti-smuggling operation. The Justice Department, which oversees the federal Drug Enforcement Agency, can operate only within a prescribed sphere of activity. The same is true of the Treasury Department, which participates in the drug war through its control of customs procedures.

Because of that, there is an expensive duplication of some activities, while other fronts are left uncovered altogether. The result, of course, is a dangerous weakening of the anti-smuggling offensive.

When members of the House Subcommittee on Government Information, Justice and Agriculture met last week in El Paso, its chairman, Rep. Glenn English, D-Okla., called for a "drug czar," who would be responsible for formulating a coordinated federal drug strategy and for seeing that the strategy was carried out.

Rep. Ronald Coleman, a Democrat from El Paso, said that without better coordination among agencies, the drug war — tough enough under ideal circumstances — will be lost.

Because it's a war we can't afford to lose, Congress and the administration should move swiftly to bring about such coordination. And a good place to start would be with the appointment of a tough, no-nonsense "czar" to head the combined agencies.

The Cincinnati Post

Cincinnati, OH, June 27, 1983

President Reagan was roundly criticized last January when he vetoed a bill passed by the lame-duck 97th Congress that would have set up a Cabinet-level "czar" to coordinate the government's war against illegal drug smuggling.

He argued that the legislation would only have added more confusion and bureaucracy to the drug-fighting effort.

This newspaper found the argument less than convincing, since that effort was already scattered among a slew of federal agencies and had just been assessed as pretty much of a failure by the General Accounting Office, Congress' investigating arm.

We're now glad to see that the president has, in effect, done what the critics have been demanding by appointing Vice President George Bush to head a new and expanded anti-drug campaign.

Bush will direct the National Narcotics Border Interdiction System, which will draw on the existing resources of federal and local crime-fighting agencies in six cities — New York, El Paso, New Orleans, Long Beach, Calif., Chicago and Miami.

The new program will utilize Central Intelligence Agency informers and surveillance by Army and Navy helicopters and will be targeted against all foreign drug traffic, not just that from Latin America.

And it won't cost the government more than it is already spending. "It is strictly a coordinating effort," said a Bush spokesman, "to bring together what the public has already paid for."

With the public paying dearly in other ways for the unceasing flow of illicit drugs into this country, we can only hope that the administration has come up with the key to stopping, or at least significantly diminishing, the traffic and that in ex-CIA chief Bush it has found the "czar" who will make it work.

St. Louis Globe-Democrat

St. Louis, MO, January 19, 1983

It is hard to see how Congress could approve a bill so obviously flawed as the crime legislation which would have created a new "drug czar" to head the government's anti-drug program.

President Reagan rightly vetoed the bill as he said "the war on crime and drugs does not need more bureaucracy in Washington."

The president said the measure also contained "an unworkable and possibly unconstitutional restraint" on federal prosecutions because it gave state and local prosecutors a veto over such cases under their authority.

Drafters of the legislation seemed to assume that the trouble in the fight against drugs is that the federal government doesn't have enough control over what goes on, a completely erroneous assumption. They would have created a drug czar with extensive powers over federal agencies, directing efforts to stem the abuse of drugs and smuggling of drugs into the U.S. He could have ordered Cabinet officials to follow his priorities.

The "drug czar" bill ignored the fact that other legislation approved at the lame duck session provided for large task forces throughout the country to go after major drug rings. The Justice Department, the FBI and other agencies involved in the new nationwide effort against drugs don't need a czar in Washington to carry out their campaign.

Past experience indicates that various czars, including a series of energy czars, often wind up being part of the problem rather than contributing to the solution.

The government is well designed to carry out its missions without superimposing czars to get in the way of regular crime-fighting agencies. Nor is there any need to cater to the whims of congressional activists who want to create new fiefdoms in the federal bureaucracy to carry out congressional policies in the executive branch.

Houston Chronicle

Houston, TX, October 8, 1984

The idea of a federal drug czar keeps popping up. Perhaps that is because it seems like an easy solution. If one person is responsible for fighting drugs, then that relieves all the rest of us of any responsibility. Talk to the czar. If the narcotics traffickers are winning, fire the czar and name a new and tougher one.

The trouble with the idea starts with the word "czar" itself. Russian emperors were called czars, and they had the final word, life or death. Then there were czars who during World War II could impose rationing and set prices. No one wants to bring back those kinds of czars.

If a drug czar were named, he would not have the kind of authority that goes with the word czar. He would be another bureaucrat, setting up an organization with secretaries, public relations men and advisers, issuing memos and begging for interdepartmental cooperation. His first priority would be to get a larger appropriation from Congress.

Early last year, Congress passed a package which among other things would have established a drug czar, a Cabinet-level position to "coordinate national efforts against drug trafficking." Even though there were favorable parts of the package, President Reagan refused to sign the bill because he questioned the worth of spending $500,000 for a drug czar. The administration chose another approach. Instead of a czar to coordinate matters, it established 12 regional task forces, hired investigators and prosecutors instead of secretaries and public relations men and achieved coordination by putting top representatives of law enforcement agencies in the same room with desks right next to one another. The result is a high degree of cooperation that extends horizontally through the federal government and vertically from the federal officials to local authorities. Up and down the line, those who are out on the streets making the arrests are saying the level of coordination has never been better. More than that, it is making a difference in the number and type of arrests being made.

Another factor that will make a difference in the war on drugs is the new legislation coming out of Congress within just the last few days. An anti-crime bill that hurts drug dealers where they are most sensitive — their pocketbooks — was passed.

Another bill passed, one sponsored by Sen. Lloyd Bentsen of Texas, will allow the Federal Aviation Administration to ground pilots convicted of drug trafficking. Sen. Bentsen said the Drug Enforcement Administration figures half the cocaine and 35 percent of the marijuana smuggled into this country arrives in airplanes, and his bill will help plug that hole.

The job of fighting the evil of narcotics isn't something to be handed off to a czar. It's an international fight. It's a federal, state and local fight. It's a fight in our schools and our homes. A "czar" can't win that fight. A society united against drugs can.

THE LOUISVILLE TIMES

Louisville, KY, December 20, 1983

While there were doubts, at first, about the Reagan administration's decision to consolidate efforts of the Drug Enforcement Administration and the Federal Bureau of Investigation in narcotics investigations, the experiment seems to be paying off.

The New York Times reports that the emphasis has shifted from arrests to convictions — a change that, ultimately, should make the federal attack on illicit drugs much more effective. If statistics compiled for the first quarter of 1983 — the most recent ones available — are a guide, convictions are running approximately 15 per cent ahead of 1982. Meanwhile, arrests appear to be roughly the same, if not slightly fewer, than last year. Law enforcement at its worst emphasizes arrests. The problem is that insufficient or illegally obtained evidence causes cases to collapse.

In addition, the new DEA director, Francis Mullen, has raised the standards for agents by now requiring a college degree. Association with the FBI, Mr. Mullins explained at a seminar earlier this year, improves drug agents' ability to unravel complex financial transactions engineered by narcotics kingpins. And with centralized, rather than regional, control, more effective use of staff has been possible.

This is not to say that the administration's war on drugs is without its flaws. The expensive, overtly political but ultimately useless spraying of marijuana plants in Eastern Kentucky and other portions of the Southeast by DEA personnel was an embarrassment. Worse were lame efforts to explain the paraquat swat teams.

Nonetheless, the broader course seems a positive one, using the existing framework of the DEA and the FBI. Congress should be skeptical of renewed efforts by Delaware Sen. Joseph Biden, who is ready to attempt once more to secure passage of legislation that would create a federal "drug czar." There are all sorts of problems with the concept — beginning with the fact that it would be a Cabinet-level position.

Although Sen. Biden says the goal is to consolidate various drug-enforcement functions in one office, the true objective seems to be the political payoff that comes from doing flashy things to combat crime. When President Reagan vetoed a crime bill last January because it provided for a "drug czar," he said the office would be counterproductive and result in duplication of existing functions.

He was right, and the attack on drugs that his administration has undertaken is on the right course. Congress would do the law-abiding public a disservice by interrupting the progress to try yet another costly experiment.

De Lorean Acquitted; Jurors Cite Entrapment, Weak Case

Former automaker John Z. De Lorean August 16, 1984 was acquitted by a federal jury in Los Angeles of eight counts connected to a scheme to distribute 55 pounds of cocaine. The 59-year-old De Lorean, if he had been convicted on the counts of drug conspiracy, possession and distribution, could have been sentenced to as many as 67 years in jail and fined up to $185,000. Unusual aspects of the much-publicized 22-week trial had included suspicion of jury tampering, admissions that government evidence had been altered, a courtroom filled with expensive electronic equipment for the playing of government videotapes and near-daily statements to the media by attorneys in the case. Government prosecutors had charged that De Lorean entered into a $24 million plot to distribute cocaine in order to raise money for his struggling De Lorean Automobile Company in Belfast, Northern Ireland. (The company was currently in receivership.)

De Lorean and his defense attorneys claimed that his prosecution was the result of an overzealous and improper investigation by ambitious federal agents. The defense claimed that De Lorean had entered talks with government agents seeking a legitimate investment and that once he found that drugs were involved he did not back out of the deal because he feared his family might be harmed. De Lorean had been arrested in October, 1982 in a Los Angeles hotel room. Videotapes made as part of the federal investigation into the case had recorded the arrest and had shown De Lorean looking at a suitcase full of cocaine and saying it was "better than gold."

Interviews with jurors after the verdict indicated that some believed the government had entrapped De Lorean into joining the drug-conspiracy. Others said that the government had not proved its drug-trafficiking case against De Lorean. Defense lawyers had avoided using the word "entrapment" during the trial, but at the end of their case requested that trial Judge Robert M. Takasugi include an explanation of entrapment in his charge to the jury. Takasugi told the jurors that in order to find De Lorean not guilty because of entrapment they must believe that he "was not ready and willing to commit the acts before he was induced to do so by government agents."

Many observers felt that the witnesses for the prosecution were in large part responsible for the unexpected verdict. The primary witness was James T. Hoffman, a convicted drug smuggler and admitted perjurer. It came to light during the course of the trial that Hoffman had sought unsuccessfully to obtain a percentage of any assets the government might obtain in the De Lorean case. Two other witnesses, government agents Benedict Tisa and John Valestra, were both forced to admit that they had altered their investigation notes. In addition, Judge Takasugi disclosed in June that some of the jurors in the case had received copies of a congressional report criticizing the kind of federal undercover "sting" operations used in the De Lorean investigation. The reports had been sent by the office of Rep. Don Edwards (D, Calif.) after receipt of a letter requesting 13 copies of the report. A grand jury was currently investigating possible jury tampering in the case.

The Hartford Courant
Hartford, CT, August 19, 1984

John Z. DeLorean might have had dreams of illegal drug profits dancing in his head when federal agents were secretly taping him in 1982, but the questions upon which his case turned were: Who put the dreams there and what triggered his greed?

There's something fundamentally objectionable about government coaxing a private citizen, with no prior criminal record, to break the law.

Members of the Los Angeles jury that acquitted Mr. DeLorean last week after a six-month trial said they found the actions of federal agents objectionable. Several believed the automaker, despite being on the verge of bankruptcy, was not "predisposed" to enter into a conspiracy to traffic in cocaine and was instead entrapped by the government. They said the state presented a faulty case weakened by the testimony of unsavory witnesses.

Justice was served, then, even if at some point Mr. DeLorean had agreed with federal agents posing as drug smugglers and dishonest businessmen to go along with the deal. The jury said the prosecution could not prove he *initiated* a crime.

There is a place for undercover law enforcement work. Sometimes the sting is the only way to crack organized crime, venal politicians or crooked judges, for example. Even then, legal scholars agree, government should conduct such operations most judiciously — using reliable agents and credible witnesses.

Mr. DeLorean is far from being a knight in shining armor, and questions about his business practices have risen in other court suits he still faces. But in this case, the jury was apparently offended by the government's uncommon zeal in pursuing him.

The Idaho STATESMAN
Boise, ID, October 21, 1983

After CBS News broadcast videotapes of former automaker John DeLorean purportedly meeting with FBI undercover agents in a staged cocaine buy, U.S. District Judge Robert Takasugi expressed doubts that DeLorean could receive a fair trial anywhere in the United States.

The visibly shaken Takasugi posponed DeLorean's trial, scheduled to begin Nov. 1, and said of CBS, "Was it truly asking too much in view of an individual's right to a fair trial to pause — a moral pause — to respectfully withhold its disclosure for just a week?"

The judge's comment raised a legitimate question. The media has an obligation to act responsibly when reporting information about criminal defendants. We'll leave it up to CBS to defend its decision to air the tapes, but must note that Takasugi himself acted questionably when he enjoined the network from broadcasting the tapes.

Takasugi's order, which three judges of the 9th Circuit Court of Appeals overturned, was blatantly unconstitutional. It violated the judicial principle of no prior restraint, which holds that the press cannot be enjoined from publishing, though it can be held responsible for what it publishes.

In their hearing on Takasugi's order, the justices repeatedly asked the lawyers to cite a case in which a court had legally restrained the press from publishing. The lawyers knew of no such case. Asked Justice Alfred Goodwin, "Where do we get the authority to tell the press how to run its shop?"

The judge's point is inarguable. The courts don't have that authority.

Later, after CBS showed the tapes, Takasugi's anguish was apparent. Balancing the constitutional right to a fair trial and the constitutional right to a free press is never easy, but the defense will have an opportunity in court to challenge the validity of the tapes and to render its judgment on their applicability. Through the jury selection process, the defense also will have the opportunity to choose jurors it feels are impartial.

To conclude that DeLorean cannot receive a fair trial is to fail to give adequate credit to the jury system. Takasugi's unconstitutional order certainly was no solution. While it's true the press must use its judgment responsibly, it must be able to use its judgment.

The Virginian-Pilot
Norfolk, VA, October 31, 1983

John Z. DeLorean, who was scheduled to go on trial this week on federal drug conspiracy charges, claims he can't obtain a fair trial because FBI videotapes purporting to show him discussing a cocaine deal have been televised.

When the defendant's attorneys and the prosecutor tried to prevent airing of the tapes by CBS and a Los Angeles station, the 9th Circuit Court of Appeals overruled the trial judge who had temporarily forbade the broadcast. That ban violated the First Amendment, the court held.

There is no question of the right of broadcasters to air the tapes, although the government was terribly negligent in allowing them to leak — a matter now under investigation.

The fashion in which CBS' Dan Rather used them, however, sensationalized their content, to Mr. DeLorean's detriment.

The tapes showed him chatting in a hotel room and examining a suitcase, which was represented as being packed with cocaine worth over $4 million. Viewers saw or heard nothing to offset the impression created by this tape except the defense attorney arguing that the tapes should not have been shown on TV.

The tape of the DeLorean meeting was inconclusive and open to interpretation. The interpretation on the tube was one-sided.

Mr. DeLorean, of course, may benefit. The judge has already granted a delay in the trial as a result. The defense may claim that he was falsely accused, perhaps entrapped, and even smeared on national television. The fact that the tapes were peddled to CBS by Hustler magazine publisher Larry Flynt, an unsympathetic figure in this caper, may even induce sympathy for the defendant.

It's great show biz. But not exactly what the authors of the Bill of Rights had in mind in calling for "a speedy and public trial."

Los Angeles Times
Los Angeles, CA, October 26, 1983

The FBI plans to use as evidence in court some grainy secret surveillance videotapes that it says show auto maker John Z. DeLorean trafficking in cocaine. The CBS network, and later other television stations, broadcast the film as news over the weekend. The events were tailor-made for a legal uproar.

U.S. District Judge Robert M. Takasugi, who will preside in the DeLorean case, has postponed the trial indefinitely, saying that CBS has interfered with the judicial process. DeLorean's attorney, Howard L. Weitzman, claims that broadcasting the videotape may "deny forever" a fair trial for his client.

The judge need not agonize over the incident, and there is nothing whatever in the record of the relationship between free speech and fair trials that gives weight to Weitzman's gloomy forecast.

To begin with, much of what transpired on the videotapes already had been reported in newspapers and on television. To argue, as did Takasugi, that the film was shown solely because of a thirst for selling news misses the point about news. Newspapers describe, discuss and, where possible, show news in photographs. Television shows news in motion. It is a difference without a distinction. In both cases a tradition as old as the country itself leans toward the fullest possible disclosure as the public's best defense against knowing only what its government or narrow interest groups want it to know.

Carried to a logical—or illogical— extreme, the argument against pre-trial publicity would lead to a British-style coverage of crime and punishment under which all such news is stifled unless it originates in a courtroom.

Under the American tradition, the public has an unobstructable view of its governments, its police, its prosecutors and its judicial system at work.

Finally, the uproar focuses not on the legal right of newspapers and television stations to exercise their own judgment in news matters without asking permission from a judge. That right has been upheld in every case in which it has arisen. The focus rather is on the stations' judgment in choosing to make the tapes public at this time—an argument that may never be resolved—and on the issue of whether DeLorean can now get a fair trial. To argue that he cannot presupposes a jury of zombies with no minds of their own and a nation of citizens who spend all their waking hours watching television, nodding in agreement with everything that they see. Nonsense.

THE SUN
Baltimore, MD, October 31, 1983

U.S. District Judge Robert Takasugi was wrong last weekend when he ordered CBS not to broadcast tapes of the events leading up to John DeLorean's arrest for alleged cocaine transactions. The Supreme Court has made it clear judges may not exercise "prior restraint" of journalists except in extreme circumstances, if at all. There may be news that journalists should not report. There may be instances in which broadcasters and newspapers may be penalized for what they report after they report it. But they may not be prevented from reporting it in the first place. That's censorship.

Judge Takasugi may be right, however, in postponing the DeLorean trial, on the grounds that the broadcast makes it more difficult to ensure a fair trial, and he is definitely right to question CBS's motives and sense of responsibility in this case. For no good reason, the network has trespassed across the line that divides aggressive, high-risk broadcast journalism from irresponsible sensationalism. And not for the first time. Last January, CBS insisted on broadcasting a report on police officers accused of brutality. In that case, as in the DeLorean case, CBS scheduled the broadcast for the very eve of the trial. (Prompting charges that it was a desire for ratings, not news judgment, that led to its scheduling decision.)

Journalists have a responsibility to present the community with news. Particularly when it comes to criminal matters, including police procedures and evidence, the community has a right to expect from its newsgatherers as much pertinent information as possible. This helps the public make up its mind about how well or poorly laws and law enforcement agents are functioning to protect the community. But there are usually ways to do that without interfering with the administration of justice. Both these stories would have been just as interesting and informative after the trial had begun, when the jurors could be prevented from watching, if need be. Journalism would not have suffered by such temporary self-restraint.

The State
Columbia, SC, October 31, 1983

THE "free press-fair trial" issue is never going to be solved to the complete satisfaction of the news and legal professions and the public.

The reason is simple: It involves a clash of two constitutional principles which are occasionally incompatible.

A defendant in a criminal case has a right to a public trial before "an impartial jury" under the Sixth Amendment. The First Amendment states that the freedom of the press shall not be abridged. But if the press disseminates news in advance of a trial that deals with guilt or innocence, the jury might be prejudiced before it hears the evidence in open court under proper judicial rules.

A classic case of this fundamental confrontation arose last week when CBS News obtained a videotape showing one-time automaker John De Lorean just before and during his arrest on drug charges. The government plans to use the tape in his trial.

Government lawyers went before a U.S. district court judge in Los Angeles and got an order blocking a broadcast of the tape. The judge was wrong. That is prior restraint. As a CBS lawyer told the court of appeals, "He has no constitutional power to do what he did." The appeals court overruled the district judge, and two Supreme Court justices let that order stand. CBS aired the tape.

In doing so, the network was plainly wrong in its judgment. Predictably, Mr. De Lorean's attorney said he would seek to have the charges against his client thrown out on the grounds that his client cannot now get a jury that has not prejudged the case.

Every journalist loves a scoop, and that is what CBS had. But a responsible journalist, it seems to us, will forego the pleasure if it chances prejudicing a case against a criminal defendant that has taken a year to build. The tape would have been available once shown in court. Any right the public has to know this information was not jeopardized. The prosecutor's case was.

Mutual restraint, when that is indicated, is the best way to handle the "free press-fair trial" issue.

Detroit Free Press
Detroit, MI,
August 18, 1984

IN DETROIT, if not in the rest of the country, the acquittal of John De Lorean on drug conspiracy charges will be read with special interest on two accounts: for itself, because Mr. De Lorean is well known here, and for the supposed contrast with the conviction the day before of two central figures in the Vista case.

Both cases involved an FBI investigation, both involved a search for the smoking gun that would prove the involvement of a key defendant in criminal acts and both followed long agony for the people involved. The De Lorean jury decided that the FBI had not produced the smoking gun. The Vista jury decided it had enough for conviction in the envelopes passed from Darralyn Bowers to William Beckham, the city's water and sewerage director, and in his testimony that he lied to the FBI when they first confronted him about the Vista sludge disposal contract.

To those who are convinced that the Beckham conviction is a racist plot, the De Lorean acquittal is the kind of thing that confirms their worst suspicions about the system. It makes doubly important that the system provide every reasonable appeal for Mr. Beckham.

The Detroit community, though, is left with the reality of the two tragedies: John De Lorean, despite his acquittal, will face continuing problems that will illustrate how the mighty have fallen. And Charles Beckham, despite the possibility of appeal, remains a convicted man.

That conviction should leave no doubt, whatever the personal obligation Mayor Young may feel to Mr. Beckham, that the city must remove him from its payroll and discontinue its payment of his legal costs. Mr. Beckham's conviction changes the equation. The mayor should step up to that, and the Detroit City Council should see that he does. The city may have some obligation to employes who get in trouble. It is not an open-ended obligation, though, and it ends with conviction. The possibility of appeal is no basis for continuing Mr. Beckham in his interim job as an aide to the mayor.

There are personal tragedies here, and we do not rejoice at the difficulties of either man. The government faces hard choices in trying to protect us against corruption and against illegal acts such as drug trafficking. Neither the De Lorean acquittal nor the Beckham conviction is proof positive of capricious government prosecution or, for that matter, of any sort of double standard. It is evidence that prosecutors, judge and jury are part of a set of human institutions that work with something less than total precision.

The trouble is, there is always a tension between broader public needs and individual rights. We can't ever know the system is going to do the right thing. But we have to live by it, feeling what empathy we may toward people who are charged with crimes, knowing that there aren't many other systems that offer more balanced guarantees to the public and to the individuals concerned.

Newsday
Long Island, NY, August 18, 1984

Every now and then, the government-controlled Soviet press makes an observation about American society that's remarkable either for its astonishing lack of understanding or for its cynical distortion of reality. But rarely has any matched a commentary by Tass, the official Soviet news agency, on the outcome of John DeLorean's trial on drug charges.

Said Tass of DeLorean's acquittal: "The U.S. courts, as a rule, stand up for the interests of big business, and DeLorean's case was no exception. The court merely disregarded a good deal of evidence testifying to his criminal actions."

"The U.S. authorities demonstrated anew with that verdict," Tass continued, "the worth of their hypocritical claims that they were out to suppress drug trafficking." And, Tass concluded, "The case of DeLorean . . . is fresh proof that the Reagan administration does not take effective measures to stamp out drug addiction, that chronic ill of U.S. society."

What Tass obviously ignores — either out of misunderstanding or a conscious effort to distort — is the fact that it wasn't the "U.S. authorities" that acquitted DeLorean. It was a jury of 12 American citizens. Actually, of course, the government — as represented by the Federal Bureau of Investigation and the Department of Justice — tried so zealously to send DeLorean to prison that, in the view of many jurors, it resorted to illegal tactics of entrapment.

Tass appears to believe that the American courts operate like those in the Soviet Union. There, if the government decides someone is guilty of a crime, that person is guilty — and no jury can decide otherwise. Maybe a Soviet expert on the American judicial system ought to remind Tass that things don't work quite that way in this country.

St. Petersburg Times
St. Petersburg, FL, August 18, 1984

There is the oft-told story, surely apocryphal, of the jury that acquitted a young man of innocent face but questionable conduct. Wagging a finger in his direction, one juror said, "But don't you ever do that again!"

Was John Z. DeLorean's acquittal some similar act of sympathy? Most likely not. From what the jurors have said about it, some were sincerely put off by the dubious background and testimony of key government witnesses. Others who might have found DeLorean guilty were outraged by the government's great efforts to spin a web for someone with no previous record of dealing in drugs. Though the entrapment defense rarely succeeds, this time it did.

DELOREAN HARDLY deserves to be lionized. There he was on the FBI's videotape describing cocaine, a dangerous drug, as "good as gold . . ." No hero, he, nor victim either.

DeLorean should be remembered instead as a symbol of two important principles. One is that jurors who reasonably doubt a defendant's guilt must vote to acquit. That puts the burden of proof where it belongs — on the government. The other is that the government cannot stoop beneath the Constitution simply to get an occasional criminal conviction. As Justice Oliver Wendell Holmes explained it, in a 1928 wiretapping case, "For my part I think it a less evil that some criminals should escape than that the government should play an ignoble part."

There's a lesson in the DeLorean verdict for all those people — such as Chief Justice Warren Burger, Justice Byron White and the Reagan administration's Justice Department — who think we no longer need to respect the Constitution so strictly. If a jury of ordinary Americans can, why can't they?

THE MILWAUKEE JOURNAL
Milwaukee, WI, August 18, 1984

The acquittal of businessman John DeLorean does not mean the government is wrong to use undercover operations in catching criminals, but the verdict should prod investigators to be more careful about how such "stings" are employed.

In interviews after the trial, jurors indicated that the verdict was based partly on the belief that DeLorean was entrapped and partly on the conclusion that the government had not actually proved DeLorean guilty of trafficking in cocaine.

DeLorean was a glamorous figure with no previous court record. Thus, when his lawyers argued that he was the innocent victim of a setup, the jurors probably were more sympathetic than they would have been in a case involving a reputed underworld operator.

In addition, the investigators weakened their case by cutting technical corners and by relying heavily on the testimony of an admitted perjurer and drug smuggler who served as undercover agent.

In a sense, the defense lawyers were able to convert the court proceedings into a hearing on the investigators' conduct rather than a debate over DeLorean's guilt or innocence. His attorneys never put him on the stand to explain why he seemingly agreed, in the presence of a videotape camera, to enter into a multi-million-dollar drug deal.

It is possible, of course, to argue with the jury's finding. Under prevailing interpretations of the law, DeLorean wasn't really entrapped unless the agent lured him into a criminal deal that he otherwise would have been unwilling to enter.

It obviously is not honorable to commit a crime even under extraordinary temptation. Yet, in a fair system of criminal justice, defendants don't have to prove themselves honorable or innocent; the prosecution has to prove them guilty, with evidence obtained by constitutional means.

To prevent the government, rather than the accused, from being made the object of any trial, law enforcement agents must be meticulous in their gathering of evidence. While a sting operation is a proper device to catch crooks on the prowl, it acquires aspects of a police-state device if its use is prompted by mere speculation that a given person is venal. The closer investigators come to acting on speculation, the more likely they are to lose in court.

The Boston Herald

Boston, MA, August 18, 1984

THE jurors in the John De Lorean case did not acquit him because they decided he was innocent of conspiring to be a big-time drug distributor. They did so because they thought the government was guilty of going much too far in the "sting" operation it used to make its case against him.

Nor did they say, in their post-trial comments, that "stings" are unjust per se — only that they were convinced this one was.

"There's not a court or judge in the country that would have acquitted De Lorean on the basis of the evidence," said legal scholar Alan Dershowitz of Harvard Law School. "DeLorean's guilt played no role in this. All the attention was focused on the government, and he was presented as a victim."

That's important, because it pinned the label of villain on the prosecution — and rightly so — for doctoring some of the evidence, backdating documents, and the like. In that sense, the government might have done more to spring DeLorean than his own lawyers did.

Yet despite occasional abuses, despite the dim view of them taken by defense attorneys and civil libertarians, "stings" — when used correctly and with proper restraint and safeguards — are legitimate investigative tactics. As Exhibit A to support that point, one need only remember the Abscam scandal which sent several members of Congress to prison for taking money from "Arab sheiks," who were actually FBI agents. In every instance, the Supreme Court dismissed the appeals of defendants that they were victims of entrapment, decided that if they were victims they were willing ones, and ordered them to begin serving their sentences.

Locally, the arrest of two public figures, Rep. Vincent Piro of Somerville and former General Services Administration official Lawrence Bretta, was the direct result of "stings" conducted by the Justice Department. Piro is scheduled for trial next month.

Without pre-judging those or any other cases, some kinds of wrongdoing — narcotics, organized crime, or corruption among them — are all but impossible to investigate by the usual methods. "Stings" are but one of several unusual — but not necessarily illegal — measures government has been allowed to take to root them out. They've been upheld when courts have been satisfied that they were properly done and that the over-riding public interest warranted their use — when, to use the words of Assistant District Attorney Charles Grimes of Essex County, their purpose has been to ferret out crime, not create it.

The DeLorean case won't deter prosecutors from using "stings" in the future, but it should make the few reckless ones more mindful of the limits beyond which they cannot go to get a conviction. If it does, justice will be served.

TULSA WORLD

Tulsa, OK, August 18, 1984

WAS industrialist John Z. De Lorean intent on crime before government undercover agents approached him with a drug deal, or was he a desperate businessman whose troubles made him susceptible to the agents' offer?

A Los Angeles jury decided in De Lorean's favor Thursday after a long trial certain to add to the controversy over the justice department "sting" operation.

Congress, already unhappy over sting operations which have netted six representatives and a senator, might be tempted to make more of the De Lorean case than it should, trying to make stings on public officeholders more difficult.

But there is a big difference in setting a trap for a private citizen like De Lorean, who appears to be ripe to commit a crime because he sees his personal and professional life crumbling, and approaching an officeholder with a bribe offer.

The predisposition of the subject, as the Los Angeles jury discovered, is the key factor in deciding whether there was entrapment.

In the case of officeholders, the predisposition angle is less important. If a bribe is offered, for example, the matter is clearcut; if it's taken, that clearly shows a "predisposition." If rejected, quite the obvious.

Federal investigators and prosecutors should certainly take a long look at their practices, some of which irritated the De Lorean jury to the point that it was willing to overlook a video tape of John De Lorean discussing a drug deal with undercover agents.

There should be no rush to pass new laws in this area. Determining the "predisposition" of a defendant is obviously a question that must be left to the discretion of a jury.

The Chattanooga Times

Chattanooga, TN, August 20, 1984

By acquitting John Z. De Lorean of all eight counts of an indictment that charged him with trafficking in cocaine, the federal court jury in Los Angeles did not just free him from the prospect of heavy fines and a lengthy prison sentence. It also delivered a stunning rebuke to the federal government's use of what the jurors, in effect, considered entrapment. The verdict does not necessarily mean the federal government will, or should, abandon all use of undercover "sting" operations. It does mean, however, that if the government hopes to avoid losing future such cases, it had better revise the tactics that resulted in Thursday's acquittal.

Mr. De Lorean, a former top executive for General Motors, quit that firm and formed his own to manufacture a futuristic sports car called, naturally, the De Lorean. But the operation, based in Ireland, soon ran into severe financial difficulties. In its indictment, handed up two years ago, the government had accused him of participating in a deal to distribute 55 pounds of cocaine; at the time, Mr. De Lorean was trying to raise $30 million to save his automobile company. The government's undercover operation, in which federal agents portrayed a dishonest banker and drug smugglers, also included hours of videotaped meetings of the agents and Mr. De Lorean.

But the government went too far in its zealous prosecution. It was that excess that prompted the jurors, in an unusual post-verdict meeting with Mr. De Lorean, his lawyers and the judge, to say that they wanted to "send a message to the Department of Justice" that "setting up" citizens to commit crimes was wrong.

Granted, Mr. De Lorean did not exhibit exemplary judgment; even his attorney conceded there had been lapses in this regard. But those lapses were overshadowed by the characters who testified for the federal government. Their general lack of credibility and truthfulness, a Michigan Law School professor observed, constituted a fatal flaw in the government's case. As a result, Mr. De Lorean's guilt or innocence became almost irrelevant. As Harvard Law School professor Alan Dershowitz told *The New York Times,* "all the attention was focused on the government, and he was presented as a victim."

That was fortunate for Mr. De Lorean, but his case, particularly the rebuke inherent in the jury's verdict, should force the government into a thorough rethinking of its tactics in the future. The government might profit from the words of former Supreme Court Justice Felix Frankfurter from a 1958 case: "No matter what the defendant's past record, or the depths to which he has sunk in the estimation of society, certain police conduct to ensnare him into further crime is not to be tolerated by an advanced society."

U.S. Drug Task Force Issues Report

The Reagan Administration's organized crime drug task force won the indictments of 1,841 people during its first 14 months, according to a study prepared by the task force released April 7, 1984. The group said it opened 535 cases against drug organizations during the period. The Reagan Administration had set up 12 drug task forces around the nation in an effort to attack drug trafficking by organized crime groups. The task forces had been funded with $127.5 million in their first year, according to the recent report. The report said the task forces had confiscated some $50 million in drug-related assets and property in 1983, that 22% of the cases opened by the task force involved heroin trafficking, 74% involved cocaine and 48% involved marijuana. "The principal defendants" indicted by the task forces, the report said, were "from the highest levels of narcotics trafficking organizations. They included physicians, bankers...public employees...drug financiers, smugglers and distributors."

But despite the Administration's claims, a series of articles in the *Wall Street Journal* surveying drug use and law enforcement suggested that the battle against drug abuse was being lost. Among the highlights of the articles was the following:

- Imports of cocaine had risen 50% over the last two years.
- Eleven states, representing about one-third of the U.S. population, had decriminalized the possession of small amounts of marijuana and police in other states made minimal efforts to arrest smokers. "Marijuana possession has been effectively decriminalized in most of the country," according to Mark Kleinman of the Harvard University Center of Criminal Justice.

The Orlando Sentinel
Orlando, FL, March 7, 1984

Congress went looking last week for the $14 million being cut from the battle against drug smugglers and found it in — of all places — Treasury Secretary Donald Regan's drapes.

While Mr. Regan was lopping a good chunk off the war on drugs, he was nailing down an extra $18.5 million for his building fund. Most of the money would come from the U.S. Customs Service's new program for using military planes to nab smugglers as they approach the coast. A big part of that program is focused off Florida. That crackdown used to be a big deal for the administration. The vice president even showed up in Florida several times to promote it.

Now Mr. Regan prefers to renovate a Treasury Department annex and install new curtains, carpet and plumbing. Some of the money also will go for upgrading telecommunications and data processing equipment and for employee merit raises.

He insists there is no link between the drug enforcement loss and his office's gain. Nevertheless, somehow priorities were rearranged so that his drapes got ahead of this part of the drug war. He says he will reconsider. He should.

THE PLAIN DEALER
Cleveland, OH, June 23, 1984

Despite claims made on behalf of the highly publicized drug smuggling task force directed by Vice President George Bush, the war on drugs is not being won. Rather, it has been hindered by government confusion, overt politicization and interagency indifference.

Drug Enforcement Administration records show that narcotics are flowing into this country at a record pace. Its good intentions notwithstanding, the task force simply has not stopped what an aide to Edward Feighan, the Lakewood Democrat who is chairman of the House Task Force on International Narcotics, calls a "cocaine glut." According to the DEA, the amount of cocaine smuggled into the country in 1983 tripled over the year previous; heroin imports doubled.

The paths these drugs take to the United States can be long and tortuous. From the growers in Indochina, South and West Asia and South America, shipments pass through the hands of international crime figures and even government officials. Recent investigations conducted by Feighan's committee have uncovered the alleged involvement of Bahamian and Bulgarian government officials along with Italian financiers and the Turkish mafia. Two Bahamian government officials have been convicted as a result.

Unfortunately, the American battle against international drug trafficking is long on desire and short on organization. This confusion is particularly evident in the Golden Triangle, a region of Indochina that includes portions of Burma, Thailand and Laos. There, the DEA's efforts are hindered by the CIA and State Department, and vice versa. As a result, the war on drugs that is supposedly being won is foundering.

A bill that would put these government activities in the hands of a centralized authority is in its second incarnation in Congress. The bill, which would create a cabinet level office to coordinate all drug enforcement activities, passed the House by a 271-27 vote in December 1982 only to be vetoed by President Reagan. The bill passed the House Judiciary Committee again two weeks ago, this time with the authority placed in the office of the vice president. The White House remains unswayed.

The White House is wrong. Fragmentation hinders drug enforcement activities. It is therefore wise to consider appointing a "drug czar" to coordinate and oversee international efforts. If the administration is worried about a bloated bureaucracy, it could review the position, say, in three years. It would doubtless find the idea to be an effective one.

THE BLADE
Toledo, OH, December 5, 1984

ONE of the best publicized activities in Washington has been the federal wars waged against the flow of illegal drugs into the United States. But in the long run the efforts seem to have been losing ones at almost every turn.

The Reagan administration is no different from its predecessors in that regard. Since 1981 federal officials have launched one counterattack after another against drug trafficking. But the campaigns, like others before them, have not halted the flow or, by many estimates, slowed it down. According to studies and first-hand reports, illicit drugs — in particular cocaine and heroin — are increasingly available in this country.

A onetime drug smuggler testified recently in Washington that sneaking large volumes of illegal substances across this nation's southern borders remains a comparatively easy task, although traffickers have grown more inventive and daring.

The enormous volume of drugs and the potential profits are attested to by the fact that Mexican officials recently seized 10,000 tons of marijuana about to be smuggled into the United States.

Bribery still works, especially in foreign countries, drug smugglers report. Also, there is a bustling but illegal farming business going on in the wilds of California, where hidden marijuana farms provide pot for domestic consumption.

Despite the failures — or only modest successes — of law-enforcement campaigns, there is no reason to abandon the drive to halt the illegal commerce. A North Carolina research institute estimated, in 1980, that drug abuse already had cost the nation $46.9 billion in lost employment and productivity, crime by addicts, and the money spent on treatment and law enforcement. The numerous instances of wasted human lives underscore the need to keep trying to enforce the law, regardless of how difficult it is.

More pressure on neighboring nations where most illegal drugs originate might help, along with more innovative — albeit costly — anti-smuggling campaigns. There will be no abrupt reversal of the flow of illegal substances into the United States, even if all levels of law enforcement keep at the task. But that does not diminish the need to keep trying.

The Birmingham News

Birmingham, AL, April 5, 1984

The federal government is claiming "solid results" in fighting the drug war. And the claim is backed by an impressive list of indictments against high-level drug dealers — a "body count," if you will, of 1,841 suppliers and distributors, money launderers and financiers.

According to a report from the Organized Drug Enforcement Task Force Program, which was created by President Reagan in 1982 but did not begin operations until almost a year ago, federal agents have penetrated 535 drug gangs in bringing about the indictments.

Attorney General William French Smith says the program represents action against entire drug networks, "not simply individual cases against random, low-level offenders." The indictments, he says, break down this way: Thirty-three percent were top leaders; 29 percent mid-level leaders; 28 percent major suppliers and distributors; 4 percent major financiers and 4 percent major money launderers.

Such results are heartily encouraging, although the indictments must be converted into convictions before it is time for too much cheerleading. Continued success cannot help but put a very large dent in illegal U.S. drug operations, however, with resulting good effects for society in general.

For it should be recognized that illegal drug activities represent not only the ruination of individual lives, but a very real danger through their effect on the economy, on financing other criminal activities and, in some cases, the subversion of law enforcement.

The war against illegal drugs, and the monstrous crime networks they engender, remains of critical importance to the future of the nation. It is to be hoped that the "body count" of drug dealers will continue to mount in the coming months.

Birmingham, AL, January 25, 1984

The FBI's uncovering this week of a international cocaine smuggling ring has perhaps not received the national attention it should have been given.

The FBI and other federal officials of course deserve commendation for their work, and it is important that prosecution continue against the 53 people who have been indicted in four cities in connection with the investigation.

The most important element of the story, however, is the sheer mass of the ring's activities. The federal charge is that the group, using the equivalent of a small air force to fly cocaine from South America and the Caribbean, imported five tons of the drug, worth about $3.8 billion.

That's five tons of a substance usually measured by drug dealers and users in ounces and grams. Its estimated value is a figure too high for most of us really to comprehend.

Agents actually seized about 2,700 pounds of the drug, estimated to have a street value of some $940 million, and reports are that large cargoes of 600 to 1,000 pounds of cocaine were flown routinely into the country. Both big-city airports and small rural strips were used by the smugglers.

And yet, there is the suggestion that a great deal more remains to be discovered in the international drug business — more tons of cocaine and other drugs, more billions of dollars in illegal proceeds.

The implications of such numbers are ominous. How much economic disruption can be brought about by billions in drug money turned to other areas?

How many law enforcement and other government officials have been subjected to corruption under the pressure of such dollars?

How much are individual lives worth in combat with billions of dollars?

The FBI's investigations, indeed, may have performed its greatest service in uncovering the dimensions of the drug problem facing the United States, as well as other countries. For it is a simply immense problem that threatens the very foundations of the nation.

The proof of the danger is, thanks to the FBI, now on display for those who care to see it.

The Star-Ledger

Newark, NJ, December 1, 1984

The Reagan Administration has sharply increased spending in an expanded drug enforcement effort to curb the flow of illicit narcotics from abroad. But despite the intensified government surveillance, there has been a significant increase in narcotics' trafficking, particularly apparent in the much wider availability of cocaine, a drug that no longer has an an elitist, cultish status.

A recent presidential report noted that, in line with a Reagan commitment when he took office, drug enforcement expenditures have been raised by a substantial 75 percent since 1981. This includes a record hike of $1.2 billion in the new fiscal year.

In the same period, a report compiled by 11 separate law enforcement agencies showed supplies of marijuana, heroin and cocaine have risen steadily. Because of its extensive use and its profitability, traffickers have been shifting to cocaine. The greatly increased availability of this drug has dramatically reduced its formerly high price. And, of course, it has encouraged wider use.

The stepped-up drug enforcement has brought about more arrests of major traffickers and bigger drug seizures. But it is depressingly evident, too, that the illegal drug trade is flourishing better than ever, clearly apparent in the abundant supplies in the clandestine drug market.

Even the most stringent enforcement efforts have not been enough to staunch the rising tide of illicit drugs coming into the United States by land, air and sea. These dismal results raise doubts that this endemic problem will ever be effectively combatted by enforcement strategies alone.

There must be a broader-based anti-drug enforcement policy, one that goes right to the foreign sources of these narcotics. These origin points are well known to American agencies—Latin America, the Middle East and Asia.

One Latin nation, Bolivia, a principal supply source of cocaine, is now actively tracking down major drug peddlers, an enforcement effort in response to U.S. urging. Similar cooperative arrangements should be negotiated with countries where drug traffickers operate, calling on them to crack down on their operations. These accords could materially help choke off supplies at the source—before they pour into the illicit drug pipelines that feed ever-increasing voracious demands in this country.

DAILY NEWS

New York, NY, June 16, 1984

The Amsterdam News' campaign to encourage citizens to get involved in the crackdown on drug traffickers got a major boost from Gov. Cuomo on Thursday, and there was also good news from Washington on the anti-drug front.

Cuomo announced the establishment of a 24-hour toll-free hot line, beginning July 1, over which people who see drug pushers plying their terrible trade will be able to report them to a central location for police action. It's a great idea, expanding on the newspaper's call for a "drop-a-dime" program to help the cops solve a problem that has reached crisis proportions. Make a note of the number—1-800-GIVE TIP—and use it.

From Washington, word came that the Reagan administration is going to spend $25 million to intensify the battle against the flow of drugs into New York City by adding 100 agents to the Customs Service and using more ships and planes to seize the stuff *before* it reaches the pushers. That's the best way to dry up supplies and put these lowlifes out of business.

THE LOUISVILLE TIMES
Louisville, KY, May 25, 1984

Francis Mullen, the director of the Drug Enforcement Administration, is widely known in Washington as a straight shooter. He is also considered a company man, so his complaints about a drug-enforcement program for which he is at least partially responsible are not to be taken lightly.

The New York Times recently reported that a memo by Mr. Mullen called a key part of the administration's fight against drugs a "liability." He warned that too much puffery could turn that effort — the Narcotic Border Interdiction System — into Mr. Reagan's "Achilles heel for drug enforcement."

The interdiction system is a network of six regional coordinating stations that employs at least 125 and utilizes staff from federal, state and local agencies. It has been a key feature of the Reagan attack on organized crime and drug trafficking, particularly because it is designed to bring together various investigative elements which formerly had little communication. Vice President Bush is chairman of its board.

The goal is sound. But the product, Mr. Mullins suggests, is not. He gets support from the General Accounting Office, which concluded after a study of 11 well-publicized cases that the chief accomplishment has been to take credit for the hard work of others. Each of the cases involved airborne drug smuggling, and, in 10 of the 11, the GAO concluded that seizure would have occurred without the interdiction system.

In addition, sharp criticism has been directed toward the effort because it has access to the military and intelligence sources, in what has heretofore been considered a civilian activity.

Because the interdiction system, in a sense, sidesteps the DEA, some will dismiss Mr. Mullins's complaints as self-serving and predictable. But his isn't isolated carping, as the GAO's findings and criticism on Capitol Hill indicate. This is especially disturbing because these doubts about the program come at a time when drug usage — especially of cocaine — is on the rise among middle-class Americans.

A survey conducted for *Time* in 1983 found that 11 per cent of adult Americans say they have sniffed cocaine; between 4 and 5 million claim to use it regularly. Of the latter, between 200,000 and 1 million are "profoundly dependent" upon it, and 45 tons of cocaine are sniffed by Americans annually. *The New York Times* reports that affluent cocaine users, no longer adequately stimulated by that drug, are switching to heroin, an even more dangerous substance because of its addictive qualities.

By emphasizing "communication" between police groups, Mr. Reagan has deflected criticism from those who seek to make a real dent in narcotics traffic. Mrs. Reagan's highly publicized educational efforts to combat drug usage among young people, while helpful, do not compensate for success on the streets and in the courtrooms.

The best news comes not from New York, Washington, Miami or any of the other hubs of drug traffic and enforcement. Rather, it comes from Colombia, where government officials, reacting to prodding from the United States, are cracking down on producers and exporters. Colombia produces 90 per cent of the cocaine sold in this country.

But reducing imports may only increase demand and competition, which can provoke more crime among users to obtain supplies. This could just add to the problems of police, thus turning up the program's "Achilles heel." More than blue smoke and mirrors are necessary if the war on drugs is to be won.

The Houston Post
Houston, TX, May 21, 1984

The seizure of two large caches of cocaine at the Port of Houston last week was a welcome victory in the battle to curb trafficking in this most popular of illicit narcotics. But we are losing more battles than we are winning in the war on illegal drugs.

The 90 pounds of cocaine confiscated by federal officers aboard a ship here Wednesday was one of the largest seizures ever made in Texas. It was followed the next day by a bust in which 63 pounds of the drug were found on another ship. The total value of the cocaine seized was estimated at $46 million.

As impressive as these seizures are, however, they are only a small part of the total amount of the drug being smuggled into this country. Most of it escapes detection. About half the total is brought in from Latin America by small private planes. It is estimated that only 1 percent of these flights are intercepted.

Much of the federal drug enforcement muscle has been concentrated in southern Florida, which used to be the destination of three-fourths of the smuggling flights. The heavy pressure on that area, however, has forced the smugglers to shift their operations westward, where thinly spread, underequipped enforcement units are unable to cope with the increased traffic.

Inadequate equipment and interagency squabbling over the division of enforcement duties and costs are hampering the government's campaign against illicit drugs. The U.S. Customs Service wants the Defense Department to take over the detection of suspected drug-smuggling aircraft, leaving Customs the job of intercepting them. But Defense, which has been giving Customs limited assistance, is resisting further involvement.

A solution to the detection problem is urgently needed. Customs has 33 planes to cover the entire area between Florida and California. And only eight of these are fast enough to catch the high-performance planes flown by many smugglers. Except in southern Florida, Customs also lacks helicopters for swift raids on smugglers and look-down radar to detect low-flying aircraft.

As long as federal agencies fail to agree on the divison of drug enforcmeent duties, as long as those agencies are shortchanged to the point that their equipment is inferior to that of the criminals they are trying to catch, we shouldn't wonder why the street price of cocaine has dropped to a third of what it was a year ago. It isn't because fewer Americans are using the stuff.

The Oregonian
Portland, OR, August 10, 1984

The Reagan administration continues to lose its self-proclaimed war on drugs. However, it continues to hallucinate, calling for more money, more weapons, more jails and more time and patience, while pretending it is winning the conflict.

Sen. Paula Hawkins, R-Fla., even has demanded flame throwers and F-16s, and Ed Koch, the Democratic mayor of New York, wants every Latin American to be strip-searched before being allowed in the country. This is frenzy, not a cool, orderly response to a serious national problem.

In a drug war, the marketplace provides the body count. When drugs are scarce, or the battle is being won, the price goes sky high. When the police are being licked, the price drops as the street supply increases.

Since President Reagan took office and ordered up the drug war, the price of a kilogram of marijuana has dropped from $1,320 a kilogram to $880, while in South Florida the glut of cocaine has dropped its price from $60,000 to $20,000 a kilogram, according to a report in The Wall Street Journal.

If the marketplace were not the best evidence of a lost war, some federal agencies supply additional testimony. The U.S. Customs Service, responsible for intercepting drug runners within the 12-mile limit, is seeking more money for more boats. Its chief recently testified that Customs is catching less than 6 percent of the thousands of smugglers' boats, most of which bring in marijuana and cocaine.

Where there is a market demand, there will be suppliers who will meet it if the price is right. So, the government must recognize the limits and often the absurdities of its polices.

The time has come to seek new tactics and, perhaps, new leaders in the drug battle that is being lost at great social and economic cost to the nation.

Attitudes about drugs can be changed as they are being changed about tobacco, called by many the most addictive drug and the drug that causes the most deaths. (The surgeon general has found its use causes 300,000 deaths annually. Compare these to the 1,800 cocaine and heroin deaths in 1983 and virtually none attributed directly to marijuana.)

Fighting the causes of addictions and trying to change attitudes among the young offer more hope than endlessly escalating the attempts to disrupt the market. If victory is not achieved early, the jails will never be adequate, nor will there ever be enough boats, planes, federal agents, troops — or flame throwers.

The Register

Santa Ana, CA, December 16, 1984

On Dec. 2, 3 and 4, *The Register* published a series of articles about a "world war" the United States government is waging against drug abuse.

In its geographical reach and expenditure of resources, in its creation of victims and in the quasi-military tactics employed by people in our government and those of some drug-producing nations, this war is more than figurative.

Like other wars with ill-conceived strategies, it has also been monumentally futile.

In a column on the opinion page at the back of this section today, Patrick Buchanan writes of the same "war." He argues that the struggle has been unsuccessful precisely because it has been only a figurative war, because there is no consensus of the public to support a real assault, partly because there is a "permissive, libertarian" attitude toward drugs on the part of "millions of Americans."

This newspaper has editorially been within the "permissive, libertarian" tradition Buchanan describes. But we have tried not to be naive about the tragic consequences of drug use for many people. We neither advocate the use of drugs nor minimize the self-destructive effects they can have. We applaud private, voluntary efforts to educate people about drugs and to treat people who lose control of themselves because of their drug choices. Nor should the violence against other human beings associated with the drug trade be tolerated.

But we also refuse to be naive about attempts to use government coercion to change individual behavior.

All the military imagery reminds us of an earlier "war" mounted by the U.S. government with a majority consensus as to its goals and chances of success against another social problem. The war on poverty, after costing billions of dollars for every conceivable variety of program, has been declared at best a standoff, even by some of its ex-generals, and at worst — we believe this is closer to the truth — a dismal failure, counterproductive to its very purposes.

The enemies in both wars — poverty then and the abuse of drugs now — are vile enemies indeed.

But the war on drugs, no less than the war on poverty, will fail because in both, the coercive force of government is aimed at individual human freedom. In that, the government is warring against human nature, a battle that cannot be won with force.

Little can be said with such certainty about the state of nature as the assertion that man is a free being. He will insist on his right to freely choose, not because his choices always make him happy or prosperous or better, but simply because he is by nature a freely-choosing being. He chooses as he breathes.

It is upon this bedrock — individual freedom — that we build our arguments both for economic and personal liberty, which are really one and the same. Individual freedom is a moral issue with us. But it is also a matter of reality: freedom is man's natural condition; maximizing freedom will increase, but not guarantee, the chances of mankind improving itself; restricting freedom will always have harmful, if sometimes unpredictable, consequences.

In the matter of drug use, we do not argue that unrestrained freedom will improve the lot of mankind. But we contend that attempts to forcibly restrict individual choices will not — cannot — eliminate, or, in the long run, even substantially reduce, self-destructive behavior. One may want to call the abuse of drugs a human weakness, but one cannot force a man to be strong.

One may have better success in forcibly removing the occasion for possibly self-destructive choices. That is really what the war on drugs is attempting — to remove the supply and thus to tamp down the demand. But, even here, the successes have been small, in relation especially to the resources that have been spent. The victories have also been temporary, because the demand for drugs makes producers risk much to get back in business or to move to a safer location. The payoff on the risk increases, predictably, when supply shortages drive up prices.

There have been other costs as well. The most measurable effect of the war on drugs has not been to reduce self-destruction among drug users but rather to increase the destructive behavior — personal violence and property crimes — of people in the drug trade against the legitimate rights of others, both users and non-users of drugs.

We do not champion the use of drugs. Morally, however, we believe each individual has the right to make such choices for himself. And because such freedom conforms to reality — to human nature, if you will — we believe that coercion will be unsuccessful in eliminating the bad choices people make, about drugs or any other behavior.

ST. LOUIS POST-DISPATCH

St. Louis, MO, December 5, 1984

"Interdicting narcotics is like stepping on a balloon full of water. If you step on one side, it tends to bubble up on the other."

Thus did Thomas Cash, special agent in charge of the U.S. Drug Enforcement Administration's Atlanta office, characterize the difficult task facing his agency. Despite the much-touted war on drug trafficking that Vice President Bush is supposed to be personally commanding, the battle isn't going very well these days for our side. *The Wall Street Journal* reports that cocaine imports are up 50 percent over the last two years and heroin is as readily available as it was in the peak drug days of the 1970s.

If anything can be learned from the experience of this extended yet ineffective crackdown, it may well be that the laws of supply and demand work just as well in underground markets as they do in legitimate business. For each of the last two years, seizures of cocaine by federal agents have amounted to some 19 tons. But the market has not dried up. Far from it, prices have even fallen owing to bumper crops of coca in South America that dumped 63 tons on the U.S. streets last year.

The most determined efforts of law enforcement agents are no match for the ingenuity, scope and motivation of the drug smugglers, whose real worry isn't how to dodge the cops, but how to stash their payoffs. According to one charter plane operator, cash payments for smuggling drugs were so great he had to buy a bill-counting machine.

What *will* work? Stiffer penalties for convicted traffickers (long jail terms rather than easily paid fines); continued international cooperation between the U.S. and the drug source countries; and, most importantly, all-out federal support for social programs of education and rehabilitation that cause the market in illicit drugs to dry up.

Nationwide Pot Sweep Launched

Attorney General Edwin Meese 3rd August 5, 1985 launched Operation Delta-9, the country's largest crackdown to date on the cultivation of marijuana. Funded by $2.9 million from the Justice Department's Drug Enforcement Administration (DEA), the three-day sweep involved 150 DEA agents and 2,200 police officials in 49 states. Rhode Island did not take part.

A crackdown on marijuana farming in 1984 had received $3.4 million in DEA funds and had resulted in 4,941 arrests and the destruction of close to 13 million marijuana plants. Almost four million of those were cultivated, the rest having grown wild.

Meese, speaking in Ozark National Forest in Arkansas, said the campaign was needed "to show that we are willing to eradicate marijuana within our own country just as we are working with other countries to eradicate crops there." The attorney general opened the program in a national forest because about 25% of U.S.-grown marijuana was believed to grow on public land.

The value of the 1984 marijuana harvest in the United States was estimated at $16.6 billion by the National Organization for the Reform of Marijuana Laws (NORML) January 7, 1985. The Washington-based group advocates the legalization of marijuana for personal use. NORML claimed that the 1984 crop had been worth a fifth again as much as the 1983 crop. It said that 25% of the 1984 harvest's 11 million pounds had been grown indoors rather than on farms, and some 75% of the crop had been an especially expensive and potent form of marijuana called sinsemilla. The lobbying group estimated the annual demand for marijuana at 20 million pounds.

But the raids hardly put a dent in the 1985 marijuana harvest. In fact, for the first time in U.S. history an illicit crop was the most valuable in the country. According to NORML, the 1985 harvest produced a record $18.6 billion, putting it slightly ahead of corn as the most valuable crop in the U.S. While one reason for marijuana making it to the number-one spot may have been the growth of the marijuana market, another reason was the decreasing price of corn. But it is somewhat unfair to compare marijuana with legal crops because marijuana is a weed that can grow anywhere and sells for $2,000 a pound. These black-market prices compare to prices in the low dollars for legal crops. In addition, marijuana is often sold directly by the farmer to the consumer. Thus there is not much difference in price between wholesale and retail, unlike legal crops where there are middlemen.

the Charleston Gazette

Charleston, WV, August 6, 1985

MARIJUANA eradication efforts are reminiscent of those 1920s newsreels of Prohibition raiders endlessly smashing bottles and dumping barrels in their futile effort to stamp out booze.

The chief difference is that, instead of rattling to the scene in Tin Lizzies, today's raiders use helicopters and the latest scientific advances.

Monday's unprecedented 50-state marijuana patch attack, code-named "Delta 9," caused the demise of many hidden pot plants and generated flattering news photos of Attorney General Edwin Meese at an Arkansas raid. But did it produce any lasting benefit?

In May the Drug Enforcement Agency drafted plans to spray up to 300 tons of poisonous paraquat — which can be harmful or fatal to humans — on pot plots in California, Kentucky, Georgia and elsewhere.

(Remember when paraquat was sprayed in Mexico in the 1970s and tainted pot was shipped to U.S. users? Johnny Carson reported it on his *Tonight* show, setting off gales of coughing among musicians in the band.)

Virginia Gov. Charles Robb recently called out the National Guard on a search-and-destroy mission against his state's marijuana patches. Californians complain that raids against bushes are becoming increasingly militaristic.

Does this Charge of the Pot Brigade really benefit America?

Look what happened in Monroe County:

Helicopter-borne officers searching for marijuana plants repeatedly buzzed the farm of Tony Giancola, a Columbia University literature graduate. The aircraft shook Giancola's home even at night. Can agents see plants in the dark?

One day last year, a chopper team saw Giancola burning brush and assumed he was destroying pot plants. (He says he was making smoke to calm his honeybees. State beekeeper Bard Montgomery says he never heard of using an open fire for that purpose.) Agents stormed in with no warrant, caused bedlam, seized Giancola and his wife at gunpoint, locked them in handcuffs, searched for more than an hour — and failed to find even one illegal leaf or root.

The officers didn't apologize. The couple sued. Case pending.

Which is worse, pot bushes on mountain farms or police blitzkriegs? Drug officers often break as many laws as they enforce. Even state police Cpl. J.D. Leffler, coordinator of marijuana eradication, admits that "all of this is bordering on constitutional violations."

America's concerns are out of balance. Marijuana is an injurious substance, like alcohol and tobacco. But beer breweries and tobacco farms are free to produce their products, while pot patches are deemed an evil that must be exorcised.

Whatever the answer to the societal problem of marijuana — if there is an answer — the tactics of Prohibition won't help today any more than they did in the 1920s.

THE KANSAS CITY STAR

Kansas City, MO, August 8, 1985

The nationwide raid recently on marijuana fields has more to do with puff than pot. For years law enforcement officers in different areas have been going to the fields this time of year to take a stand against marijuana. Making a national pageant with Attorney General Edwin Meese III pulling up a few token plants in Arkansas isn't going to do much more real eradication than the purely localized ones did. Especially when everyone, from the news media to the entrepreneurs, are alerted a week in advance.

Little lies like the one involving Kansas further mock the operation. The state didn't participate in the great coordinated sweep. But the Drug Enforcement Administration said it did. Whether that was done through error or contrivance, the agency hurt its own credibility.

Lack of enthusiasm for this federal showmanship doesn't equal a clean bill of health for marijuana or approval of growing the stuff on bottom land. Children and teenagers particularly risk serious health problems with it and although its notoriety is more subdued, use of the chemical among the young is higher now than it was in the heyday of the drug counterculture in the 1960s. Moreover, marijuana is illegal.

But making a circus out of enforcement is a poor way to deal with a problem especially when profits and abuse of more deadly drugs are out of control. DEA has said it needs 40,000 agents to curtail the flow of drugs like heroin and cocaine into this country. There are 1,900 worldwide. The illegal narcotics trade is a $110-billion annual business but the federal drug abuse budget totals only $1.5 billion.

Personal appearances by bigwigs in designer clothes at student assemblies are no substitutes for commitment of substance to the war against drug abuse. Such circuses undermine everyone's faith in law enforcement. And the criminals' fear.

The Miami Herald
Miami, FL, August 17, 1985

WHEN law-enforcement officials conduct a raid on the site of a suspected illegal activity, the idea is to surprise the culprits in the act of breaking the law. Many a planned police raid has fizzled when the culprits received advance warning from a friendly tipster, but it's a rarity when that tip-off comes from the law enforcers themselves.

Yet that's exactly what the U.S. Department of Justice did four days prior to the initiation of the much-touted Delta-9 project — a nationwide crackdown on marijuana producers. First, Justice Department officials held an embargoed press conference, which the reporters involved honored. But at the same time, "sources" within the Department leaked the crackdown plans. Then, Attorney General Edwin Meese announced plans to attend one of the raids and invited a full media contingent to accompany him on this photo opportunity.

That's no way to run a complex, long-planned, inter-agency, multistate, *surprise* crackdown on marijuana producers. And several states' top law-enforcement officials said so, including Florida Department of Law Enforcement (FDLE) Commissioner Robert Dempsey. Mr. Dempsey rightly criticized the Justice Department's premature reporting of its plans as possibly endangering police officers, not to mention allowing some marijuana growers to harvest their crops early, thus escaping detection.

Florida's participation in the Delta-9 project was downplayed deliberately. The FDLE's search-and-destroy raids have been quite successful so far this year, according to Mr. Dempsey, and one reason is the secrecy surrounding the raids. The Delta-9/FDLE action resulted in 11 arrests and the discovery of approximately 3,500 pot plants at 157 sites in 13 counties. Not a bad day's work, but how much bigger might the raiders' take have been if growers hadn't been forewarned by the U.S. Department of Justice?

The Orlando Sentinel
Orlando, FL, August 11, 1985

Never mind that it hardly put a dent in the drug problem. Drug agents nationwide went on a much ballyhooed search-and-destroy mission last week for marijuana. Accompanied by Attorney General Edwin Meese, the agents burned thousands of plants and made hundreds of arrests. In Florida, agents arrested 11 people and uprooted about 3,500 plants.

The problem: You don't win wars with a one-week, highly publicized skirmish. Indeed, these short sprints seem to be the problem lately when it comes to drugs. Too many people are going for the publicity, and no one is organizing a coherent plan.

While Mr. Meese was out looking at marijuana, Florida Sen. Paula Hawkins was pushing to get $350,000 in tax dollars to form an international task force to talk about the drug problem. The committee would have room for seven U.S. senators. What would it do? Nothing except give lawmakers TV time. Better the money go for more drug agents, as drugs come into this country in record numbers and at record low prices.

Mr. Meese and Sen. Hawkins would be better off spending their time studying recent reports from the General Accounting Office, Congress' investigative arm. It has found serious problems in the war against drugs.

This year it looked at the National Narcotics Border Interdiction System. That's a fancy name for a program that began three years ago in Miami to nab drugs at the border as part of Vice President George Bush's task force on drugs. Now the program has been extended to five other cities. The idea was to get the U.S. Customs Service, the military, the Coast Guard, the Drug Enforcement Administration and other police agencies together to stop the drug flow.

But the program is a flop, says GAO. It has stopped very few drugs at the borders. The system isn't doing such a bad job in Miami because that city has added such a vast system of prosecutors, judges and law enforcement officials that are necessary for battling drugs. The problems came in trying to expand it to the other areas that aren't so prepared. The El Paso, Texas, office, for instance, stopped only three planes last year. Furthermore, GAO investigators found that many of the seizures were attributed to just plain luck.

One of the problems? This war on drugs doesn't have a general. A lot of people are running around with their own ideas about how to reduce the flow of drugs, but no one is in charge. Around the country, for example, the narcotics interdiction operations are headed by different agencies. That's incredibly confusing. In some states, Customs Service officials head the effort, in other states it's the Coast Guard, others the DEA. Who's in charge?

These latest marijuana raids organized by the attorney general are only more examples of poor coordination in this war. Local police already eradicate marijuana fields. In Florida so far this year police have seized almost 43,000 plants in such raids and made 159 arrests.

The GAO report did offer one idea for battling the drug war more effectively. It suggested that the federal government create a Cabinet-level position to coordinate it. Well, there already is a Cabinet-level person who should be doing that: Attorney General Edwin Meese.

He doesn't have control over the military and Customs Service, but Mr. Meese can use his power and influence to coordinate a meaningful war on drugs. And that means doing more than watching police burn marijuana plants.

The Washington Post
Washington, DC, August 9, 1985

WHEN YOU SEE a picture of Attorney General Edwin Meese squinting at marijuana plants seized in a raid in the Ozark National Forest, you may be tempted to conclude, as one critic of the marijuana laws did, that Operation Delta-9—last Monday's 50-state raid of which the Ozark operation was part—was "just good propaganda." Certainly Mr. Meese understands that it is probably impossible to stamp out marijuana entirely. It is easily grown and in considerable demand. Possession and use of marijuana in small amounts is a minor offense now in most states.

Even so, we think Mr. Meese and his 2,200 federal, state and local comrades were not engaged in a quixotic enterprise. For one thing, while this country asks its Latin neighbors to take politically costly steps to stamp out their drug business, it behooves Americans to do something visible and major about their own. And if marijuana use is common, there is good evidence—about as good as is possible, considering that the activity is illegal—that marijuana use is less common in the 15-to-25 age group than it was a few years ago, and it may very well be less common in older age groups as well.

So the predictions commonly made by marijuana advocates in the 1970s that the habit would become well-nigh universal have not come to pass. A dozen years ago you could not refute claims that marijuana smoking was harmless, and you had to concede that some of the claims made against it were exaggerated. But now, after a decade in which perhaps 30 million Americans have smoked marijuana, evidence of harm—harm on the order of that caused by tobacco and alcohol—is accumulating. It would not be surprising, then, in a nation where cigarette and liquor consumption is declining, if marijuana consumption were declining too.

In the 1970s it was said that marijuana, like alcohol, could not effectively be prohibited. But it was forgotten that, in the century up to repeal, alcohol use was vastly reduced in the United States, partly by legal prohibition, more by persuasion and the power of ideas. Alcohol use increased after repeal, but to nothing like the early 19th century levels. Now it seems that the country has reached an equilibrium on marijuana. Americans know it's unhealthy and use it less often. And they insist, properly, on enforcing the law against commercial production and distribution. Mr. Meese's raid in the Ozarks and Delta-9 serve a useful purpose not just in making the business of marijuana less secure but in underlining Americans' intention that this law should be enforced.

The Louisville Times
Louisville, KY,
August 13, 1985

"Operation Delta-9" — the not-so-secret raid by federal and state drug agents against the nation's marijuana fields — is being hailed as a success, but one wonders for whom.

It was a publicity plus for Atty. Gen. Ed Meese, whose badly tarnished image may have been improved by his declaration of war on pot. "This is the largest (anti-marijuana) campaign yet," he noted, "in terms of numbers of states participating, in terms of the number of plants seized, in terms of the number of plots investigated, in terms of the number of people arrested."

Indeed, every state but Rhode Island (which so far as anyone could ascertain has no marijuana plants) was a target and the raiders killed at least 340,000 plants and made 175 arrests, according to the U. S. Drug Enforcement Administration. (At least 11 per cent of the plants were found in Kentucky.)

And, to that extent, the raid was a triumph in that it means some reduction in the crop and, ultimately, less of the illegal weed on the market. Since marijuana is the drug with which many youngsters are introduced to narcotics, limiting the supply is beneficial.

But the public must also wonder whether the raiders would have been more successful if news about Delta-9 had not been leaked a week in advance. Mr. Meese was baffled that the operation was as successful as it was. "You have to feel that some of these people either don't read or can't read," he said.

However, the attorney general's contribution to the result is superficial. Most of these raids would have occurred anyway because of state and federal enforcement efforts already in place. Kentucky this year has already eradicated about five times as many plants as the 30,000 killed last week.

Then there's this item to limit the merriment: While the Delta-9 squads were on the march, a *New York Times* story last week reported that federal drug and border agents have been overwhelmed by the unprecedented influx of cocaine. And a report this summer by the General Accounting Office concluded that the Justice Department's attack on drug traffic has not had much effect. That strategy was the brainchild of Mr. Meese's predecessor, William French Smith

It is important to note that — in the case of cocaine, at least — federal agents are intercepting more than ever. The drug agency's statistics show that in the first six months of 1985, just in south Florida, 13,000 kilograms of cocaine were seized. Compare that to a total of 4,400 kilograms seized nationwide in 1982.

Nevertheless, the Reagan administration has fumbled badly in its attempt to crack down on narcotics, which are gushing into this country by land, sea and air. One major area — pressing Latin American governments to act against growers — has been a dud. That's not surprising given the general ignorance about that region in the current White House.

So no matter how much Mr. Meese glows about the Delta-9 harvest, the folks who are smiling even more are those who buy or sell illegal drugs.

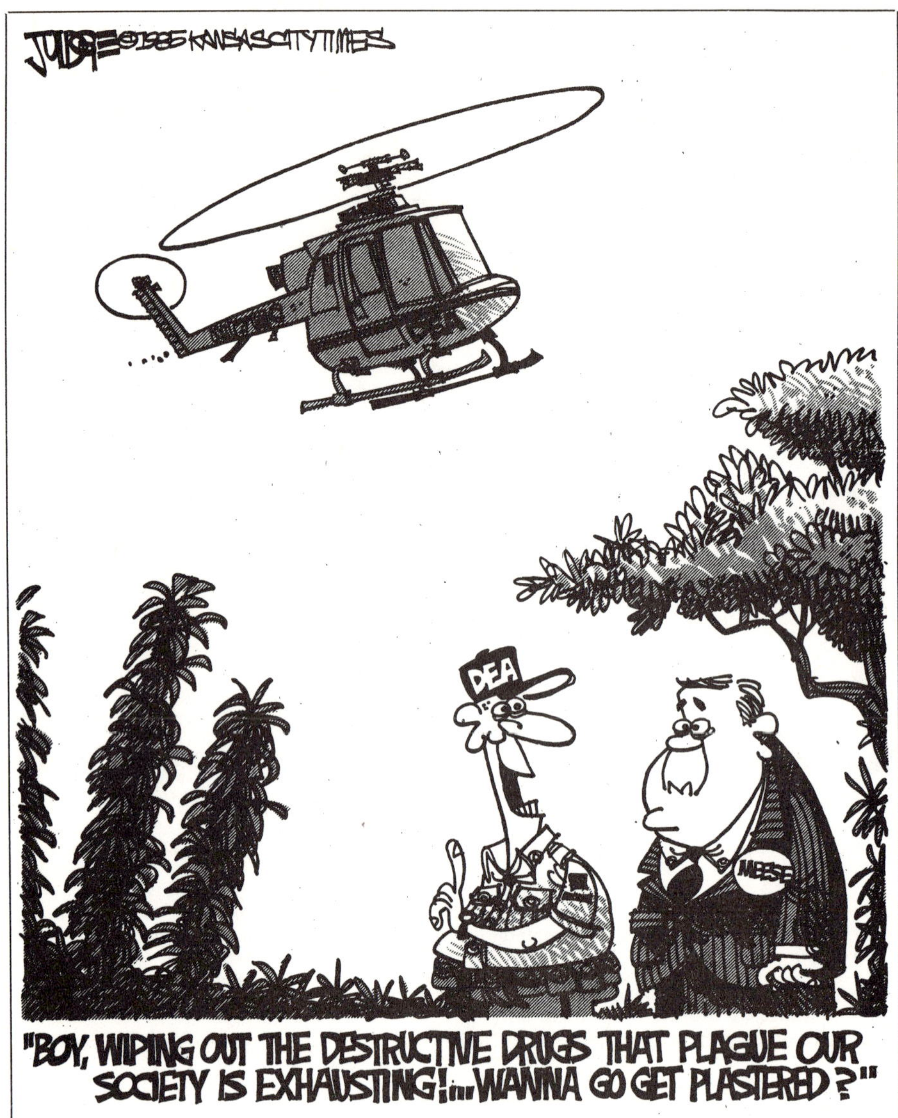

The Boston Globe
Boston, MA, August 7, 1985

It is reassuring to know that Attorney General Edwin Meese has taken charge of a three-day mission to send the domestic marijuana crop up in flames, and to arrest every suspected grower caught in a web cast by 2200 federal and state law enforcement officers.

Meese, in the style of J. Edgar Hoover, dramatized the importance of the project by going into the field. Only bad weather in Arkansas kept him from taking machete in hand and slogging into the Ozark National Forest to cut down marijuana plants. Meese had to watch from a helicopter as others performed the task.

The early signs are that the mission, known as Operation Delta-9, will be successful. On Monday – the first day – 105,058 marijuana plants were uprooted. Fifty-four persons were arrested, and 16 weapons were seized. Meese's goal is the destruction of 250,000 plants. Local officials in almost every state are gladly participating.

Meese's decision to oversee Operation Delta-9 may involve recent Justice Department decisions. He has had to explain why "career people" in the Justice Department dropped an investigation of Teamsters president Jackie Pressler. Federal prosecutors in Cleveland had recommended that Pressler be indicted on charges of authorizing union payments to "ghost employees."

Meese also had to explain why no one at E.F. Hutton was charged after the company pleaded guilty to 2000 counts of wire and mail fraud.

Citizens can be sure that there will be no deals with the cultivators of dope; they will be prosecuted to the fullest extent of the law. The "career people" will not make deals for information. There will be no need for Meese to have to explain why no one was charged and why no one went to jail.

This time things will be different. Although white-collar criminals often elude justice, Meese is proving his intolerance of crime by relentlessly pursuing the cultivators of pot.

The Hartford Courant
Hartford, CT, August 8, 1985

The U.S. Justice Department's nationwide crackdown on marijuana farms was valuable mostly for the publicity it created.

Under the direction of U.S. Attorney General Edwin Meese III, 2,500 federal, state and local officers destroyed millions of marijuana plants in recent days.

In Connecticut, officials couldn't find any in an aerial search, but a drug enforcement agent said "we're sending a message that we will not tolerate marijuana cultivation."

Not tolerating marijuana cultivation and stamping out marijuana are two different things, of course. The foray this week claimed only an infinitesimal amount of the marijuana growing wild or under cultivation in this country. Farmers probably mow or burn more marijuana each year — treating it as a nuisance — than Mr. Meese's agents are ever likely to see.

The Meese-led marijuana raids bring to mind the anti-alcohol crusade of Carrie A. Nation at the turn of the century. Ms. Nation, with a hatchet in one hand and a Bible in the other, smashed whiskey bottles and closed the saloons in Medicine Lodge, Kan., before turning her wrath on "wet" states across the country.

Ms. Nation didn't vanquish alcohol by breaking all the bottles in her sight, and Mr. Meese won't eliminate marijuana use by conducting highly publicized raids. They both treated the symptom, not the problem.

Law enforcement dollars are best spent in attacking abusers and pushers, rather than a weed whose seeds are carried by the wind.

The Detroit News
Detroit, MI, August 7, 1985

Midsummer is the height of the agricultural growing season. It's also a slow time for news. So if your goal is to get the maximum publicity for a few marijuana raids, this is a good time to run them. That goes a long way toward explaining what Atty. Gen. Ed Meese, the federal Drug Enforcement Agency (DEA), and the Justice Department are doing right now with their well-staged campaign to eradicate America's homegrown dope.

Make no mistake about it. These *Miami Vice*-type stunts — police 'copters out in the Ozarks, feds sniffing through New Hampshire blueberry patches, Iowa's waving wheat and Michigan's sweet corn fields with dogs, guns, and blazing TV cameras — make good theater. But they're not likely to have a serious impact on marijuana cultivation.

They will have even less impact on the amount of pot consumed in the United States. DEA officials estimate that 14,000 metric tons of the stuff are smoked annually, which at the very least indicates a tremendous market demand. The domestically grown variety accounts for an estimated 12 to 25 percent of that market. There is now no state in the union that doesn't grow dope. It is far too lucrative a cash crop for many otherwise legitimate farmers to resist. The 1984 marijuana crop in Michigan was estimated at $250 million.

In fact, it's pretty clear that the war on drugs is being lost. The street price of domestic commercial pot is $45-$65 per ounce; more potent domestic sensimilla goes for $100-$175 per ounce. Those prices have not risen at all during the Reagan administration's highly publicized anti-drug campaign, indicating that that supply is greater than ever before.

So, Ed, the time may have come to mellow out a little and consider other ways of dealing with marijuana. Charging around the country like Eliot Ness may be fun, and it may even discourage some marijuana cultivation for awhile, but it's likely to have about the same long-term effect on pot that Ness had on booze. Surveys indicate 70 million, or 35 percent of the public, have tried pot. Approximately 18 percent of the population use it regularly: nine out of every 10 users is an adult.

Where so many people disobey a law, that law becomes a mockery and the credibility of the law in general suffers. What's needed is a serious debate on whether we wouldn't be better off simply legalizing marijuana.

Some people fear that legalizing it will cause use to increase, especially among teen-agers. Actually, there is much evidence that the "natural" level of marijuana use has been reached. National surveys of high school students have shown an actual decrease in use for the past few years, even though 85 percent of high school seniors claim they can get some dope if they want it. There has also been an increase in disapproval of those who do use drugs.

Though common sense tells us that no drug — including aspirin or alcohol or caffeine — is entirely benign, there are levels of risk, some of which are tolerable. There is no credible evidence that small amounts of marijuana are any more harmful than equal amounts of alcohol. Nor is it credible for the administration to try to create guilt by association, by calling pot "the gateway drug" — the use of which leads to more serious substance abuse. Most people who drink a beer now and then don't become alcoholics. Most people who get stoned now and then don't become heroin addicts.

In any case, it's a little late for such scare tactics. Attempting to ban marijuana has only driven it underground, where criminal elements control its production, distribution, and use. Decriminalizing marijuana, it can be argued, would free up police and courts for more serious work. It would also take the profit out of drug hustling, which entices many youths out of school and onto the streets.

Legalizing marijuana flies in the face of much-received wisdom about "morality" and the evils of drugs. It also begs the question of what to do about more serious drugs, such as heroin, cocaine, and the newer "manufactured" chemicals. But as we watch the price of pot decline at the same time taxpayer-financed operations to suppress it soar (Monday's raids cost the feds a reported $250,000), we think it's time to seriously consider legalizing it.

The Hutchinson News
Hutchinson, KS, August 7, 1985

Shades of Vern Miller!

Attorney General Edwin Meese has taken a breather from his arduous duties in Washington and headed to the hills of Arkansas to look at pot.

Early reports are that the attorney general discovered a couple of truckloads of confiscated marijuana in Harrison, Ark., which is not exactly the sticks, but close to it in those Ozark hills.

If the president had jetted off to Dogpatch, you would have described the event as a "photo opportunity." Theatrics have become government, with America's affection for illusion of activity, even if there isn't any.

To be sure, the attorney general has the spare time available to focus a national effort at finding marijuana. He and his staff aren't worrying about complex legal issues such as the E.F. Hutton case (in which all the white-collar criminals were ignored).

Marijuana bashing is simple. Folks can understand that much easier than check kiting.

If Mr. Meese follows the script first devised in Kansas a few years ago, his next activity should be easily forecast. He'll be jumping out of the trunk of a car, en route to apprehending a miserable malefactor.

Well, since he's the U.S. attorney general, maybe he'll decide to jump out the back door of a helicopter.

The Dispatch
Columbus, OH, August 10, 1985

The recent federal, state and local crackdown on illegal marijuana fields across the country may not stop all the growing of the banned plant, but it will put the growers on notice that the risks they take are growing with each day.

More than 2,000 law enforcement officers took part in raids which included every state in the nation. They destroyed an estimated 60,000 plants and arrested more than a score of persons.

The need for such dramatic action is demonstrated by the facts. In 1980, about 5 percent of the marijuana smoked in the United States was grown in this country. Now the figure has jumped to 12 percent, authorities said, in the wake of some success in slowing the illegal import of the crop from foreign lands.

We salute all those who joined in the raids.

U.S. Issues World Drug Report; Opium and Pot Down, Coca Up

The United States State Department February 14, 1985 issued its annual report on world production of illegal drugs. The study found that despite U.S. efforts, many nations receiving U.S. foreign aid were still producing and exporting large amounts of illegal drugs. A 1983 U.S. law had threatened narcotics-exporting countries with foreign aid cutoffs. But the State Department report found that in 1984 narcotics output had gone up in seven of the 10 major drug-producing countries with which the U.S. had relations. The U.S. gave aid to all seven. The report expressed dissatisfaction with the efforts by many foreign governments to combat the problem. Bolivia's campaign to curb the cocaine trade, for instance, was called "a major disappointment." Two countries that before had not been regarded as significant drug producers increased their output dramatically. Belize rose to become the fourth-largest supplier of marijuana to the U.S. Ecuador became possibly the world's third-largest exporter of coca leaf. Both received U.S. aid. The report cautioned that "much of the production data should be considered preliminary, some even speculative." However, the report traced the outlines of worldwide drug output.

Sen. Paula Hawkins (R, Fla.), the chief sponsor of the 1983 law, said: "I am going to put a hold on the aid to all the countries that have not made progress." Rep. Dante Fascell (D, Fla.), chairman of the House Foreign Affairs Committee, said: "The bottom line is that...the war is being lost."

Nancy Reagan April 24-25, 1985 hosted an international meeting of first ladies concerned about teenage drug abuse. The 18 participants, counting Mrs. Reagan, listened to government officials and private antidrug activists, as well as contributed their own views on the problem. The meeting began in the White House and continued the next day in Atlanta. There the first ladies attended an international conference held by the private Parent Resources Institute for Drug Education.

The Wichita Eagle-Beacon

Wichita, KS, August 29, 1985

THE much-heralded "war on drugs" started with the assumption the drug enemy could be identified and routed. More than two decades and many billions of law enforcement dollars later, the war is far from being won, and it's becoming increasingly clear the enemy includes ourselves.

Americans take a wide assortment of legal drugs to combat everything from headaches to "nerves" to obesity. In addition to that, 20 million Americans regularly use illegal drugs — from marijuana to cocaine — for "recreational" purposes. Cocaine use has reached epidemic proportions, despite the clear dangers of the drug. Do Americans really care about stopping drug abuse?

Most do. It's easier, though, to accept drug use as an inevitability — especially since drug laws have had little success in stemming the flow of illegal drugs into this country. Many Hollywood movies these days have what's become almost an obligatory pot-smoking scene. It's similar to the way movies glamorized cigarette-smoking for an earlier generation. The message to kids is this: It's cool to smoke pot — everybody does it.

Further, many minor drug offenses have been decriminalized as enforcement efforts concentrate on the Mr. Bigs. Unfortunately, this has created a perception among some that it's all right to use drugs, as long as you don't get caught dealing them.

In fact, some observers, including conservative William F. Buckley Jr., have decided the war isn't worth it — that drugs should be legalized, thereby bringing them under federal regulation and reducing related crime. What these people don't admit is that with increased availability, drug use — particularly among young people — would soar.

Giving up isn't the answer. Attorney General Edwin Meese has stepped up the federal anti-drug war lately, undertaking high-visibility raids and working more closely with law officials in drug-producing countries. Although he admits the war is far from won, "we're not losing it, and that's a change from what has happened."

Above all, attitudes must change if America is to make any headway against drug use. That takes public education. First Lady Nancy Reagan has been very effective in this area, raising teen-agers' awareness about the dangers of drug abuse. But much more could be done.

Attitudes can change — witness the enormous turnaround in public perceptions of drunk driving and cigarette smoking. What is lacking is the commitment from parents and the public. Americans must take a clear stand: Drug use is not acceptable.

The Courier-Journal

Louisville, KY, April 14, 1985

IT'S REASSURING that Attorney General Edwin Meese has disavowed reports that the federal war on drugs is about to start concentrating on users. As law violators who also finance the drug trade with dollars, they obviously should be discouraged in any way possible. But the government's drug-enforcement resources already are stretched thin. It should leave to state and local police the job of chasing the users, so it can focus instead on battling drug traffickers.

A Justice Department official broached the idea of a federal crackdown on users last week. Despite enforcement efforts, he said, "people are out there using these drugs, and we have not broken that (demand) curve."

It's true that drug abuse has continued to increase. But the federal government is better equipped to cope with the criminal conspiracies, global commerce and enormous flow of money that mark the drug traffic.

It's no easy task. The federal drug enforcement effort, which gobbles up $1.2 billion a year, has had its successes. But officials acknowledge it is far from cutting off the supply of drugs from Latin America and elsewhere. Thus, according to the Justice Department's second annual Organized Crime Drug Enforcement report, cocaine imports continue to rise, from 69 metric tons in 1983 to an estimated 90 metric tons last year.

This difficulty was underscored two months ago by the murders of a U.S. Drug Enforcement agent and a pilot who were working in Mexico. Now, with the arrests of two alleged kingpins in the Mexican drug trade, the influence that drug bosses have over police and other government officials in that country seems increasingly clear. Indeed, U.S. officials feel that, without their demands for a serious investigation, the Mexican police might have ignored the killings.

Closer to home, there's ample evidence that trafficking across state lines is best left to federal officials. Organized crime's presence in the drug trade makes the federal role even more important. So does the growing evidence that some banks, unwittingly or not, have gotten involved. The use of Miami banks to launder billions in illicit profits is a well-publicized example, but the conduct of banks elsewhere also has raised suspicions. The Bank of Boston, for instance, pleaded guilty to federal charges of failing to report $1.22 billion in international cash transactions that investigators believe was a money-laundering operation.

Certainly, all levels of government must be concerned about catching and punishing abusers, and prevention programs must be encouraged. But switching the federal government's emphasis from traffickers to users would be like using the homicide squad to give out parking tickets. The real hoodlums would have a field day.

The Record

Hackensack, NJ, July 23, 1985

Every day, it seems, we read of another major drug bust that nets quantities of cocaine or heroin worth many millions on the street. Contemporary legend is made of the stretch Mercedes, the streaking powerboats, and the 20-room mansions acquired by drug dealers from the profits of their trade.

Congress has given federal judges special powers to bring stiff sentences against these predators. But now its General Accounting Office reports that the courts are surprisingly reluctant to use at least one of those powers: the power to confiscate the drug dealers' ill-gotten booty. Though major drug traffickers receive average prison sentences of 10 years, twice as long as the average for all federal offenders, the average fine for the 244 most serious drug offenders was just $60,000 — less than the price of one of those Mercedes. For all major traffickers, the average fine imposed was less than one third of the maximum allowed by law.

Congress has now directed judges to re-think this practice. Its Comprehensive Crime Control Act, which took effect after data collection for this study was completed, gives judges three new monetary weapons: forfeiture of profits from drug trafficking; restitution to victims, where practicable; and uniform maximum fines of $250,000 per criminal count. Drafters of the law say these harsh provisions grow out of Congress's determination to penalize drug dealers as painfully as possible.

Why should drug dealers pay heavier fines than other offenders? Because drug dealers are different. The distribution of dangerous drugs has produced illicit wealth for which there is no precedent in world history. The cost of drug-related law enforcement is staggering, but even higher are the costs of victimization — in the robberies and burglaries to support drug habits, in medical treatment and support for addicts and their benighted children, in ruined lives. Judges should be taking from drug traffickers every nickel that the law allows.

THE MILWAUKEE JOURNAL

Milwaukee, WI, July 14, 1985

The old Nancy was seen as a kind of latter-day Marie Antoinette. Elegantly coiffed and expensively dressed, she collected $1 million from rich friends to buy new china for the White House while her husband, the president, was hacking away at programs for the poor. She was the woman who gazed worshipfully at her husband during his speeches and who confounded feminists with her insistence that her life began "the day I met Ronnie."

The new Nancy crusades against drug abuse among the young, promotes voluntary child care and (if certain news accounts are accurate) coaxes her husband to cool down his Cold War rhetoric and warm up to Gorbachev. She is said to be the president's unofficial personnel manager and the primary force behind a string of White House purges, including those of Alexander Haig and William Clark.

The parallel retooling of Mrs. Reagan's image from that of clotheshorse to workhorse, and from demure helpmate to influential adviser, is one of the more intriguing metamorphoses of the electronic age.

A cynic might conclude that the Nancy *d'autrefois* was the real one and that the *nouvelle* Nancy is simply the creation of White House media handlers. A more charitable view is that Mrs. Reagan herself has grown in her role. Wherever the truth lies (probably somewhere in between), it's clear that the public, as shown by opinion polls, likes the new model better than the old.

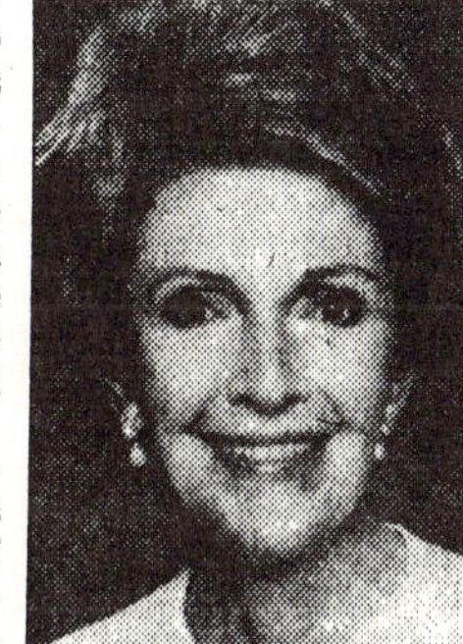
Nancy Reagan

That says something about changing perceptions of women and of first ladies in particular. The term itself has a quaint, 19th century ring — reminiscent of a time when women were expected to be mere appendages of their men. Long before there was an organized women's movement, Eleanor Roosevelt broke the first-lady mold, charting an independent course of social activism and concern.

Her successors have had to contend not only with the daunting example set by Mrs. Roosevelt but also with Americans' ambivalence toward the job. In the waning years of the 20th century, the public, it seems, expects a first lady to be something more than ornamental but something less than assertive. When a first lady gets really pushy and, say, sits in on cabinet meetings, as Rosalynn Carter did, people start sniping, "Who elected her, anyway?"

Perhaps the transformation of Nancy Reagan will inspire a more realistic view of this job — a job that, like that of homemaker, too often goes unappreciated and unrewarded, yet helps shape institutions (the family, the presidency).

Considering the influence that Mrs. Reagan has on her husband, voters in future elections might remember that marriage, like many a presidency, is indeed a partnership; that partners influence each other's judgment and behavior; and that the character and attitudes of a candidate's spouse are surely more important than what she (or he) wears.

Even more fascinating to ponder are the expectations that Americans may have when they finally elect a woman president. Will her spouse, if she has one, be known as the "first gentleman"? The "presidential consort"? Will he be expected to look distinguished and hold his tongue? Will he lie about his age? Or, as we suspect, will all such questions at last be irrelevant?

The Providence Journal

Providence, RI, December 5, 1985

Society's war against illicit drugs unquestionably is an uphill battle. The narcotics racket is so profitable that no matter how often pushers are arrested, others quickly take their place. If this unholy succession is to be stopped, it requires not only continued tough law enforcement, but also tough sentences for those caught and convicted. Federal Judge Bruce M. Selya sets a good example of how the courts should act in such cases.

For about the past year, Judge Selya has been coming down hard in U.S. District Court in Providence on those found guilty there of drug trafficking. In one instance, he administered a heavier penalty than even the prosecution had recommended. Earlier this year, the judge gave a big-time cocaine dealer the maximum sentence of 20 years imprisonment. Last week, he imposed similar jail time on two more cocaine pushers, with an additional five years for one of them who was a repeat offender. Stiff penalties of this sort, regularly administered, may yet put a crimp in the drug trade.

That such punishment fits the crime cannot be disputed. As Judge Selya told the defendant to whom he gave the 25-year term, "You have placed yourself at center stage in the ongoing tragedy of widespread drug distribution which is eating away at the fabric of our society." Those willing to poison their own community and the nation for personal profit hardly can be dealt with too harshly.

Difficult though it has proven to stem the drug tide in America, authorities must keep working at it. If they are to be successful, they will need the same judicial backup Judge Selya has given them from all other courts and judges as well.

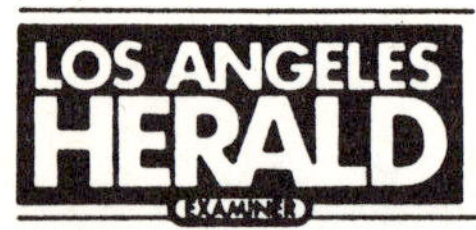

*Los Angeles, CA,
April 3, 1985*

For years now the government has been going after narcotics rings and ringleaders. Faced with insurmountable odds, particularly in combating cocaine trade, the federal drug-busters are considering the revival of an old approach — the prosecution of drug users. Our hearts don't go out to drug abusers, ingrained and accepted though their habits may have become at various levels of our society; those who are involved in any part of the illegal drug traffic deserve to feel the full weight of the law.

Nevertheless, the idea of setting out to imprison some users — even, say, high-profile users — in the hopes that others will learn from the example has a familiar and disturbing ring. Didn't the country experiment with this approach during Prohibition, only to find it a notable failure? Even in the unlikely event that people might change their attitudes and behavior this time around, we have some other concerns. The government's resources in the battle against drugs are limited. It is not at all clear that diverting manpower to focus on users would make a dent in the drug trade, or prove cost-effective in the long run. Finally, such a system could result in unequal enforcement of the law, a violation of our constitutional protections.

We'd rather see the feds channel any extra resources they have into educating young people about the dangers of drug abuse. Further partnerships between law enforcement and the schools — like the promising DARE program developed between the LAPD and the Los Angeles school district — would do more to break the vicious drug cycle than targeting a handful of citizens.

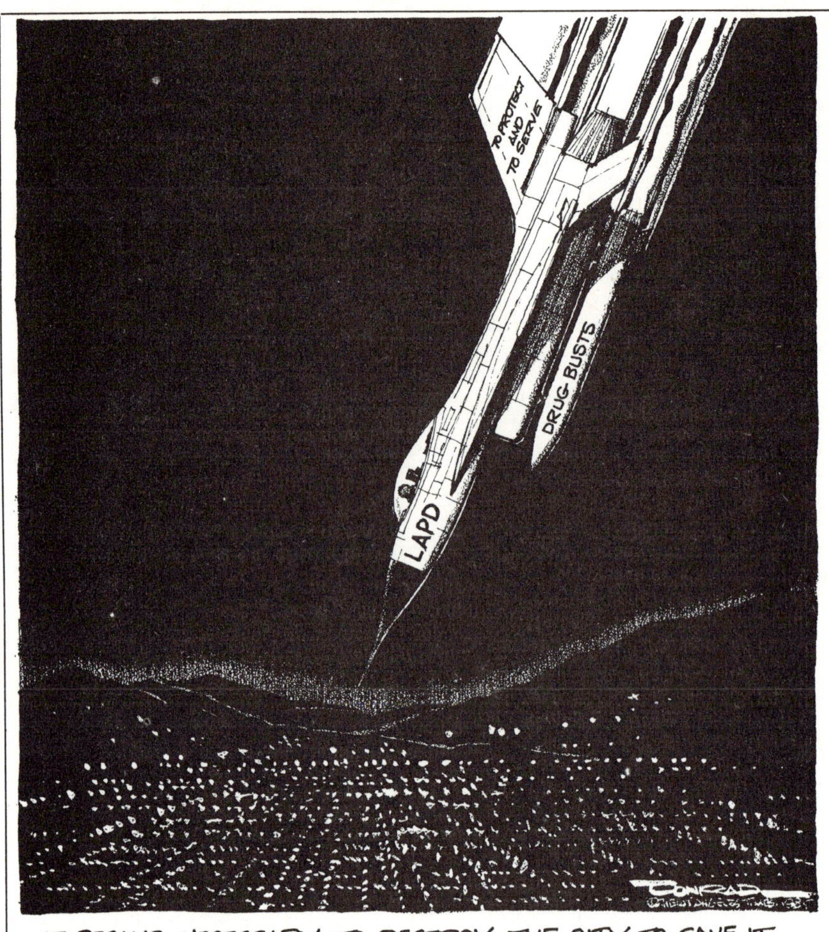

IT BECAME NECESSARY TO DESTROY THE CITY TO SAVE IT.

The Washington Post

Washington, DC, June 10, 1985

THE WASHINGTON AREA'S war on drugs would be helped substantially by greater cooperation among the narcotics officers in our area police departments. D.C. Del. Walter E. Fauntroy and Rep. Stan Parris (R-Va.) have announced plans to seek congressional approval to create a regional group to help local police work together against drugs. There is much to be done.

Such cooperation already exists to a certain extent. The federal Drug Enforcement Administration works with area police departments in a PCP task force. The Fairfax and Arlington county police departments are, with Alexandria authorities, also involved in a Northern Virginia task force on drugs that includes the Virginia State police and authorities from more distant Virginia localities. The value of cooperation in the sharing of information and other matters was shown laste week when Howard County undercover narcotics officers made several large purchases of PCP. With the cooperation of Prince George's police and the DEA, several local arrests were made involving a nationwide PCP distribution ring.

But questions are raised by the idea of creating a regional body to combat drug trafficking. What exactly would it or should it do? How will it address the problem that arises when neighboring police departments argue over whether it is the city's drug crime that affects the suburbs, or vice versa?

There has already been some griping over a statement by Mr. Fauntroy that the suburbs are becoming the place where the PCP is being manufactured and where the heroin and cocaine are cut. Suburban police say that is wrong and that the drug criminals from the city are the problem. If the proposed regional authority does anything to still such arguments, it would be beneficial.

The narcotics officers of our local jurisdictions also have some ideas that the proposed body might focus on. In Northern Virginia, police officials say they want more federal involvement to combat drug trafficking. Specifically, they want a continuing presence of FBI agents and/or DEA agents in the Virginia suburbs. In suburban Maryland, police want legislation passed that would enable them to use the drug money they confiscate in raids to finance investigations. Montgomery County police seized $130,000 in drug raids last year, which could have been used to buy surveillance equipment and unmarked cars. Suburban police also want to see tougher sentencing in the District.

Some of this cooperation could be accomplished without legislation, but a congressionally approved body might develop uniform sentences and perhaps add needed funds to aid local police departments. A regional group that would focus on these areas is a good idea.

THE ATLANTA CONSTITUTION
Atlanta, GA, April 3, 1985

The federal government will risk the promising progress it appears to have begun making against major drug smuggling and distribution operations if it now turns its attention to individual and, often, casual users.

Yet hints of just such a unwise turn are accumulating at the highest levels of federal law enforcement. Attorney General Edwin Meese recently let on, in the standard Washington trial-balloon manner, that such a policy change might be in the offing. Now Charles Blau, head of the Organized Crime Drug Enforcement Task Force, has said that prosecution of small-time users of marijuana and other drugs should be stepped up.

Meese was quite right, of course, when he made the point that drug buys, even small and occasional ones, build up to the violence and corruption that has come to mark the big-time drug commerce. That is especially so in the case of cocaine, whose mega-profits set off wars.

But, as the saying goes, those who don't remember history are doomed to repeat it.

Law enforcement got nowhere against the drug trade in the 1960s when it was obsessed with busting users. The preoccupation allowed police departments to run up towering arrest records, while in fact accomplishing nothing but adding misery, often out of all proportion to the offense, to the lives of individuals, typically youths.

Assessments of the federal drug-enforcement program vary, but it seems fair to conclude that after a few years spent getting the act together, the effort is beginning to make a dent in some major production, supply and distribution operations — and, crucially, in the trade's money-handling. Any federal attention to small-time users necessarily would be at the cost of time and effort against the Mr. Bigs. This is one area in which the Reagan administration ought to stick to its supply-side policy.

The Birmingham News
Birmingham, AL, March 24, 1985

When officials of the federal Drug Enforcement Administration presented their 1986 budget request to Sen. Jeremiah Denton's subcommittee on security and terrorism, they asked for $345.6 million.

That amount, when compared to the vast resources available to drug traffickers and the billions of dollars to be made in the international drug trade, is like "trying to fight a forest fire with a glass of water," Denton said.

Sen. Howell Heflin, on another occasion, put it another way. "We must approach this situation as if it were a war," he said.

The senators are right. The invasion of drugs into this country is a crisis that threatens our economy, our political system, our law enforcement and our very way of life.

It is a war we must win.

Consider a few of the acts of war: Drug dealers kidnapped and killed a U.S. drug agent in Mexico. They put a price on the former DEA chief's head. After a joint U.S.-Colombian crackdown on cocaine smuggling, they exploded a bomb outside the U.S. embassy and reportedly threatened to kill one American for every Colombian extradited to the U.S. to face drug charges. They have put a bounty on DEA agents.

Consider a few of the consequences for our society: The huge sums of money generated by the drug trade are distorting the economy of south Florida. Politicians and law enforcement officials are corrupted. The cancer is spreading through all the Gulf Coast states, including Alabama. Just last week, a former FBI agent who had been assigned to spy on drug smugglers pleaded guilty to working for a smuggling ring.

Consider the threat to our national security: Denton's committee is looking into information that suggests "a strong bond has been forged between drug traffickers and terrorists," he said. Secretary of State George Shultz said earlier this month that both Cuba and Nicaragua are linked to international drug trafficking.

Those are just some of the threats posed by the business of smuggling drugs into this country. Even more tragic are the consequences, especially for our young people, of using these drugs once they arrive. Too many young lives are ruined or lost.

If we are to win this war, we must fight it on two fronts. We must dry up the supply, and we must stop the demand.

As long as Americans are willing to pay big money for drugs, someone will take the risk to bring them in. Parents have to be involved enough in their children's lives to help steer them away from drugs, and to chase the pushers from the schools and playgrounds.

At least some in Hollywood seem to be recognizing that glamorizing drugs and alcohol in movies and on television is destructive for our society, and they told a congressional panel that the entertainment world is trying to send the message that it is no longer "in" to get high.

This awakening, if that's what it is, is long overdue and should be encouraged.

Meanwhile, the government must attack the source of the drug problem. We must insist that drug-producing countries crack down on drug dealers, even if it means applying the kind of pressure diplomats are reluctant to use.

Why should we be giving aid to a country whose citizens are killing our young people? This is war, and a government that tolerates our enemies — the drug dealers — is not our friend.

Also, we must step up our own enforcement efforts, including use of the military to protect our borders. The legal safeguards that keep the military from policing our streets should not keep them from becoming involved in this war.

We must match the sophisticated arsenals of our enemies. The use of radar aircraft to patrol the Mobile Corridor, as suggested by a number of Southern senators, is one step that can be taken.

Above all, we must make a strong national commitment to bring the drug problem under control. The cost of winning the war may be high, but the cost of losing is intolerable.

el diario / la prensa
New York, NY, January 28, 1985

Combatting drugs is a noble effort; sweeping them under the rug is not. Yet that has been precisely the effect of the city's highly publicized "Operation Pressure Point" on the Lower East Side.

While many politicians have been lavish in their praise, local residents and community leaders who witnessed the sweep, in which hundreds of dealers were arrested, point out that the dramatic round-ups simply forced the dealers from one part of the neighborhood to another, in the process producing several undesirable changes in the way they conduct their business.

Because of the heavy police presence during the first weeks of the operation, many dealers moved their operations off the street and into apartment buildings, where they now harass and intimidate tenants, including families with young children who are easy prey for drugs. Police Commissioner Ward admits that the city has little recourse once the dealers are indoors, which means that the drug trade may now actually be in a better position than it was before.

The real beneficiaries of the much praised operation would appear to be the landlords and real estate brokers who now feel free to charge upwards of $1000 a month for apartments east of Avenue B, which affluent young whites once viewed as the dividing line between this life and the beyond. Sadly, instead of helping to eradicate the use of drugs in a community whose life blood has been sucked away by them, Operation Pressure Point has served to herald the city's intent to "gentrify" a primarily Hispanic neighborhood and to ignore the needs of those who already live there.

Drug addiction is an illness, not a crime. It often leads to crime, but that is very different. And to treat the crime without treating the underlying illness, as Operation Pressure Point tried to do, creates a lot of expectations that can not be fulfilled. There is great concern in this country about the cost in lives and productivity of such preventable diseases as cancer, strokes and heart attacks. Police raids are not an answer to those diseases; they will be just as futile with the problem of drugs. No, the struggle to loose the grip of addiction does not belong on the streets. The real pressure point lies deep within the heart of this society which, as Representative Charles Rangel has long argued, is still far too willing to sedate vast stretches of its population.

Crime Panel Urges Testing of Government Employees

The President's Commission on Organized Crime March 3, 1986 issued a report on the federal government's effort against illegal narcotics. The paper was the first in a series on the fight against organized crime. Drug trafficking, the paper said, was "the most serious problem presented by organized crime in this country." The panel said narcotics dealings accounted for 40% of United States mob activity and each year generated illegal profits of $110 billion. The commission contended that the fight against drugs had to target users as well as traffickers. Accordingly, it called for "suitable testing programs" to monitor federal employees and also recommended that state governments and private companies adopt such programs. Those suggestions soon enbroiled the commission in controversy.

Attorney General Edwin Meese 3rd March 4 defended as legal the crime panel's idea of testing federal employees and screening prospective employers for drug use. The American Civil Liberties Union March 3 had attacked the plan as an invasion of privacy. A spokesman for the American Federation of Government Employees, representing about 700,000 federal workers, said: "We oppose the witch-hunt mentality. Wholesale drug testing, we believe, would violate the Fourth Amendment." Meese told reporters the same day that employee drug testing could constitutionally be considered an invasion of privacy "because it's something the employee consents to as a condition of employment. Meese said drug testing to screen federal job applicants would in many cases be "a very reasonable step." But he cautioned that the screening's usefulness had to be weighed against its "impact [on] and acceptance by employees." Proponents of all drug tests argued that even off-duty drug use cost an employer heavily on absenteeism, health benefits and diminished efficiency. Opponents said that claim had never been proven and contended as well that the commonly-used EMIT urinalysis test, developed by the Syntex Corp., was unreliable.

The Boston Herald

Boston, MA, March 7, 1986

THE President's Commission on Organized Crime has recommended wide-spread drug testing of federal employees and contractors. Despite the objections of certain misguided civil libertarians, it's a sound proposal.

As part of a wider program of education and enhanced enforcement, the commission urged mandatory testing of all federal workers, as well as employees of businesses which contract with the government. Rodney Smith, the commission's deputy director, cautioned that individuals who use drugs, regularly or occasionally, should not be "packing parachutes or building airplanes."

The panel's recommendation drew the predictable response from the American Civil Liberties Union. Such a program would be "very irresponsible" and an "unwarranted invasion of the privacy of millions of workers," an ACLU spokesman charged.

Terms like "invasion of privacy" simply are not applicable to this situation. No one has a constitutional right to government employment. If one wants to work for the federal establishment, particularly in a sensitive area, he or she must be willing to abide by necessary standards.

That we have a drug problem in this country is undeniable. There are an estimated 20 million Americans who use marijuana regularly, five to six million cocaine users, and half-a-million heroin addicts. It's probable that some of them are in the federal work force.

Of course, testing should be done sensibly. For instance, we question the need to screen the file clerk in the Department of Education or the janitor in Health and Human Services for drug use.

But those workers performing security or safety functions — among them air traffic controllers, the crews of missile silos and Border Patrol officers — may reasonably be expected to submit to such tests.

When the well-being of millions is at stake, the public interest must take precedence over privacy.

The TENNESSEAN

Nashville, TN, March 11, 1986

IT's bad enough to hear a presidential commission recommend Big Brother treatment for millions of citizens. But it's worse to hear the attorney general endorse the idea.

Early last week, the President's Commission on Organized Crime recommended that mandatory drugs tests be given to all federal workers, employees of companies with government contracts, and applicants for federal jobs. The recommendation does not just cover employees who might be naturally exposed to drugs — like the Drug Enforcement Administration, or the Federal Bureau of Investigation — but all federal jobs.

Since the commission's recommendation made no omissions, one must assume that it wants candidates for Congress, federal judges, ambassadors, and cabinet members to also undergo the testing.

The commission recommendation also encourages private corporations to do the same.

Attorney General Edwin Meese, the nation's chief defender of the Constitution, was quick to defend this recommendation. He said that by definition, the drug testing would not constitute unreasonable search, and instead, it would be something that a "person consents to for the privilege of applying for the employment." Last year, the attorney general suggested giving federal employees the "privilege" of taking a polygraph test.

Fortunately, the recommendation was not easily swallowed in all corners. Rep. Pat Schroeder, chairman of the House civil service subcommittee, called it "idiotic," and Rep. Don Edwards, D-Calif. described it as much more Russian than American. Rep. Steny Hoyer, D-Md., wondered how Secretary of State George Shultz, who said he would not take a polygraph test, would react to the notion that he take a urinalysis.

The commission logic is elusive. Yes, organized crime exists. Yes, it is tied to the illegal drug traffic. But how does a wholesale sweep, at an enormous cost, of millions of innocent Americans get to the root of this country's drug problem? And would it be worth violating the civil rights of millions of innocent public servants? Of course not — not in this country.

Granted, the commission on organized crime did not have the easiest topic. But to imply, as the commission does by its recommendation, that testing all federal employees for the use of marijuana, heroin, or cocaine is going to clean up "The Syndicate" is really stretching it. ∎

THE DENVER POST

Denver, CO, March 5, 1986

DRUG ABUSE is a real and growing danger. But the Presidential Commission on Organized Crime has gone overboard in recommending wholesale drug tests of all federal employees.

We support the commission's recommendation to step up drug-abuse prevention and treatment programs and to make expanded use of military surveillance technologies to track international drug smugglers. But besides urging wholesale drug tests for federal employees, the commission also urged private employers to use such dragnets. Finally, it recommended requiring them from companies who do business with the federal government — a category loose enough to cover most American workers.

Instead of trying to set standards for private employers, the commission would have been wiser to learn from them. Private employers generally are resisting the mass disruption and invasion of privacy which the commission's proposed dragnet would cause. But they are not taking the drug problem lightly, either.

Many private firms, including such diverse and famous names as the New York Times, IBM and General Motors, test job applicants for drug use before they are hired. Many firms also ask employees to take drug tests if the employee is involved in a work-related accident, or if a supervisor or fellow employee suspects the employee is unfit for work.

Those are reasonable standards for public and private employers alike. The only places where random checks without reasonable cause should be permitted are in super-sensitive jobs involving public safety or national security, such as air-traffic controllers, armed military personnel, CIA employees and the like.

A federal testing program modeled along these four principles would be defensible. But a mass witch hunt of federal employees in the name of depriving drug traffickers of a market would be as futile as it is insulting.

Birmingham Post-Herald

Birmingham, AL, March 8, 1986

The President's Commission on Organized Crime has recommended testing American workers for illegal narcotics as a way to reduce drug use and combat organized crime.

How many employees the commission wants tested is unclear. The panel's final report to President Reagan proposed mandatory testing of all federal workers and those who work for federal contractors, and it suggested other employers consider such programs.

After vigorous protests arose in Congress and elsewhere, commission spokesmen began to hedge, even acknowledging that the testing recommendation had not been seen by commission members before the staff inserted it in the report.

The chairman, federal appeals court Judge Irving Kaufman, said such testing should be "used very selectively" and only in "appropriate cases."

The commission was wise to backtrack. It would be serious overkill to subject all or most American workers to drug tests.

Such wholesale intrusion into the privacy of individuals probably wouldn't pass constitutional muster. But even if it did, it smacks too much of police state tactics.

The commission apparently has fallen back on drug testing because other methods have not reduced drug use or the flow of illegal narcotics into the country. It evidently believes that if jobs were on the line, drug demand would dry up.

Admittedly, the drug problem in the United States is alarming. The commission estimates 20 million Americans regularly use marijuana, about 6 million regularly use cocaine, and a half million are addicted to heroin.

Even so, we cannot accept the notion that the only way to combat illegal narcotics is to subject every American worker, or even every federal employee, to drug tests.

There are other ways, and the commission mentioned several. Among other things, it suggested easier legal access to electronic surveillance of suspected suppliers, more cooperation from the armed forces in catching drug smugglers, a reduction or elimination of foreign aid to countries from which drugs are sent to the United States, more money for educational programs to convince Americans not to use drugs, and repeal of state laws that decriminalize possession of marijuana.

Particularly galling is that law enforcement officials know who the overlords of organized crime are, as well as many of the underlings, and yet most of the criminals of the dope trade are out on the streets. When they do get hauled into court, the result too often is a slap on the wrist.

Every new president and Congress promise a "war" on drugs and crime. The "wars" have been fought haphazardly at best.

A better effort needs to be made to march the dope peddlers into jail before suggesting that 110 million workers, most of whom have done nothing wrong, be marched into drug-testing centers.

The Chattanooga Times

Chattanooga, TN, March 8, 1986

Let's agree that the use of marijuana, cocaine, heroin and other addictive drugs is a terrible thing. Illegal drugs — and some that are legal yet still abused regularly — exact a fearsome toll on society. The cost in ruined lives, crime, loss of life and the corruption of public officials is impossible to calculate. But what is it about drug trafficking that prompts the almost casual resort to measures that punish the innocent and the guilty alike, and hang the damage to constitutional liberties?

A prime example of that occurred this week with a report by the President's Commission on Organized Crime. The commission, having concluded that law enforcement agencies are failing to reduce drug trafficking in the United States, recommended a national program to require most working Americans to submit to drug testing. The fact that upwards of 30 million Americans use drugs is a serious national problem. But it's not bad enough to justify this Orwellian intrusion into the lives of others who don't.

The commission did suggest several other ways of dealing with rampant drug use in our society. It recommended stiffer penalties for those convicted of using drugs, even in small amounts. It said law enforcement agencies should have access to expanded court-ordered electronic surveillance of suspects, and called for increased federal spending on programs to persuade Americans not to use drugs.

The last proposal may seem naive in this age of reduced federal spending across the board, but the commission would finance such programs through the seizure and forfeiture of drug traffickers' assets. Federal authorities seized nearly $450 million in such assets in 1984 but by law only $20 million went to law enforcement agencies. The rest went to the general treasury. The commission recommends lifting the $20 million ceiling.

Good enough. There is undoubtedly much more that can be done to impede drug trafficking. But that can be done without trifling with the constitutional freedoms of millions of innocent men and women. Yet that could be the exact result of the commission's drug testing recommendations.

The commission proposed testing of all federal employees, and urged the federal government not to award contracts to employers that do not begin similar programs. Finally, it suggested that all private employers seriously consider testing their own employees. Why the resort to such methods? The chairman of the commission, federal appeals Judge Irving Kaufman said the body's investigation has convinced him that "law enforcement has been tested to its utmost." And he added: "But let's face it, it hasn't succeeded. So let's try something else. Let's try testing."

In other words, the crooks are winning, so let's penalize millions of Americans, the innocent and the guilty alike, by forcing them to submit to drug tests.

The apparent rationale is that widespread testing would diminish the market for illegal drugs, thereby making it unprofitable for the huge apparatus that imports and sells the substances. That's a desirable goal, but one that the commission's recommendations is unlikely to achieve — while diminishing the constitutional protections so essential to the enjoyment of liberty.

The Des Moines Register

Des Moines, IA,
March 12, 1986

A special presidential commission has declared illegal drug trafficking to be the nation's most serious organized-crime problem. So serious, in fact, that the commission proposes eliminating whole segments of the Bill of Rights to take care of it.

If the commission's recommendations were carried out, all employers could shake down their employees regularly, make them submit to blood or urine tests, perhaps, and bring drug-sniffing hounds into offices and locker rooms. And the armed forces would be pressed into the domestic battle against drug abuse.

It's no wonder the Reagan administration does some crazy things, what with such crazy proposals from commissions chosen to look into national problems.

Sure, there is a drug problem, but let's not get carried away with the cure. After all, there is a strong American tradition that one is presumed innocent until proved guilty, and that unreasonable searches are illegal. Wholesale, indiscriminate tests of employees for evidence of drug abuse are gross violations of both traditions.

If that isn't bad enough, the commission would have the military get involved in domestic law enforcement — a step the nation has thus far wisely avoided.

It's worrisome enough having the FBI around, a secretive national police force with a record of keeping a furtive eye on citizens whose "crimes" are no more than taking part in civil-rights and anti-war protests.

Having the Army prowling around the country, too — conducting office-by-office checks for illicit drugs, perhaps? — is a horrifying prospect.

Every once in a while, the Reagan administration reminds us why it's a good idea for citizens to be ever on the alert for problem-solutions that contain the seeds for the destruction of this democratic republic.

The Arizona Republic

Phoenix, AZ, March 12, 1986

A presidential commission is recommending a national program to test workers for drug use.

It is an idea born of exasperation, but one which probably will die in the courts, if it is not killed by the large financial and other costs involved.

The Commission on Organized Crime says the government should begin by testing all 700,000 federal employees, and recommends that Washington not offer federal contracts to firms which refuse to start similar testing.

The commission bases its views on the magnitude of the nation's drug problems. It estimates 20 million Americans regularly use marijuana; 5 million to 6 million are addicted to cocaine and 500,000 are on heroin.

Drug trafficking is said to account for 40 percent of the country's criminal activity.

Illegal drugs are the No. 1 menace facing the American people. The fact that the threat is constantly increasing despite stepped-up law enforcement efforts is all the more alarming.

It is understandable that any group commissioned by the president with such responsibility would react with strong countermeasures.

Yet, a program that arbitrarily forces people to prove their innocence — with no clear evidence to suggest the use of drugs or any case-by-case provision — not only is against the spirit of the law, but probably unconstitutional as well.

The commission's report is also vague. It does not explain how tests would be conducted, how the plan would be financed or the penalties for workers found using drugs. Moreover, it has been noted that current tests are not always accurate.

If such a program were implemented, the courts would be further overcrowded, and so would prisons. More probation officers and other law enforcement officials would be needed.

This is not to argue against any of that. The rising seriousness of the problem is a warning sign that such drastic measures may be needed.

However, the effects and costs of the proposal must be more carefully considered before another runaway social program is created.

There is a lot to be said about drug prevention programs — especially in education — which have not been adequately used. Also, more can be done legally, such as court-ordered electronic surveillance of suspects as well as tougher banking and tax laws.

Trite as it may sound, the plan needs more study. Yet, society is clearly sounding a distress signal in a storm. The nation can ignore the call only at its peril.

THE PLAIN DEALER

Cleveland, OH, March 9, 1986

Recognition from the federal government that drug trafficking is a major and growing problem is long overdue. The war against illicit drug-dealing that feeds millions of dollars into terrorist and organized criminal coffers is far from won.

However, the President's Commission on Organized Crime wrongly implies that enforcement cannot work when it proposes widespread drug-testing of American workers. Not only would employer testing imperil individual freedoms and rights, and violate constitutional guarantees for government workers, it would give the government another excuse to cut back on drug enforcement.

Already, Coast Guard interdiction of drugs has fallen off because routine patrols have been cut back under the budget ax. A special air-force interdiction program of the U.S. Customs Service on the Mexican border is targeted for severe cuts in the latest Reagan budget.

The administration says it has added more drug-fighting funds and struck new accords with Latin American supplier nations to fight the narcotics menace. But cutting funds for crucial sea and land border patrols seems a poor trade-off.

The surging level of the drug trade, bedeviling enforcement agents, is a tough problem but not an intractable one. It can be handled using traditional forms of law enforcement, which go after criminals and not the general public.

Stopping rental cars driven by dark-skinned drivers in their early 30s, who might weave slightly on the freeway, may yield a 25% drug-bust rate for one Florida patrolman, as was claimed recently. But that's not comforting for those who happen to fit the general racial and social description. The Fourth Amendment to the Constitution is supposed to guard against unreasonable search and seizure.

The worker search proposals are no different, just infinitely more far-reaching. In the private sector, where the Bill of Rights does not apply in employer-worker relations, drug testing is increasingly common. Only in a few places, such as San Francisco, is it outlawed. The price in lost civil liberties for the society is too high to justify the marginal returns.

The obvious law enforcement answer is a significant increase in border patrols, and stronger programs to head off illicit narcotics before they hit U.S. shores. The commission's call for an aid cutoff to nations that fail to take required steps against drug traffickers, as required under at least one congressional amendment, is warranted.

But beefing up border patrols is one thing; declaring drugs a "national security" menace and giving the U.S. armed forces a chief role in fighting trafficking is another. Although the Marines, Coast Guard and Navy now all aid in border patrols, Defense Secretary Caspar Weinberger rightly has opposed widening their role. The armed forces should have one priority—national defense.

The president's commission noted how paltry basic drug education is in the schools, and called for major new funding in that area. Media awareness campaigns can work, as the ads on liquor and drunken driving have shown. Another move, directly opposed by the commission, would be to decriminalize marijuana, which siphons off drug enforcement funds but is not—despite some studies to the contrary—the pernicious, addictive, dangerous narcotic that cocaine, heroin or the other controlled substances are.

But the best way to combat the problem is through increased public support. That support won't be forthcoming if the government accepts commission recommendations that could restrict individual freedoms.

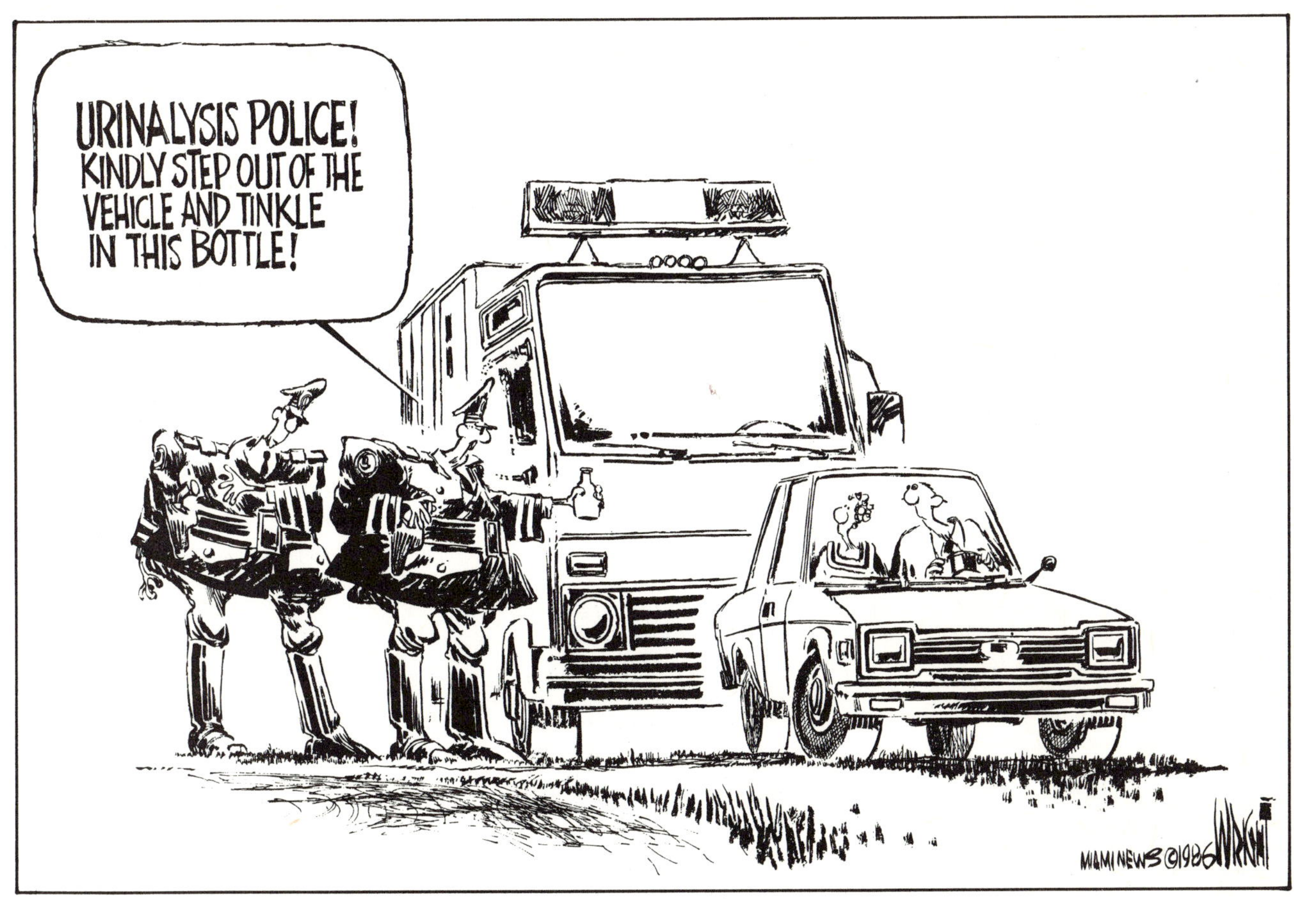

CHARLESTON EVENING POST

Charleston, SC, March 10, 1986

The President's Commission on Organized Crime justifies its call for drug tests for most of the workforce on the grounds that the U.S. drug problem has become a threat to national security. If drug abuse has reached that stage, some drastic measures are in order. There still is plenty of room to wonder, however, if the situation is so grave as to warrant turning a basic American tenet on its ear.

That's what some of the commission's recommendations would do were they implemented. The commission has urged mandatory drug-testing for all federal employees and of workers hired by contractors with federal contracts (with the threat of contract cut-offs if contractors do not adopt effective screening programs). It has urged that state and local governments, as well as private businesses, require workers to submit to periodic tests for illegal drugs. In effect, such testing would require workers to prove their innocence, and that's not the way the American system is supposed to work. Tradition holds that innocence is presumed until guilt is proved in a court of law.

The president of the American Federation of Government Employees contends that mandatory testing for drug use "is the equivalent to illegal search and seizure" — a violation of a constitutional right. That is not much of an exaggeration, if indeed it is any exaggeration at all. "Probable cause" should figure prominently in any plan for drug tests for employees, in government or private sector.

Certainly a case can be made for drug tests for those in sensitive or high-risk jobs (in government and out). Certainly a case can be made for stiff employment regulations that provide for the discharge of any employee who shows up for work under the influence of drugs. And certainly a case can be made for employer assistance in establishing drug counseling and rehabilitation services for workers. But all other possible drug countermeasures should be considered — and tried — before government or employer reports to countermeasures that impinge on citizen liberties.

The Houston Post

Houston, TX, March 6, 1986

Big Brother is knocking at the door a couple of years behind schedule, but he certainly seems to want in. For proof, look no further than Monday's proposal by the President's Commission on Organized Crime. It urges that most of the working U.S. population be tested for drug use. The idea is so flawed, it is hardly surprising that on Tuesday the panel's chairman tried to backpedal, saying against all evidence that widespread testing wasn't intended.

If nothing else, it is a sacred tenet of our legal system that a person is innocent until proven guilty. Besides, under the Constitution's Fourth and Fifth Amendments, people are protected against unreasonable searches and seizures, and are guaranteed due process of law. The commission's major recommendations, if followed, would knock these cornerstones of the law asunder.

Too, the proposal is so unworkable that it could be viewed as a joke, were not the civil-liberties implications so abhorrent. The laboratory procedures are of questionable accuracy. Besides, the report makes no mention of who would underwrite such a massive testing program, or how we would keep the nation's workplace running if all people possessing small amounts of drugs were prosecuted to the full extent of the law. Forget, for a moment, whether such prosecution is desirable in theory: In the late 1960s and early '70s we tried this, and our judicial and law enforcement systems nearly collapsed under the burden. There is no reason to believe a new effort would yield a different result.

If the federal government's estimate is accurate, 20 million Americans — one out of 12 among us — regularly use marijuana. How can anyone suppose we could cope administratively with that sort of convict population, whether in jail or on probation?

Are drugs in the workplace desirable? Certainly not, and one might add that that includes alcohol, our most abused drug. Will we ever eliminate the abuse of these substances? Again, certainly not — human nature being what it is.

But what hope there is for trimming drug use may lie in a couple of lesser facets of the panel's findings. One urges curtailing aid to foreign nations that do not reduce their narcotics crops. Another is increased public education, something that first lady Nancy Reagan seems to understand already without benefit of any study.

We hope that when the report's sections on the broader aspects of organized crime emerge, they will prove more helpful. The part that came out Monday was shockingly unoriginal. With minor exceptions, it was a waste of time and taxpayers' money.

Reagan Declares National War on Drugs

President Ronald Reagan August 4, 1986 declared a "national mobilization" against illegal drugs, a problem that in the past few months had become a top national concern. In a bow to his wife's highly publicized campaign against drug abuse, Reagan said that "starting today, Nancy's crusade to deprive drug peddlers and suppliers their customers becomes America's crusade." The President listed goals ranging from stopping smugglers to treating abusers, but he laid most emphasis on using both government and private groups "to pressure the user at school and in the workplace to straighten up, get clean." Reagan offered no details on how he would accomplish his goals or how much money it would take. Questioned by reporters, he answered that details would wait until "the near future. This is chapter one," the President said, "more to come."

Republican legislators were reportedly pressing the White House to come up with detailed legislation before the Democrats could seize the drug issue for the fall elections. But the Administration was said to have already spent weeks debating the matter intensely. Newspaper accounts said White House Chief of Staff Donald Regan wanted a bill ready for quick unveiling. Attorney General Edwin Meese 3rd was said to be against the idea.

Many drug-abuse experts and clinics were reported to be skeptical of the chances that substantial concrete action would follow Reagan's announcement. Cutbacks in the federal budget under his administration were widely blamed for the overburdening of treatment centers.

One move Reagan set out in his announcement was mandatory drug testing of federal employees who held sensitive posts in law enforcement, national security, safety and public health. He said mandatory testing was justified in any job "where employees have the health and the safety of others in their hands," and he urged that "voluntary" testing also be considered outside the government. To show the way, Reagan underwent urinalysis Aug. 9. The idea of the President submitting to urinalysis sparked some queasy humor around the capital such as a *Washington Post* headline heralding "Jar Wars."

SYRACUSE HERALD-JOURNAL

Syracuse, NY, August 5, 1986

President Reagan's proposal that members of his Cabinet be tested for drug use ranks right up there with Sen. Alfonse D'Amato's much-publicized drug "buy" in New York City.

In other words, it promises to be a huge public relations spectacle with no meaning whatsoever. Set an example? What does he take us for? Does the president really believe that if this squeaky-clean collection of stuffed shirts allows their blood to be tested for the presence of foreign materials (we'll guarantee they won't do you-know-what in a bottle), that the dealers are going to close down operations in the Bronx?

And that malarkey about the death sentence for dealing drugs. Now seriously, folks. Even if he could get a majority of Americans to accept the death penalty for anything (for all we know, maybe he could), we New Yorkers could give him an earful about how tough penalties — remember the Rockefeller drug laws? — take drugs, druggies and dealers off the streets.

Think about it for a minute: If you're a cop and you catch some small-time dealer — for instance those two Australians who were hanged in Malaysia a couple of weeks ago for possession of a couple of ounces — would you think twice about making the bust, knowing he was going to get the chair?

We're not saying anybody should go easy on drugs and dealing, particularly on those who are raking in millions at the top end of the delivery system, but we seriously question whether tougher laws are more appropriate than proper enforcement of the laws we have now and better interdiction of the drug supplies coming into this country.

You know, the president talks a good game against drugs, and he seems prepared to go for the headline-grabbers, such as testing his Cabinet — even sending troops to Bolivia (a move we applauded, by the way, as better than no action at all) — but he has not shown any inclination to beef up the U.S. Drug Enforcement Agency, the federal agency with the authority and responsibility to stop drugs from coming across our borders.

In fact, he has done just the opposite; he has cut the DEA's funding to the point where it hasn't a prayer of doing the job entrusted to it. Does that sound like a president with a determination to put an end to the drug problem in this country? To us, it doesn't.

It sounds more like a politician who is willing to turn the spotlight on glamorous, perhaps even politically popular moves, while at the same time gutting the front-line agency, the agency that does the work while he grabs the headlines with meaningless gestures.

THE ARIZONA REPUBLIC

Phoenix, AZ, August 15, 1986

WHETHER the highly publicized urine tests of President Reagan, Vice President Bush and 78 White House aides are classified as a reaction or an impetus to public awareness about drug abuse, the message is the same: Drug abuse is a serious threat to the well-being of our nation.

It is estimated that 50 million Americans have experimented with illegal drugs of some form. Twenty million Americans reportedly use marijuana regularly; 5 million to 6 million use cocaine; and a half-million are addicted to heroin. Drug users reportedly commit at least 40 percent of the nation's crimes.

Public outrage over drug use is rising along with the crime rate. According to a recent *Newsweek* poll, more than two-thirds of Americans favor prosecution for possession of even small amounts of marijuana compared with 43 percent just six years ago. The poll also found support for periodic screening.

Drug testing is but one part — albeit a highly controversial one — in the overall battle plan, both public and private, for the war on drugs. Substance testing already is a fact of life in certain private industries, and support is gaining for the mandatory testing of those in "sensitive" occupations — airline pilots, air traffic controllers, police officers, for example.

But some questions remain — not the least of which concerns the cost of administering such a comprehensive program — about drug testing on a widespread scale, including the reliability, confidentiality and constitutionality of such tests. Critical public policy answers must be forthcoming before such testing can be justified on any across-the-board basis.

There is no quick-fix or simple, single treatment for America's drug epidemic. Drug testing, education, treatment, interdiction of sources, control of supply and vigorous prosecution of law violators are but individual components of an overall strategy that may lead to an acceptable remission, if not a cure.

The real answer to the drug abuse problem may be forthcoming only when the public attitude shifts with the equal force of social condemnation against both users and suppliers. Encouragingly, there are signs that shift already is under way.

The Boston Herald

Boston, MA, August 10, 1986

EVEN the raw statistics are alarming. According to federal figures, there are some 5 million regular cocaine users in this country and as many as 24 million Americans have tried the stuff.

Some 30 percent of all college students have tried cocaine and 42 percent admit to having tried marijuana.

Another 500,000 Americans are heroin addicts.

It's a problem for schools, right down to the grade school level. It's a problem in the workplace — whether that be the assembly line or Silicon Valley or Wall Street. It's a problem in the sports world, which has lost too many of its promising young stars, and in the entertainment world, where too many careers and lives have been put on the line by drug abuse.

And now there's the growing realization that drug raids, even those that hit at the coca crop itself, only address half the problem — the supply side — but never really touch the other half — the demand side.

There's no doubt about the good intentions which drive both the White House and Capitol Hill in their truly national effort to combat the menace which narcotics have become to all Americans.

Our own war, the Alliance Against Drugs, was declared by Gov. Michael Dukakis some 20 months ago — and since that time upwards of 220 cities and towns have *voluntarily* enlisted in it.

The Alliance brings parents, police, educators, athletes, the media, medical personnel, other professions, and young people together in a cooperative effort to cut the trafficking in dope by reducing the demand for it. The federal Drug Enforcement Administration has become sufficiently impressed by the concept to offer to spread information about it to other states trying to launch their own attack on drugs. The DEA doesn't back dud ideas.

That's not to say the war has been won here. Far from it. Only two years ago a survey of 5,000 high school students found that 90 percent had taken drugs and/or liquor; 60 percent had used hard drugs; and 30 percent started using them when they were 12 — or younger. The same survey also showed that the traffic cut across all levels and neighborhoods of society; its victims came from cities and suburbs alike, from wealthy families as well as poor ones, from private as well as public schools.

But we are making progress. One reason for that has been the acceptance by the state of what the kids told them — that if young people were to be saved from drugs they had to be taught about its dangers in every grade from kindergarten on. Waiting until high school to educate them was too late — because by that time most of them had already flirted with narcotics and many had become hooked.

Out of all this has developed a statewide effort in which The Herald, WBZ-TV, and the Bank of Boston have enlisted as working partners with those who drafted and/or joined the Alliance. Briefly, the Alliance is doing these five things in cities and towns which volunteer to be part of it:

● Establishing a K through 12 anti-drug curriculum in the schools.

● Re-evaluating school discipline codes to deal effectively with students who use drugs and/or liquor, or who supply them to their classmates.

● Influencing local superintendents of schools and police chiefs to sign written memos of understanding spelling out exactly what each must do in proceeding against offenders. (This is intended to head off possible "turf wars" between educators and police.)

● Identifying treatment programs and centers in each city or town where kids who need help can receive it without difficulty or delay.

● Setting up community advisory groups of adults and youths alike, as well as all the professions cited above, in all communities to guide the Alliance and help reach its goals.

All this is aimed at teaching our children from their earliest years not only about the danger of drugs but the wisdom and necessity of avoiding them throughout their lives. That should, and we believe will, cut the demand for drugs. We believe all this is excellent, and are proud to be part of it. We urge other private interests and businesses to enlist in it too, in whatever way they can assist it most. And we wholeheartedly endorse its adoption by other states.

This war can't be fought to a stalemate; it's got to be waged by all until a complete and lasting victory is achieved. That will take a while, to be sure. But it's worth every ounce of sweat, effort, persistence, and dedication we possess. Enlist in it, please.

Edmonton Journal

Edmonton, Alta., August 7, 1986

Ronald Reagan has finally shifted the emphasis on his war on drugs from the supplier to the user, where it belongs.

But just how he plans to purge the U.S. of this "deeply disruptive and corrosive evil" is not clear.

In fact, Reagan's call for a major offensive against drug abuse is long on rhetoric and short on detail. Apart from his predilection for nationwide mandatory drug testing — a scary proposal that conjures up Orwellian nightmares — Reagan is vague on the programs and financing needed to fight drugs such as heroin, cocaine and crack.

His challenge is to address the reasons Americans take drugs; to treat the problem and not just the symptom.

That's not an easy task. Drug abuse affects every segment of society — from the unemployed, poverty-stricken junkie to the trendy yuppie. One person may take drugs to escape the reality of poverty; another for entertainment. Yet drug addiction has a way of making all its victims equal.

The U.S. government has a role to play in promoting public awareness and discussion of the dangers of drug abuse. But a lasting solution lies in changing society's attitudes, in dispelling the atmosphere of "public acquiescence" which Reagan says sustains drug abuse.

Charleston Evening Post

Charleston, SC, August 12, 1986

Secretary of State George Shultz said last year he would quit his job rather than take a government lie-detector test. Fortunately, it never came to that. But Mr. Shultz has agreed to participate in a voluntary White House drug program which involves a urinalysis. His sensibilities aren't as offended. Neither are ours.

A spokesman for Mr. Shultz explained that the secretary views drug testing as a much more reliable scientific tool than a lie-detector. What's more, the spokesman noted, the process is relatively non-intrusive. Let's even concede the possibility that mistakes will be made. The results will be kept confidential. Certainly there will be an opportunity to check and double-check. The goal is to provide help, not to send staffers packing.

The skeptics doubtless will point to a few well-publicized horror stories from the military side as evidence of how the test results can be skewed. We'll agree a case doubtless can be made for the proposition that there is no perfect system. But not even the most ardent civil libertarians would argue that the occasional error justifies abandoning all drug detection programs. There seems to be a consensus that those in certain critical jobs — including private, government-regulated industries such as the airlines — have to expect checks on whether they are operating with impaired judgment.

But more and more private employers — newspapers included — have become alarmed by the danger posed by drug-using employees. More and more are making drug-free test results a condition of employment. Certainly both private and public employers have every right to establish such a condition as long as it is administered uniformly. The tougher question is how and when to require tests of employees who were hired before such programs were initiated.

There was a time when testing of all employees wasn't even worth considering. The number of abusers simply didn't justify unnecessarily irritating good employees and kicking up the privacy issue. But no more. Drugs are being used in grade schools and on Wall Street. The odds are that if society had taken a tougher stand sooner, or a president had gotten at the head of the parade earlier, there'd be less need for such drastic steps now.

Military schools are tough on drugs not only because of their disciplined regimen but because an officer with a drug problem isn't going to escape detection long. Liberal arts colleges doubtless would be far less permissive on the subject if their graduates increasingly failed to pass the drug-free entrance tests in the marketplace.

Detroit Free Press

Detroit, MI,
August 31, 1986

AS IMPORTANT as it is to reduce the demand for illegal drugs and provide more treatment programs for abusers, those steps are only part of the solution to the drug problem in this country — which, if not growing, at least now is receiving the attention it always merited.

Early headline-grabbing presidential initiatives, such as drug testing of federal workers, suggested that Mr. Reagan's new war on drugs was too narrowly focused. Such a war will have to be fought simultaneously on several fronts; the flow of illicit drugs will have to be reduced if the war is ever to be won.

Attorney General Edwin Meese's announcement that the United States and Mexico would co-operate in a drug interdiction effort along the border is a hopeful sign. But the recent arrest and torture of a U.S. narcotics agent in Mexico shows very clearly that the bulk of the burden will be the United States' for the foreseeable future.

Stepped-up law-enforcement efforts won't come cheaply. They already cost nearly $1.8 billion, and the Congress, the president and the American people must be willing to foot a still higher bill to put the drug traffickers out of business.

Political bickering also must not be allowed to defeat the federal government's war on drugs. About 80 pieces of drug-related legislation are now pending on Capitol Hill, and a partisan battle is shaping up over how much money to devote to all aspects — enforcement, education, treatment, research — of the expanded federal anti-drug program.

The president's approach — which is being called a war of words by some — is to devote relatively little new money. House Democrats, on the other hand, are at work on a plan that may involve up to $3 billion.

In an era of desire for deficit reduction, the Democrats' figures seem unrealistically steep. But growing public commitment to eradicating what the president himself has called a "corrosive evil" that is "victimizing us all" suggests that a middle course must be found.

ST. LOUIS POST-DISPATCH

St. Louis, MO, August 20, 1986

"Just say no," is President Reagan's answer to those tempted to abuse drugs. The advice is cheap, harmless and probably ineffective. But some other anti-drug comments from the president are not nearly as harmless and are catching on in a disturbing way. In Hawkins, Texas, for instance, the school district is requiring that students in grades six through 12 pass drug tests this fall before being allowed to sing in the school chorus, join the marching band or play varsity football.

The school's superintendent, Coleman Stanfield, reports that 325 students have decided to participate in these school activities and will be required to submit urine samples that will be tested for 19 drugs, including cocaine, marijuana, steroids and amphetamines. "This isn't punishment," the superintendent says. "We're just trying to give the students another reason to say no to drugs."

Punishment or not, the action has frightening overtones of police-state practices that have no place in a society where a presumption of innocence is a cherished freedom. Unfortunately, this scare approach got its start when Mr. Reagan submitted to a drug test and acted as if his example was a magic wand that would turn the nation into a "drug-free" society.

Hawkins school officials promise that no student will be suspended on the basis of test results. But how long will the test results be kept in a student's file, and what happens in the event law enforcement officials subpoena the information to find out which students are drug users?

Parents should demand that the school board and school officials in Hawkins "just say no" to Mr. Reagan's quick fix or to other cheap solutions to a problem that offers no easy answers and is likely to be costly to solve.

The San Diego Union

San Diego, CA, August 11, 1986

"It's like a pharmacy, with 24-hour service. Everybody comes here to buy," says recreation supervisor Neal Petties about Mountain View Park. Ben Tukufu of the San Diego Street Youth Program says that selling, in a reference to the corner convenience store, "is in the 7-Eleven mode in the neighborhood." Horribly, the business that both men refer to is drug traffic.

Most Americans are aware that endemic drug use has become a national scourge. The problem's magnitude is to be seen in the recent sweep by U.S. soldiers into Bolivian jungles and in the deaths of star athletes Len Bias and Don Rogers. Yet, even with the immense amount of publicity, energy, and resources directed against drug trafficking, drugs have never been more available or lower priced. As Messrs. Petties and Tukufu warn, one need not look beyond our community to realize this.

Part of the problem stems from a fundamental mistake in law-enforcement strategies. Traditionally, big drug dealers have been targeted in an effort to cut off and isolate the street-corner sellers. But experience is showing that fighting the supply source is a losing strategy. Moreover, it has worked at cross-purposes with another sad fact of drug activity — drug-related crime.

Imagine, for instance, that strenuous law-enforcement efforts result in confiscation of 40 percent of the drugs entering the country. What does this accomplish? It means the price of drugs on the street will rise. And so will crime as addicts are forced to steal more to pay for their habit. Worse, by focusing much of their efforts on major drug dealers, law-enforcement officials have unintentionally but effectively decriminalized the use of drugs.

Equally discouraging is that a vast amount of drugs are produced inside the United States. California Attorney General John Van de Kamp asserts, for example, that there are about 800 clandestine drug labs in California and that the state "is drowning in homemade drugs."

Getting at the drug source is only half of this intractable problem. That's why it's time go after demand, the other half of the equation. As U.S. Attorney Peter Nunez correctly points out, "The public must be reacquainted with the idea that drug use is against the law." His office is developing a program with this in mind. Presently, those persons at the border who are carrying small amounts of narcotics are fined and their drugs confiscated. The U.S. Attorney's office wants to end this administrative slap-on-the-hand and, with the help of U.S. Customs and the Drug Enforcement Agency, aggressively prosecute these cases.

A key component of this plan involves confiscation of a suspect's car. The federal forfeiture statute allows seizure of an automobile if it is used in the purchase, sale, transportation, or concealment of cocaine. Automobile forfeiture has been a valuable tool for narcotics enforcement in New York City and should be particularly effective in the highly mobile society of Southern California.

Another law-enforcement innovation that targets the drug user is the "Eleven Five Fifty" program established by the National City Police Department. Patrol officers look for heroin addicts, who commit an inordinate amount of crime to feed their more than $100-a-day habit. If a suspect is under the influence of heroin, he is arrested, and if convicted, receives a mandatory 90-day sentence. Such punishment has produced remarkable results. There was a 33 percent reduction in burglaries and robberies following the program's introduction in 1984. Chief Wayne Fowler asserts the program is still doing well.

Given drug manufacturing techniques and the huge profit in trafficking, there will never be an end to the supply of drugs. But confiscation and arrest send the message to drug users that their habits — which are sapping the moral and physical vigor of America — will no longer be tolerated.

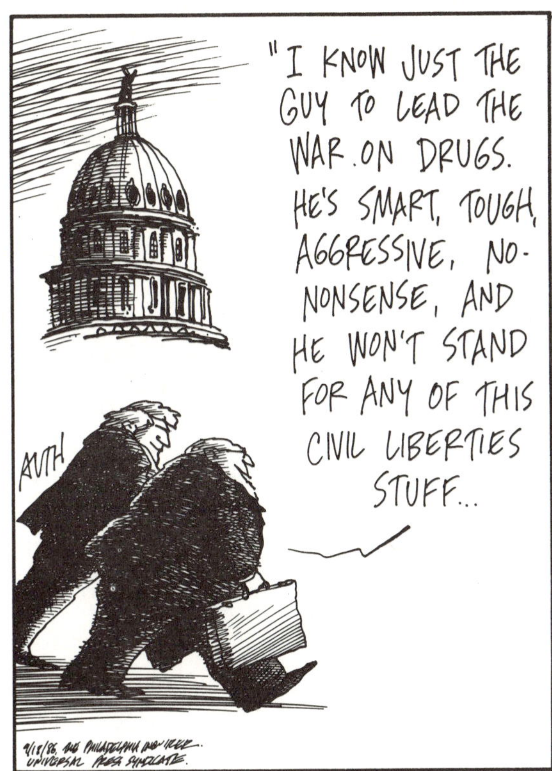

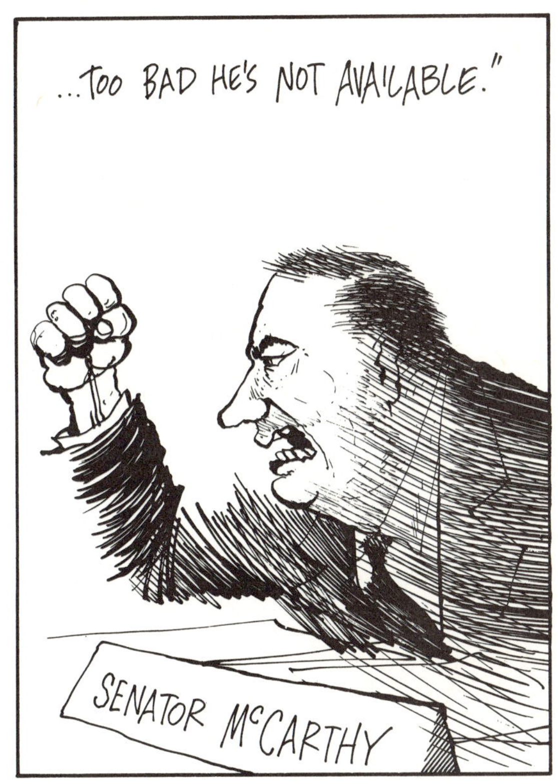

CHARLESTON EVENING POST
Charleston, SC, August 28, 1986

This country's campaign against drugs is becoming more politicized. As a consequence, it might be wise to take with a grain of salt what a Democratic congressman and a New York City police official told governors recently convened at Hilton Head. It would be unwise, however, to dismiss their comments out of hand.

Rep. Glenn English of Oklahoma, chairman of a government operations subcommittee, said the war on drugs is going badly because the Reagan administration is not committing the resources necessary to turn the tide of battle. Administration budget cuts, Rep. English said, have led to a shortage of personnel and equipment, including aircraft and fast boats needed to detect and intercept smugglers. Noting that 60 percent of the cocaine shipped to this country arrives by air, he said, "We have only two detector aircraft to patrol the border in the Southwest. You could fly an aircraft as big as this hotel across that border and not be detected."

Francis C. Hall, commander of the New York Police Department's narcotics division, labeled federal efforts to interdict drug shipments a complete failure. "In my 33 years of police work," he said, "I've never seen anything like what I'm seeing on the streets of New York right now. They're selling cocaine in front of the cardinal's house on Fifth Avenue."

That sort of talk might fit into the same category of "rhetoric" that Rep. English accuses the administration of engaging in. If even some of the talk is accurate, however, it suggests that stemming the flow of narcotics into this country is just as difficult — or more difficult — as ever. It suggests, too, that more attention should be given to other targets, such as reducing the demand for drugs. In drug trafficking, as in legal activities in the marketplace, demand dictates supply.

Reducing demand wouldn't be easy, either. It would have its costs, too. It would require a massive public education campaign on the dangers of drugs. It would require cooperative efforts of schools, churches, anti-drug agencies and the media — especially television. In the end, discouraging demands by changing attitudes could be less costly than beefing up interception efforts, and as effective.

Sunday News Journal
Wilmington, DE, July 13, 1986

NANCY REAGAN made fighting drug abuse her major cause from the day she and her husband moved into the White House. As Mrs. Reagan points out in the Sunday Forum on the opposite page, some successes have been scored.

But they are overshadowed by new and growing problems, primarily lower price and greater availability of cocaine. Nationally, emergency room admissions due to cocaine-related problems have doubled in the last three years and deaths from cocaine-complications have tripled since 1983.

Delaware is not immune to drug-related problems. Children as young as 15 are in residential alcoholism treatment programs. A 12-bed residential treatment program for those addicted to drugs other than alcohol has a waiting list of 30.

Mrs. Reagan is right. American society as a whole must gear up to prove its intolerance of drug abuse. Families, schools, religious organizations, employers, professional organizations — everyone — must join in that effort.

Just as a parent immediately punishes a child who crosses a street without looking, so parents must exert discipline at the first sign of drug abuse. Schools must not tolerate drug use; employers have to intervene as soon as a problem is detected. At the same time, there must be community resources to help the beginning abuser stop before a habit is formed.

The only sure-fire cure for drug abuse is prevention — meaning not to get involved in drug use. Next best, is to intervene before a habit is formed. After that, treatments are lengthy, costly and not necessarily successful.

Lack of stiff and swift punishment for drug dealers is a problem.

To date, there has been more concern about protecting the civil rights of the abuser than protecting the abused, meaning those lured into drugs, family members of abusers and victims of crimes committed by abusers. The challenge to Americans is how to channel the full force of the laws against drug abusers without doing permanent damage to civil rights.

Chicago Tribune

Chicago, IL, August 7, 1986

The multibillion-dollar traffic in drugs has become a hot topic for Congress and the Reagan administration. This being an election year, it may be that their chief concern is how to get the most votes out of the issue. Still, whatever triggered it, this sudden interest is welcome if it improves the chances for action.

President Reagan unveiled a dramatic program this week for a "drug-free America." Its six points include moves to eliminate drug use from all federal agencies and pressure on federal contractors to follow suit; tougher enforcement of drug laws on high school and college campuses, along with expanded education programs; continuing military and other action against drugs in coordination with foreign governments; and "prompt and severe punishment for drug peddlers, the big guys and the little guys." Mr. Reagan even has mentioned a death penalty for drug pushers; as he told an interviewer, "I know they deserve it."

Even before this, leaders of both parties are scrambling to be identified with antidrug legislation. Republicans in the House and Democrats in the Senate have set up their own "task forces" to investigate drugs. House Speaker Thomas O'Neill and his majority leader, Rep. Jim Wright of Texas, have announced a "bipartisan" effort to fight drug abuse, though their Republican colleagues suspect it will be bipartisan in the Democrats' favor.

The congressional flurry apparently was set off by a poll showing that drug abuse is an intense public concern, second only to the deficit. Congress' reaction is welcome; the danger is that members will see the drug menace as a "safe" campaign plank rather than an urgent reality.

Hard drug use is a plague—an epidemic whose victims destroy their lives. Regardless of how soon they die, addicts leave themselves little to live for beyond the next fix. They are pretty well neutralized as citizens and human beings with skills, talents, potentialities; their lives are trapped in a cramped cycle of chemical need and gratification.

Mr. Reagan's talk about a death penalty for pushers is hyperbole, of course. But drug pushers are such dangerous characters that they deserve almost any punishment society is willing to give them.

Compared to these criminals, the vulture is an admirable creature; it feeds only on things already dead. The pusher feeds on ruined lives, and the more lives he ruins, the wealthier he gets. An effective penalty for drug pushing must be heavy enough to outweigh its enormous profits.

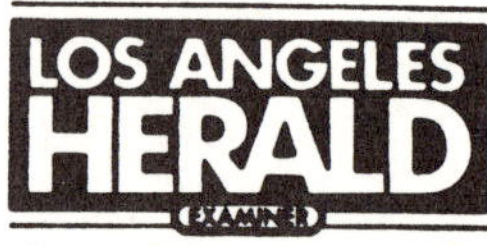

Los Angeles, CA, August 6, 1986

The flourish with which President Reagan this week called for a "national mobilization" against narcotics abuse couldn't hide the fact that he doesn't really know how to fight the drug war or how to pay for such a full-scale effort.

The president's plan includes a call for a crackdown on the drug trade. But the feds already spend $1.8 billion annually 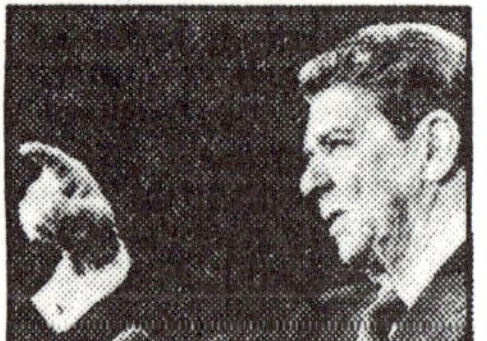 trying to stem the sale of narcotics, and with the current budget constraints, the administration isn't likely to come up with funding for a more aggressive attack.

Likewise, Reagan proposed increasing the amount of available drug treatment programs, despite his budget policy that has reduced spending for treatment and research from $260 million a year to $60 million.

Perhaps the president will be able to marshal the will to reverse that trend. Otherwise, his anti-drug progam doesn't seem to offer much beyond tactics that have already been proposed, and found lacking.

For example, he calls for testing, which, we've pointed out before, invades people's privacy, is often unreliable and could force people to use other legal drugs if it succeeds in deterring them from narcotics.

Reagan also suggests more education, which is indeed an important tool to discourage drug use. The request of 338 House members yesterday that the TV networks use their stars to discourage drug use is a good move, but the messages have to offer honest cautions.

Unfortunately, the core of the administration's efforts is Nancy Reagan's high-profile project that serves up scare-stories. The horrors of crack, heroin and other drugs are increasingly well-known. But trying to frighten people away from marijuana, for instance, by claiming it always leads to heroin use undermines the first lady's credibility.

This country will never totally eliminate drug use. But it can do a better job of dealing with the problem by providing adequate treatment facilities for abusers and offering legitimate warnings about drugs.

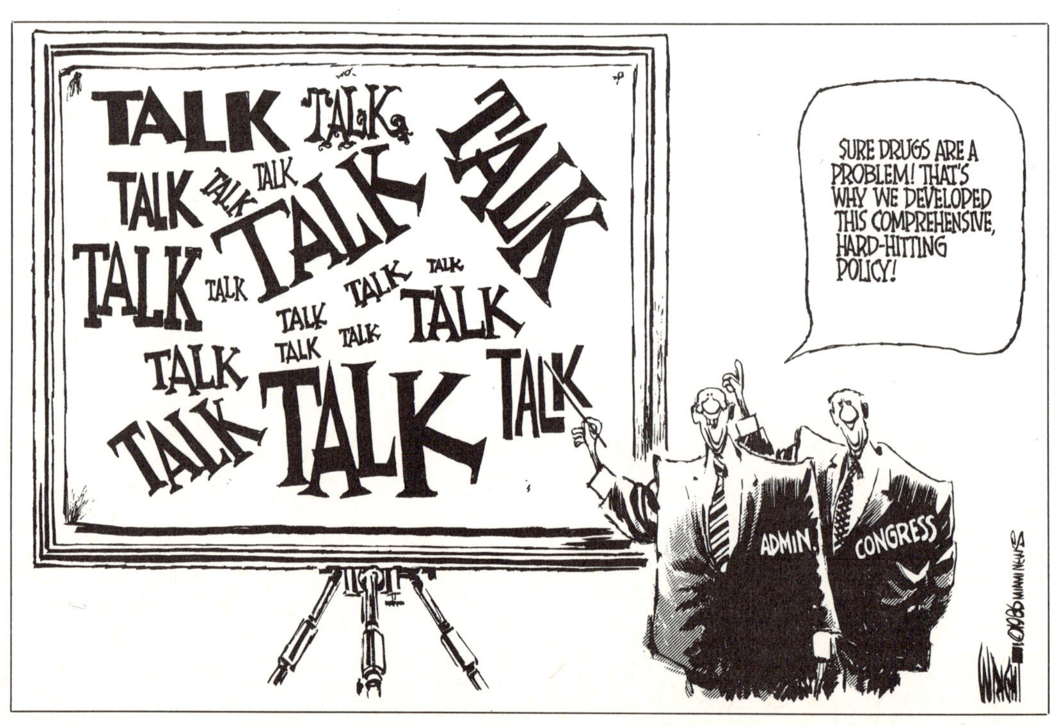

Chicago Defender
Chicago, IL, May 27, 1986

America can win the war against drugs. It is a tough battle, but we can beat narcotics.

The Just Say No to Drugs (JSND) campaign, which recently culminated in a highly successful week of promotions, rallies and marches and are prime examples of how our people can unite and positively confront a common enemy.

In this vein, President and Nancy Reagan deserve credit for their highly visible and enduring attacks on illicit drug use. Mrs. Reagan has been on a minor crusade against dope, and her statements have alerted many individuals about the pitfalls of drug use.

This gets us to the reason why JSND and The National Federation of Parents (NFP, who are promoting drug-free proms) are so important. Leaders and volunteers of the organizations share information about how narcotics depress, maim and kill individuals and try to convince people that a non-drug life is both possible and preferable.

Mrs. Reagan understands the devastation dope causes. It, therefore, pleased us when Mrs. Reagan asked approximately 2,000 Washington D.C. students, who were visiting the White House, "What should you do when someone offers you drugs?" and the kids shouted back "Just say no!"

The ideology of just saying no is very important because the great majority of drug users were not forced to try them. Most of them got into drugs through: peer pressure; a desire to be cool, relaxed or laid back; a wish to get instantaneous happiness; to avoid depression; to get quick kicks for avoiding boredom; and a number of other reasons.

Also, thousands of Americans use drugs as a result of the tensions and general day-to-day experiences they faced during the Vietnam War.

So most individivuals have a choice about whether they will use drugs. We realize that the choice for many will not be an easy one. Peer pressure is tough on a youngster but drug abuse is tougher.

The JSND and MFP campaigns are educating and sensitizing thousands across America. Such efforts are desperately needed because too many persons, young and old, get involved in narcotic use through a bizarre combination of curiosity and ignorance. Many of them don't understand that drugs, like quicksand, look harmless, but can sink a person before he or she realizes it.

These simple-sounding, intensely executed and potentially effective efforts of the JSND, NFP, and other drug fighters throughout the country, illustrate that mainstream America is choosing to stem the tide caused by the ocean of narcotics currently in use. People are becoming more aware that they can drown in the flowing filth.

Therefore, we must get to the student's minds before the pushers do. In cooperation with JSND, the people in Boise, Idaho for example, are trying to do just that. To educate youngsters on drug abuse there, adults showed them a rattlesnake and told them that narcotics use was like being asked to pick up the snake.

There are some similarities but the rattler, at least, gives a warning before it strikes.

WINSTON-SALEM JOURNAL
Winston-Salem, NC, September 17, 1986

When they made their highly personal and emotional appeal to end drug abuse in America on Sunday night, President Reagan and his wife Nancy made a nice picture. Was anything wrong with it?

"Nice" is the best word. It was perhaps too nice, and sweet, and corny, for the first volley in a drug war. Or for an address by the leader of the U.S. government to his fellow citizens. A kind-hearted, well-meaning, old couple gave us a sermonette on drugs. Then the man, remembering his profession and perhaps a practical need to justify to the television networks his use of their valuable time, promised that the government would do *something*. A multi-point program would be announced Monday.

Then again, said our president, government couldn't solve the problem, addiction being individual, medical, personal and work-related. Drug abuse is a moral question as well, as the first lady allowed. But is it truly a public and political question? Is it a governmental matter? One for the state and the head of state to concern themselves with in a major way? One presumes a crusade is a major undertaking, and that is what Reagan has promised us.

No one rational doubts the truth of what the Reagans say about drugs, that the problem runs deep. Even those who say the numbers are down from what they were two years ago would not contest that "the drug problem" remains at epidemic levels in some segments of our society: That it is a killing cancer. That it would be good if athletes and television stars led the way by saying they are, or are becoming, clean. All this said, however, what can the president of the United States do about drugs that cannot otherwise be done? What does Ronald Reagan add to the efforts of private groups, or the secretary of health and welfare, or the long-standing and admirable public-education campaign of his wife? Isn't this the fellow who believes in minimal government, in the private sector and individual responsibility?

Certainly there is nothing objectionable in government backing a "Just Say No" drive. Lady Bird Johnson was for highway beautification and endeavored to get the nation to cease littering. President Kennedy backed fitness. Drug abuse is more important in human terms than either of those causes, but it is similarly tangential to public business and to national government. Which can do some positive things. But this is a case where Reagan rhetoric fits reality: The real work is for families, health professionals, individual persons. Insofar as it is a public matter, it is proper work for a first lady or first man. It is *not* the proper work of a president.

The president risks demeaning his office, the dignity of which he was elected to restore. He devalues it. Has no one at the White House noticed that all of the tough talk and military buildup of the last six years could not prevent a foreign power from snapping an American citizen off the streets and holding him for diplomatic ransom? Has anyone there thought that a president might engage in a crusade to lower unemployment or to save American heavy industry?

The first ladyship is rather like an American version of the modern English monarchs. It is honorific, symbolic and familial. The presidency is supposed to be different. You get the feeling that this president would rather be a monarch than a CEO, ruling instead of governing — presiding over the state as a benevolent father but taking no active part.

Crusade has a pleasing kingly sound to it. Ike saw his efforts in politics as a crusade. Like Richard the Lionhearted. Ronald Reagan can't resist the noble call of the trumpet; to arms he goes even when one crusade contradicts another. In a crusade one can be tough and good.

One is also reminded of Jimmy Carter's famous address on energy in the 1970s. He wore a sweater and sat by the fire and he said we were talking "the moral equivalent of war." He had no concrete action in mind as it turned out, and little real evidence, but he wanted to get us onto the right plane of consciousness. Liberals in America can't be overtly monarchical, so they assume the posture of the all-knowing psychologist.

Both the monarch and the shrink are variations on an odd new theme in statecraft. Few of us seem to believe government can do anything practical to ease people's way, but there is universal faith in the ability of the state to purify society. Hence the unemployed citizen wants for labor and bread but may rest easily at night knowing he has not helped Pieter Botha today; that he can donate as much to a presidential candidate as a "fat cat;" that he will not get lung cancer riding the airlines; and that he shall meet no communists selling all-beef chili dogs along the Southern Texas border.

House Backs National Assault on Narcotics

The House of Representatives September 11, 1986 approved a sweeping legislative package targeting the problem of illegal drugs. Backed by both the Democratic and Republican leadership, the bill passed 392 to 16. Speaker of the House, Thomas (Tip) O'Neil (D, Mass.) had called for preparation of the bill less than two months before when public feeling against drugs was running high throughout the country. Senate Democrats had unveiled a similar bill before the House vote, while the Reagan Administration and Senate Republicans were each working on packages of their own. The House bill was expected to cost as much as $6 billion over the next several years. It would provide new funds for local and federal enforcement of drug laws, as well as for state and local programs to counsel drug abusers and educate the public on the dangers of narcotics. The bill would also stiffen trafficking penalties and give prosecutors new tools to fight money laundering. In addition, it would provide for economic sanctions against drug-exporting nations that did not try to eradicate their drug crops.

The bill's three most sweeping and controversial provisions were amendments proposed by House Republicans. The measures attracted the special ire of civil libertarians. One amendment, for instance, would require the Defense Department to use whatever military resources where needed "to halt the unlawful penetration of United States borders by aircraft and vessels carrying narcotics." Normally, the United States allows no role for the military in law enforcement. Another amendment would allow prosecutors to use illegally acquired evidence in some drug trials so long as the officials who had gathered the evidence had not realized they were breaking the law. Under the so-called exclusionary rule, courts normally bar evidence that has been gathered in violation of the defendant's constitutional rights. In all, 31 amendments were attached to the bill. Describing the voting, Rep. Brian Donnelly (D, Mass.) said, "It's a mob mentality in there. It's just become the single biggest issue in the country." Donnelly added that he supported the measures being adopted.

The Washington Times

Washington, DC, September 17, 1986

Drugs are the consensus issue *du jour*, and the issue has moved up a gear in the past week. Some solid proposals are on the table, but every so often one is reminded of the movie director who shouted at a peripatetic but ineffective aide-de-camp: "Don't just *do* something, *stand* there!"

The House bill contains several good elements — the death penalty for drug-related murders, mandatory sentences for pushers, etc. Other parts are silly, e.g., ordering the military to halt importation of drugs in 45 days. If that sort of fiat works, let's order the police to stop crime in 45 days or, for that matter, get the preachers to eradicate sin. Also, under this sort of legislation, Congress would assume some of the functions of commander-in-chief, powers reserved by the Constitution to the president.

Speaking of whom, Ronald Reagan's testing program has deepened the significance of the observation that drugs are our No. 1 problem. Does his proposal collide with the Fourth Amendment's prohibition against "unreasonable searches and seizures"? In all likelihood it does. The National Treasury Employees Union charges, without much exaggeration, that "invasive tests will be imposed despite the fact that there is no documented problem of drug abuse amongst the federal work force."

In an effort to sidestep constitutional strictures, the administration says that (a) employees in offices where testing is ordered are to have 60 days' warning, (b) a positive first test is to entail only a second test, and (c) a positive second test is to lead, not to dismissal, but to counseling.

Yet the Fourth Amendment is unambiguous. It prohibits all searches undertaken without "probable cause," by which the Framers meant something more specific than the mere occurrence of crime. And nothing in the Fourth Amendment suggests that this requirement may be waived if the authorities give sufficient notice.

Weighing one thing with another, it seems doubtful that the courts will affirm blanket drug testing except in those especially sensitive occupations — air traffic controllers, for example — where lives are at stake and where submitting to periodic drug tests may be regarded as a reasonable condition of employment.

The administration seems to be gambling that compulsory drug testing will be approved, willy-nilly, and bets to this effect should be and probably will be lost.

EVENING EXPRESS

Portland, ME, September 30, 1986

Congress ought not to get carried away in its zeal to mount a full-scale "war" on drugs.

To be sure, drug abuse is a big problem in this country and it is important that steps be taken to combat it.

But too many members of Congress, seeing in all this a hot election-year issue, have indicated too great a willingness to trample fundamental rights and protections underfoot along the way.

Among other proposals from both Congress and the White House, there have been calls for widespread drug-testing both in and out of government, death-penalty provisions, relaxation of the rule against the use of illegally obtained evidence and expanded use of the military in fighting the drug market.

Defense Secretary Caspar Weinberger spoke out last weekend against a House-approved bill which, in part, calls for the military to seal U.S. borders against drug smuggling. The defense secretary rightly characterized the provision as "absurd."

Weinberger pointed out that thousands of airplanes cross the borders of the United States each day and that it would be impossible, short of firing upon them, to determine "what's inside each one of them."

Weinberger and others have pointed out what should be obvious to our elected representatives — that the primary mission of the U.S. military is defending the nation against armed enemy attack.

Fortunately, the Senate has been a bit more coolheaded than the House in this matter. The military amendment in the Senate version of the anti-drug initiative was rejected late last week 72-14.

As big a threat as drug abuse may be, it is fundamentally a domestic police problem. The military simply ought not to be involved in this particular "war."

The Pittsburgh PRESS

Pittsburgh, PA, September 18, 1986

Although President and Nancy Reagan didn't sign the declaration of war until Sunday night, the battlewagons have been rolling for some time in this country.

The mood of the nation is quite clear. Drugs are the nation's contemporary Pearl Harbor and an efficient and destructive war machine must be built, much the same as it was after Dec. 7, 1941.

But the architects of the machine that we need so desperately to combat the enemy need to recognize that a war wagon is more than a bandwagon. A war wagon is designed to fight, to fight hard and long, to destroy with calculated firepower. A bandwagon is nothing more than a blaring decoration, a gaudy showcase addition to a parade that appeases the masses, rather than satisfying their needs.

Distressingly, a large portion of the emphasis in government right now is in saddling up the bandwagon horses, much more ready to prance, rather than shaping up the war wagon horses, which take more time to be made battle-ready.

In Washington, the House last week, with the Nov. 4 election parade in mind, was determined to show its resolve against dealers in narcotics.

Legislation was approved that would, among other things:

• Authorize the death penalty for anyone involved in a continuing criminal enterprise who intentionally causes the death of another person.

• Order mandatory life imprisonment for anyone over age 21 who sells a dangerous drug to a child or teenager on or near school grounds.

• Allow the introduction of illegally obtained evidence in criminal trials in cases in which a police officer otherwise "acting in good faith" seizes the material without a search warrant.

In Harrisburg this week, Attorney General LeRoy Zimmerman called upon the Legislature to enact mandatory prison terms for the delivery of drugs, especially to children.

Mr. Zimmerman, for instance, would like to see a mandatory minimum term of five years for supplying marijuana, 10 years for cocaine and 15 years for heroin.

Under present law, there are no mandatory minimums for drug dealers but there are maximum terms, 10 years for marijuana and cocaine and 30 years for heroin. The only mandatory minimum term under present law is for the manufacture of methamphetamines, that only for two years.

We share the mood of the country and agree that the war must start in earnest. And we recognize that the proposals in Washington and Harrisburg are in response to that mood.

But we are reluctant to endorse the battle plans that are being drawn. They smack of knee-jerk reaction when what is needed is a change in attack philosophy, from hysterical haste to thoughtful thrust.

In the case of authorizing the introduction in trial of illegally seized evidence, for instance, we agree with Rep. Peter Rodino, D-N.J., who said "We started with a war against drugs — now it seems to me the attack is on the Constitution."

Mr. Zimmerman's proposals, though far more sensible, also need to be examined. If they are enacted in haste, without regard to the effect on already overcrowded jails, their impact could be devastating.

Drugs, indeed, are a cancer that has invaded the country.

It is necessary, though, that the war against them must be waged the way it is being waged against cancer. With solid, unyielding, well-financed and well-researched methods.

In the war against drugs, ultimate and total victory, the kind that President Roosevelt foresaw when he asked Congress to declare war in 1941, must be the goal.

THE BLADE

Toledo, OH, September 18, 1986

THE U.S. House last week whipped itself into an election-year frenzy over anti-drug legislation. Its performance, designed primarily as good theater for the benefit of voters, falls far short of representing a solution to the drug problem.

What the House passed is a Christmas tree loaded with controversial, and in some cases possibly unconstitutional, proposals that will cost as much as $4 billion over three years.

The legislation would allow U.S. military forces to arrest drug smugglers, reinstate the death penalty for certain drug dealers, permit use of improperly seized evidence, and create a $1.3 billion bonanza for state and local drug fighters.

The measure is timely in the war against drug abuse. But the White House, the Defense Department, and senators who will have to vote on the bill have discovered troubling flaws in it. Allowing the military to work as a law-enforcement agency, for example, is a distortion of its fundamental role, and loosening the rules concerning evidence guarantees an extended Senate fight and possibly a filibuster from liberals.

A few days after the bill was passed President Reagan, in unveiling his plan to attack drug abuse, ordered drug testing for 1.1 million federal employees. That approach is raising questions as to whether it amounts to invasion of privacy.

No one questions the need for tougher policies on all levels to discourage drug smuggling and drug abuse. The recent deaths of two star athletes plus the growing incidence of "crack," a highly dangerous cocaine derivative, have underscored the insidious nature of drug abuse and the moral depravity of persons who make a living by peddling harmful substances.

Throwing every possible federal dollar and every conceivable punitive and investigative measure at the problem will make some inroads, but it will not solve it. The remedies offered by the House and Mr. Reagan will assure headlines, but more time, care, and selectivity would have been more desirable.

St. Louis Review

St. Louis, MO, September 19, 1986

A lot of news passes through the pages of our newspapers and magazines. Tidbits of news are thrown our way by radio and television. Shoppers at the checkout counter thumb the tabloid crazies for something just a bit more bizarre. Some of this news is obviously of greater and more lasting importance in the daily lives of all of us. In this category we would locate the current anti-drug campaign now raging throughout our country on all fronts.

Within recent days we have seen both President and Mrs. Reagan on national television decrying drugs and announcing plans to battle this problem. We have helicopters and troops closing down Bolivian drug production at the risk of bankrupting that impoverished country. The House of Representatives has passed a bill to spend $4 billion fighting drugs and providing the death penalty for drug-related murder and life prison terms for people convicted a second time of selling drugs to children.

We are witnessing a powerful campaign being mounted on all sides to battle the dangers and costs of drug abuse on the personal, corporate and political levels. For those of us who lived through the 60s and 70s, who heard of the marvels of drugs from everyone from the kid on the corner to Cheech and Chong this is a new world. The pendulum really does swing from one extreme to the other. Those who claim that public morality changes with elections are proven right.

We have abhorred the permissive public attitudes about drugs the last 20 years. On the other hand when we suddenly hear all this hullabaloo and read that drug-related testing might be required to apply for and to keep jobs in many civilian industries we wonder a bit. Public morality is badly in need of improvement, but when dealing with practices which affect people as deeply and with as much impact as drugs do our national policies and corporate rules need to be carefully thought out.

If drug tests are not reliable and if the results are not evaluated by well-trained and intelligent personnel the whole process is easily able to destroy innocent lives and careers can easily be ruined. A wise person might stand back and ponder the long-range results and implications of some of these proposed measures. We need some time to work these points through, both personally and politically.

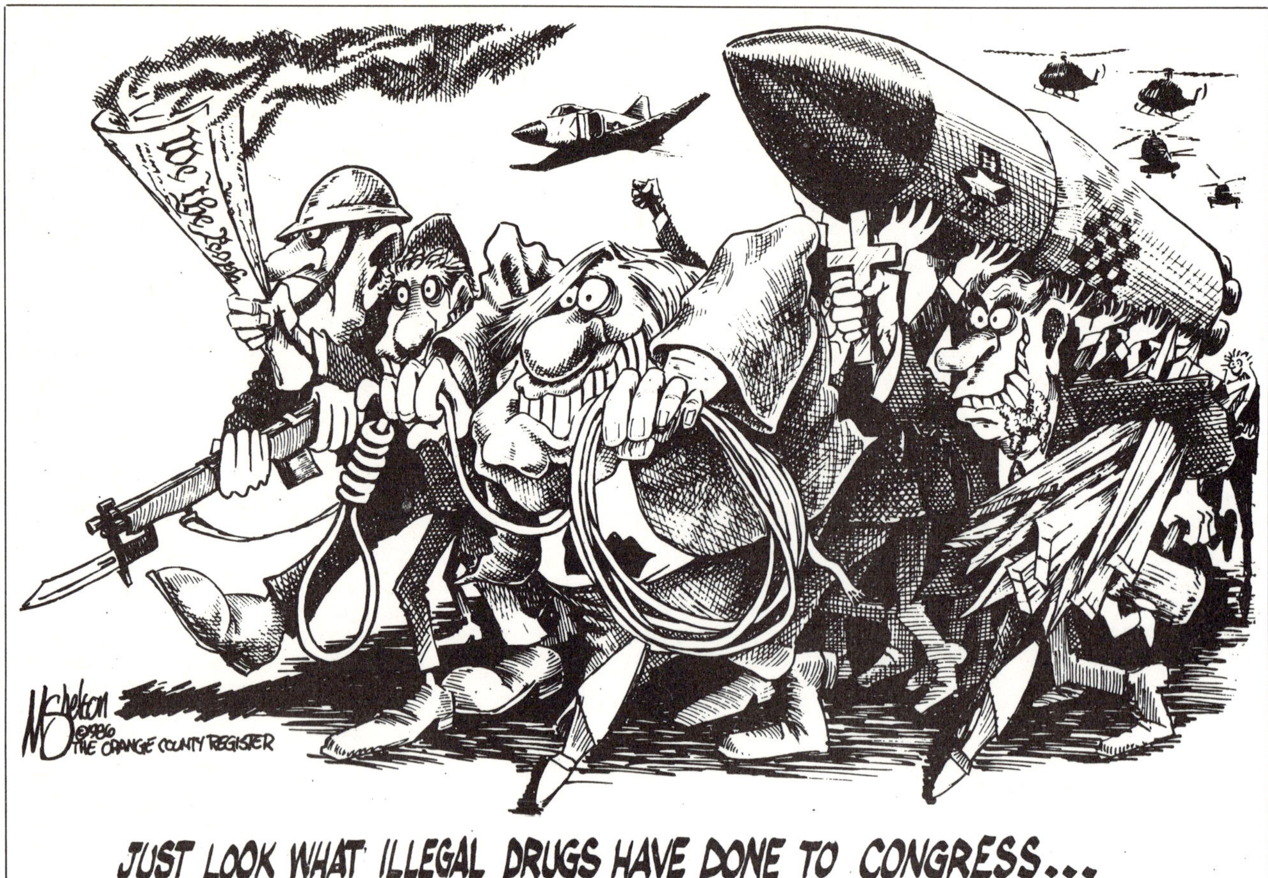

LAS VEGAS REVIEW-JOURNAL

Las Vegas, NV, September 16, 1986

Drugs, drugs, drugs. That's all you hear these days.

The Congress has whipped itself into a frenzy over this issue. Democrats and Republicans alike last week were stumbling all over one another to lead charge against illegal drugs.

Only a few took note that the Constitution was getting trampled underfoot. But the prevailing attitude seemed to be that the Bill of Rights is expendable — that the war on drugs is more important than any outdated guarantees of civil liberty.

The latest war on drugs is under way. On some fronts the war is a good war, a war that's overdue — one that can attack this grave national problem of drug abuse. But it is fraught with dangers, not the least of which is the danger that civil liberties will be an early casualty.

There was no stopping the steamroller. With the elections coming up in November, Congressmen — indeed politicians at all levels — have seen the public opinion polls and have embraced this war on drugs with a passion that has blinded many to the very real constitutional issues involved.

The latest Time magazine survey, conducted by Yankelovich, Clancy, Shulmann last week, indicates that 75 percent of the American public believes that drug abuse is a serious problem in the United States.

That kind of overwhelming public concern is powerful political fodder in a campaign year. As November approaches, no politician can afford to be characterized as being "soft on drugs."

Polls have shown time and time again that relatively few Americans know what the Bill of Rights contains, what freedoms they are guaranteed. Yet, as the polls indicate, most Americans do have an awareness of the drug problem, and are possessed of a gut reaction that something must be done. Congressmen know this, and many seem willing to brush aside very serious questions of civil liberty in their frontal assault on drugs.

So Congress last week overwhelming — 392-16 — approved a drug bill that toys dangerously with the Constitution. The bill would pump new billions into the war on drugs.

But the bill also contains an amendment that would allow police to use illegally obtained evidence in court, and never mind the Fourth Amendment to the Constitution. Another amendment would expand the use of American armed forces to interdict drug traffickers — and never mind the dangerous implications that wide-scale use of the military in domestic affairs entails.

Both Nevada Congressmen — Harry Reid, the Democrat, and Barbara Vucanovich, the Republican — voted both for the bill and the amendments.

Now President Reagan has ordered the heads of every federal government agency to establish drug-testing programs for "employees in sensitive positions." This may mean mandatory urinalysis for more than 1 million federal workers — and never mind the Fourth and Fifth Amendments to the Constitution.

With the flurry of legislation and executive orders emanating from Washington, one gets the impression that this nation is facing a drug crisis of unprecedented proportions. No question, drug abuse is noxious and widespread.

But is it suddenly of runaway proportions? The government's own figures say the number of heroin users in the United States has stabilized at about 500,000. Marijuana use among high school students is now at 5 percent — about half what it was in 1978, according to government surveys. The number of cocaine users has remained stable since 1979 and remains at about 4.3 million.

Obviously these figures — stable or not — are unacceptable. The tragic waste and pain visited upon the chronic cocaine user or heroin addict or crack user and his family represent needless suffering. And it is the duty of this society to curtail that suffering — to eliminate it, if possible.

More money for drug education in the schools, more money for treatment centers for the victims of drug abuse, harsh sentences for those who push chemical death, the creation of — as Nancy Reagan puts it, an attitude of intolerance for drug abuse — all these are welcome developments in the effort to rid this nation of the spirit-stifling plague of drugs.

But that noble end does not justify the use of any means to achieve it. Who would be the vanquished if basic constitutional rights are victims of this war?

The Houston Post

Houston, TX, September 15, 1986

The House of Representatives got a little carried away in its zeal to crack down on drug trafficking. Of course, it's less than two months until Election Day. But the brass-knuckles bill the lawmakers passed 392-16 accurately reflects public exasperation with the failure to stem the tide of illegal narcotics sweeping the nation.

We have no quarrel with the bill's requirement that the armed forces be used to guard our borders against drug smugglers. Opponents argue that the military should not be involved in civilian law enforcement. But if we won't give our civilian police agencies the resources to do the job, the military is our only option. After all, aren't U.S. troops and equipment helping the Bolivian government in its fight against cocaine traffickers?

The bill's stiffer penalties for drug offenders, including death for "killer drug dealers," impress us as making the punishment fit the crime. But it bends the "exclusionary rule" too far when it permits the use of improperly obtained evidence in some warrantless searches. That provision is not confined to drug-related cases.

Our chief reservation about the measure is that it may cost more than it is worth. It authorizes spending $2 billion-plus for drug treatment, law enforcement and other programs. Winning the war on drugs isn't going to be cheap, but the problem won't be solved by throwing money at it. And the House hasn't yet said where it plans to get the funds in this era of huge deficits.

Besides the House bill, the Senate and the Reagan administration are preparing anti-drug measures. Out of all this proposed legislation should come a tougher, more realistic battle plan against the illicit drug menace. It is too pervasive and too deeply entrenched to yield to a quick fix.

Rocky Mountain News

Denver, CO, September 18, 1986

FEW sights are as unedifying as packs of Washington politicians baying in pursuit of an issue less than two months before an election. The spectacle is on now and its title is "Our War Against Drugs."

Quite simply, the idea is that this will help a candidate to declare on the hustings: "I voted against drug abuse." And thus no lack of money or risk of bad law will stop the president and Congress from rushing through a drug bill.

To her credit, at least one member of the Colorado delegation has resisted the stampede. Rep. Pat Schroeder has taken a close look at President Reagan's plan to test tens of thousands of federal workers for drugs and found it wanting. Given the scope of testing sought by the president, she says, the program could cost $300 million and not the $56 million Reagan has suggested.

For that much money Congress could double the size of the U.S. Drug Enforcement Agency, Schroeder argues.

Why the high cost? In part because the president has defined employees in "sensitive" jobs — those eligible for drug tests — as people dealing with national security or classified information, those appointed by the president, those whose work affects public health or safety, and those whose position requires "a high degree of trust and confidence." By such standards, over a million workers might be required to hand over a urine specimen for analysis.

The tests themselves won't be the only cost, either. Treatment will follow for some employees and many others will no doubt file lawsuits whether or not they're guilty.

And for what purpose will all this money be spent and suspicion generated? There is no evidence that drug abuse is growing among federal workers. Quite the contrary. Since the use of all illegal substances except cocaine has been on the decline nationally for the past five or six years — despite hysterical statements to the contrary by politicians — use among federal workers has probably been declining, too. Unfortunately, our elected officials are several years late in launching their crusade.

This is not to argue against all drug tests. There *are* sensitive jobs — those involving spying and intelligence, for example — where the government should not risk having a single employee dependent on drugs. Moreover, tests for drugs should be required whenever probable cause exists that an employee has been using them.

Blanket testing of the sort proposed by Reagan, however, is an overreaction so long as most drug use is on the wane. Among other things, widespread mandatory tests would poison the work atmosphere, submit innocent employees to personal indignity and foster the notion that employers may indiscriminately probe into the personal life of their workers.

To be fair, Congress hasn't been much more restrained in its approach to the drug problem. Some bits and pieces in congressional proposals could be useful, such as cracking down on launderers of drug profits and continuing to educate youths on narcotics' dangers. But other provisions are wasteful or useless: A White House conference on drugs (yes, another one), a study on drug-use and highway safety (it causes accidents) and appointment of an anti-drug "czar" (our last czar was for energy and we promptly got gasoline lines).

A more sensible way to crack down on drugs is to insist on heavier penalties for dealers and some categories of users; beef up border patrols, treatment programs and educational efforts; and continue to marshall peer pressure in all social settings, from school to executive parties. Drug use is undoubtedly a scourge in the United States, but progress against it has already begun. Further success doesn't depend on the draconian solutions now advocated.

Los Angeles Times

Los Angeles, CA, September 16, 1986

Topic A on the nation's agenda these days is drug abuse, with Congress and the White House falling all over each other to get in on the act. Maybe even some good will come of it.

But when Congress acts in haste in response to a perceived emergency and with an election near, it frequently acts in error. Frenzy rarely helps sound decision-making, particularly in legislative bodies.

The latest evidence of this is the anti-drug bill that the House of Representatives approved last week by a lopsided margin. Even though many members knew that parts of the bill were seriously wrong, only 16 congressmen were willing to risk the wrath of their constituents by voting against it. More of them should have, for the measure contains provisions that are anathema to our country's respect for civil liberties and to the proper role of the military in a civilian government. Besides, there is scant evidence that the extreme measures would work.

The widespread use of narcotics and other illegal drugs is a deeply troubling problem. Citizens are calling on the government to do *something*, and the House responded by passing a bill to stiffen penalties for drug-related crimes, to provide more manpower and equipment for the fight against drug smuggling and to increase drug education and treatment. A good case can be made for reinforcing drug-related education and police functions. But the members of the House could not stop there. They accepted in addition panic amendments that pose more danger than they would prevent.

Among the most glaring excesses is a mandate for the Pentagon to use military forces to guard the country's borders to stop smuggling. This idea flies in the face of a long and appropriate tradition, backed by law, that the armed forces should not be involved in civilian law enforcement.

Another part of the bill would allow the use of illegally obtained evidence at drug trials as long as the police made a "good-faith" effort to follow the law—a flagrant challenge to protections of the Constitution. A "good-faith" exception to the exclusionary rule of evidence is a loophole so large that nearly everything can pass through it, jettisoning the Fourth Amendment protection against unreasonable searches and seizures.

Furthermore, the House bill would authorize the death penalty for drug smuggling that intentionally caused a death. What that means is anybody's guess. But the political expediency of intruding extreme and controversial elements into this piece of legislation could serve only to divert the police and the courts from the pursuit and punishment of drug marketers.

Meantime, the Reagans' address to the nation Sunday night will help draw attention to the dangers of drug use. The President and Mrs. Reagan were right to say that the problem can be solved only by eliminating the demand, not by police work. Yet this Administration has cut the funds for drug education and treatment. It seems to have chosen widespread testing over other programs that might work.

The causes of drug use are deep and complex, and eradication must be mounted at many levels. Voters will not confuse expedient solutions and theatrics of extreme measures with the steady, costly kinds of program that will eventually bring this problem under control.

President, First Lady Urge Antidrug Crusade

President Ronald Reagan and his wife, Nancy, September 14, 1986 broadcast a television and radio appeal for a "national crusade" against drug abuse. It was the first time Reagan and his wife had delivered a joint television address during Reagan's presidency. Narcotics abuse inspired a recent surge in national concern. The talk came a day before Reagan unveiled a legislative package of antidrug proposals. President Reagan said the government would "continue to act aggressively" against the narcotics problem, but that "nothing would be more effective than for Americans simply to quit using illegal drugs." He called for "a massive change in national attitudes" toward drugs. Mrs. Reagan said: "There's no normal middle ground. Indifference is not an option. We want you to help create an outspoken intolerance for drug use." Adding a personal appeal to young people, she declared: "Just say 'yes' to life. And when it comes to drugs and alcohol, just say 'no.'" "Just say 'no'" is the slogan of the antidrug publicity campaign Mrs. Reagan launched after coming to the White House. The drive is aimed at preventing future drug abuse by appealing to children aged seven to 14. By one count, the drive had spurred the establishment of 10,000 clubs, in which at least 200,000 children have pledged not to use drugs. However, government spending for antidrug education and prevention programs had fallen by 5% under the Reagan Administration, the *New York Times* reported Sept. 14, 1986. *Time* magazine reported in its Sept. 15, 1986 issue that the Department of Education spent so little on the matter there was no record of the funds.

The Chattanooga Times

Chattanooga, TN, September 19, 1986

By making a televised appeal for a nationwide crusade against illegal drugs, President and Mrs. Reagan lent the force and prestige of their respective positions to a serious social problem and provided educational leadership as well. To the extent that the appeal energizes efforts around the country to combat a problem that victimizes young and old alike, the Reagans' joint speech will be especially valuable.

The president outlined several goals, including schools and workplaces that are free of drugs, expanded efforts in the research and treatment of drug abuse and tougher punishment for those who deal in drugs. Another prime goal was the effort to make the public more aware of the consequences of illegal drug use. That will probably be easier to accomplish, given the response by Congress and the White House to the drug problem, not to mention the numerous reports by the press.

Predictably, some complained that the Reagans' White House speech was political. That's true to an extent, but the same can be said of the congressional measures being pushed by Republicans and Democrats. But although the use of politics to promote a matter of public concern is not entirely wrong in and of itself, there is always the danger that political excess can subvert dispassionate consideration of the issue. For example, in the announcement Tuesday of his candidacy for the Republican presidential nomination, former Delaware Gov. Pierre S. du Pont called for mandatory drug testing of all teen-agers, a dumb idea if there ever was one.

Mr. Reagan didn't go that far after his television speech, but he did sign an executive order requiring mandatory drug tests for all federal employees in sensitive positions. Members of the military and other security agencies are already subject to such tests. It's anybody's guess, however, how many government employees will actually be tested, since the president's order leaves that decision to the heads of government agencies.

The inherent ambiguity of the president's order suggests it is vulnerable to constitutional challenge, and indeed some lower court decisions have already held that mandatory tests for public employees are unconstitutional. The reason is simple: Such tests force individuals, whether or not they are suspected of drug abuse, to prove their innocence.

We are seeing the application of that kind of thinking here in Chattanooga. Responding to a letter from the firemen's union requesting a suspension of mandatory, across-the-board drug testing for firefighters without guidelines, Fire and Police Commissioner Tom Kennedy said the tests were begun because of "problems" of drug use. But instead of testing only those suspected of drug use, the requirement was imposed on all.

It won't be easy to make a dent in the drug abuse problem, but it can be done without sacrificing our civil liberties. The proposed increase in spending for antidrug efforts would strengthen law enforcement and reinvigorate drug education and treatment programs which the administration reduced in 1981. More promising than increased spending and new programs, however, is the president's assertion that "we seek a massive change in national attitudes (to) separate the drugs from the customer." Whether that is accomplished by education, peer pressure ("Just say no") or law enforcement, the hope is that it can be done without succumbing to counterproductive measures.

The Evening Telegram

St. John's, Nfld.
September 17, 1986

When the President of the United States and the Prime Minister of Canada say drug use is an epidemic and call for a crusade against drug use, then it is obvious North American society has a drug problem.

President Ronald Reagan and his wife Nancy appeared on national television in the U.S. Sunday to appeal to Americans to fight drug abuse.

Monday morning, the president signed an order making drug tests mandatory for federal employees; last week, the House of Representatives ordered the U.S. military to intercept drugs at the nation's borders and called for the death penalty for drug dealers.

Sunday, Prime Minister Brian Mulroney promised "important" legislation to deal with drug abuse in Canada.

Drug abuse is a serious problem in North America.

There has been scandal after scandal in professional sports over drug abuse.

Two federal crown corporations screen job applicants for drug use. Other Canadian companies have drug and alcohol treatment programs for employees.

An estimated 25 per cent of U.S. firms have mandatory drug-testing programs; more companies are considering such programs.

Tougher laws, drug testing programs, use of the military to stop smuggling and the death penalty for dealers do not address the problem of why people use drugs.

What is it about North American society that encourages, or persuades, people to use illegal drugs?

The answer to that question is as important as the legal efforts to curb illegal drug use.

Until it is answered, there will always be a problem with use of illegal drugs.

THE CHRISTIAN SCIENCE MONITOR
Boston, MA, September 16, 1986

THE speech from the White House on Sunday night is an example of the kind of moral direction the President and, in this case, the First Lady, Mrs. Reagan, can provide in the nettlesome matter of drug abuse.

Particularly heartening is Mrs. Reagan's focus on individual responsibility, on fostering development in young people — especially of the strength to say no. She rightly insists that young people have too much going for them, and are too much needed, to waste their lives on drugs. Speaking of drug criminals, she said, "It's up to us to change attitudes and simply dry up their markets."

Meanwhile, the drug issue has become such a political wildfire across the country that what is most needed at the moment is some calm consideration of what measures need to be taken to fight the drug menace. In a midterm election campaign lacking in serious partisan issues, calm consideration is unfortunately in short supply.

The omnibus antidrug bill moving through the House of Representatives includes a number of constructive tactics, notably increased funding for drug rehabilitation centers. But last week the House also approved floor amendments allowing for use of the military to interdict drugs at the borders, of illegally obtained evidence in trials of accused drug dealers, and of the death penalty for some drug-linked murders.

These suggestions are troubling. Illegal evidence in the case of an accused drug dealer is no less illegal than such evidence in the case of an accused serial killer. The tradition — and law — keeping the military out of civilian law enforcement have deep roots in the American system, along with other civil liberties provisions.

Having clear principles such as these thought through in advance often prevents one from making a foolish or wrong decision in the heat of the moment. The scene in Washington right now seems to be precisely one of those heated moments when the system needs all the principles it's got. And as for the death penalty, it can be sanctioned for drug dealers no more than it can for those found guilty of other heinous crimes.

And the reasons for opposing the death penalty — or the involvement of the military or mass urinalysis or whatever — have nothing to do with not taking the drug problem seriously.

Clearly, drugs are extracting an unacceptable toll, not only from direct victims such as basketball star Len Bias, but from society as a whole, including anyone who pays an insurance premium higher than it would be without drug-related crime.

The reports that drug use is actually on the decline are welcome news and help provide a useful perspective; those who need help, however, still need it.

Hence the continuing need for not only moral leadership from the White House, but also sensible steps like increased funding for treatment programs.

It would be unfortunate if the manufactured version of the crisis — the campaign-season furor — were allowed to get in the way of taking serious steps to deal with the actual problem.

The Afro American
Baltimore, MD, September 27, 1986

Now that the initial shock and bewilderment over President Reagan's ordering of mandatory drug tests for some federal employees has waned, the implementation of the order won't happen for at least some six months.

The constitutionality of the order must first be determined, then the guidelines written, and money allocated, and after all this, the various departments must give employees a two-month notice before beginning random tests.

So it would seem, as many have pointed out, that this entire drug-testing maneuver is a "top of the head" reaction to the drug problem facing the country today. It does, however, signal a shift in policy.

Initially, the drug pushers and suppliers were the major thrust of the Drug Enforcement operation — drug testing moves it over to a concentration on the users. This is not unlike the Volstead Act enforcement of Prohibition in the 20s — and it was a total failure.

Politicians all across the country have leaped aboard the publicity bandwagon, singing huzzahs for drug testing. They are trumpeting that they have taken the test and are challenging opponents to do likewise.

The actuality is that no politician would make such a claim, unless he was absolutely sure he would pass. However, is drug testing the answer? We doubt it. An example of the rationale can be observed in the case of prostitution, wherein the "john" was to be arrested as a user.

It hasn't worked either — and neither will this highly publicized drug-testing of federal workers.

THE ANN ARBOR NEWS
Ann Arbor, MI, September 16, 1986

One of the tragedies of addiction is that dependency on a product or substance that comes in a package represents such a frightening example of squandered potential and loss of freedom.

In the meantime, a great hoax is being perpetrated on the user. Addiction fools him into thinking his mind and body can withstand the insult of drug ingestion when in fact both are slowly being wasted. Pleasure enhancement via drugs is ultimately victimization.

It is because so many young people are being victimized by drug dependency that various personalities from President Reagan to a growling Mr. T are trying to get the attention of young Americans. The war on drugs is getting serious.

It should; the manufacture and demand of illicit drugs is a growth industry. No sooner does use of one drug decline than another, more potentially dangerous one takes its place. Synthetic drugs replace the home-grown variety. High-potency "crack" is now the drug of choice among thrill-seekers looking for a new experience.

Drug-running is a billion-dollar business into which organized crime has sunk its hooks. If the country is going to wage an ultimately successful war against drugs, the crime angle alone argues for a powerful effort involving a corresponding outlay of dollars and personnel.

Good intentions won't suffice. Voluntary drug-testing by national leaders such as President Reagan and Vice President George Bush may have some symbolic value, but it doesn't dent the drug traffic.

If there is big money involved in moving drugs from source to user via the crime connection, then big money is needed to hire agents, set up drug buys and do the myriad number of things to make this war a winning effort. Fact-oriented, non-hysterical drug education programs are part of this all-out war.

Unfortunately, the administration which now has declared war on drugs opted from the beginning to treat the supply side but not the demand side. Washington has tried to secure our borders against the traffic in drug's raw materials without doing more to help the drug abuser.

For example, the Department of Education's budget for programs to combat drug abuse declined from $14 million in 1981 to just $2.9 million in 1985. During this same period dollars for enforcement were way up.

While all of us as parents and concerned Americans should support the war against illegal drugs, it's important to keep the drug issue in perspective.

For one thing, drug wars are nothing new. National assaults on drug use began with Prohibition.

No substance is more abused, causes more heartache and is responsible for more deaths annually than alcohol. Just because alcohol is legal and somehow more respectable doesn't make its abuse any less dangerous, as any set of statistics or broken home can testify.

It's also important that an effective war on drugs be focused on the pushers and suppliers, without trapping a lot of innocent people. We need to crack down on organized crime and the drug rings with confiscations and arrests. In our enthusiasm to wipe out illegal drugs, we should take care not to sign away our freedoms. Worthwhile social policy is not implemented at the expense of our civil liberties.

It is worrisome, for example, that there is some support at the state level for expanding wiretapping privileges as a tool to catch drug kingpins. Without electronic surveillance, it's very difficult to make a case against big-time drug operators, Attorney General Frank Kelley said.

While that may be true, expansion of the wiretap law should be considered very carefully. The potential for misuse is considerable. Michigan's experience with the Red Squad list is an object lesson in police power abuse.

Ultimately, the war on drugs may be won with generous funding of drug education and drug abuse treatment and rehabilitation programs. Sustained public education campaigns have effected a change in public attitudes about smoking, drinking and drunk driving. That strategy is worth applying to drugs as well.

DESERET NEWS
Salt Lake City, UT
September 16/17, 1986

No one wants to see this nation's youth ravaged by drugs. The nation joins President and Mrs. Reagan in calling for a comprehensive effort to limit drug abuse by reducing both supply and demand.

White House backing for a reasoned, determined anti-drug push is welcome and comes as no surprise to those who have seen Mrs. Reagan's dedication to the issue over the past five years. President Reagan's ordering of mandatory drug tests for federal employees in sensitive jobs is a dramatic demonstration that he means business.

But voters are not naive. They recognize that drugs are not the nation's only problem. They know that hastily thrown together, election-year legislation, such as the House passed last week, that threaten constitutional guarantees are not the answer to a vicious, deeply ingrained national problem.

They're not ready to jettison carefully worked-out rules of evidence and let police use any illegal methods they please to convict someone, as long as the suspected crime involves drugs.

They're not ready to send soldiers rushing to the borders to start arresting suspected smugglers without some consideration of the implications of this blurring of military and police functions. Wisely, the administration has strongly opposed this measure in its present form.

They're not averse to using the death penalty in certain cases, but they want the gravity of the offenses and the standards of proof involved to be commensurate with those in other capital cases.

They're not aware that handing out life sentences without parole to every person convicted twice of selling drugs to minors would require a mind-boggling increase in prison cells.

In Utah, for example, voters haven't forgotten that the state prison is already filled to overflowing, and that new laws giving all drug users inflexible, mandatory punishments would mean more pressure on a system that is already turning prisoners out early.

Drug offenders are not the only dangers to society: Sex offenders released from prison without treatment because of lack of money for programs are also a cause to get up in arms about. Crime-fighting dollars must be allocated with a view to the entire problem.

Politicians say they're often pressured by special interest groups to cast votes based on emotions without consideration of the larger context and the general public good. In this case, it appears to be the public that is maintaining some perspective and the lawmakers who need to get their emotions under control.

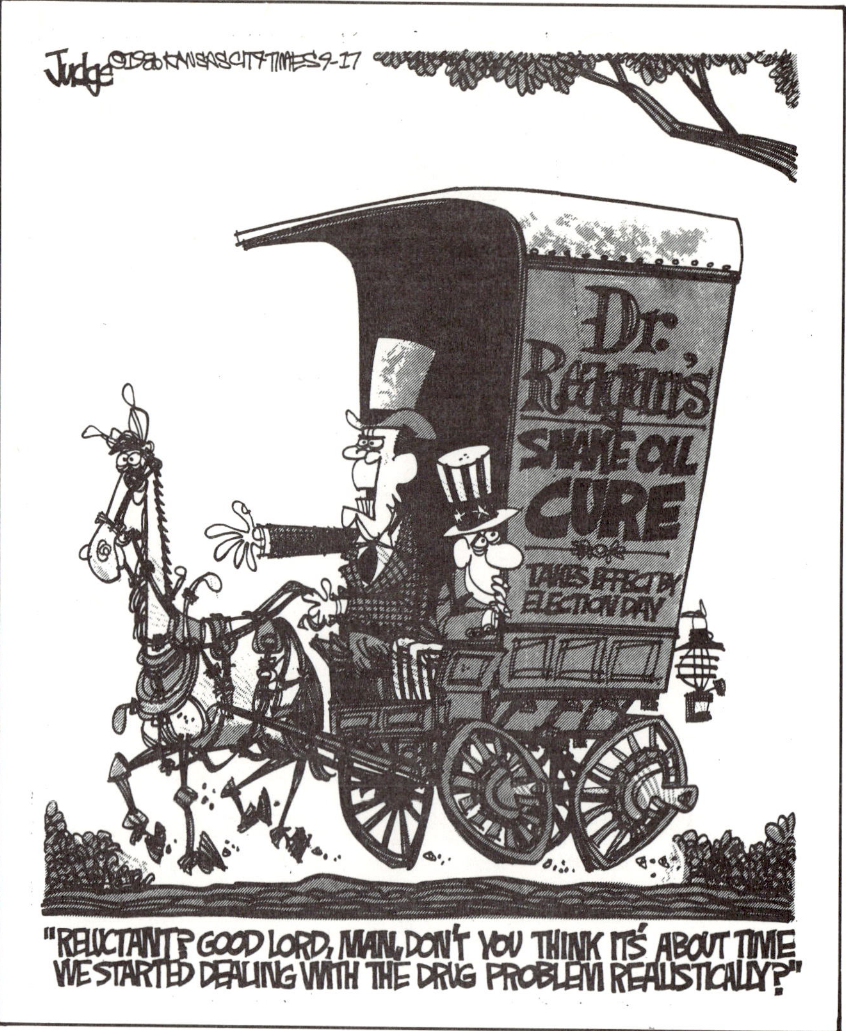

The Kansas City Times
Kansas City, MO, September 18, 1986

One plain truth about President Reagan's drug initiative is that no one knows if it will make much difference. Right now, that seems to be about the only thing anyone knows for sure about America's latest crisis.

Mr. Reagan, after wrestling about a campaign to counter the ones developed in Congress and launching his effort in a television performance, proposes nearly $900 million in additional federal funds to deal with the problem. The largest part, $500 million, will go for enforcement. Treatment and education also are to get new money.

Cynicism abounds because the initiatives are smack in the middle of fierce partisan politics. There are differences in the congressional and presidential proposals, but people are confused about what's real and what's illusion. This one won't work because there's not enough money, some critics proclaim. Another proposal won't because emphasis is on users rather than sellers, or sellers instead of producers, or Americans rather than foreign suppliers.

Nonetheless, on this issue the administration has taken the first step of leadership although it has made two major mistakes. The first is taking money to pay for it away from other programs. There's no excess.

Making mandatory testing of certain federal employees the centerpiece is another. It's a spot of drama that would at best barely dent the drug epidemic. But in light of the unreliability of testing now, it's a futile exercise. Damage to the innocent and the issue of invasion of privacy will spawn a whole new layer of litigation.

The only hope for resuming control in the streets is statesmanship. Elected officials and government specialists should know that concentrated attacks must be made on the many faces of the enemy. Throwing everything against one would be a waste. Round up drug smugglers at the borders, but let addicts suffer unto death? Imprison pushers for long terms; but do nothing to strengthen children against drugs? It is a circle of demon tails with no one part uglier than the one before.

Mr. and Mrs. Reagan know this. Now the country waits for leadership with a generosity of spirit on multiple fronts.

The Union Leader

Manchester, NH, September 16, 1986

If there are, anywhere, citizens who remain blissfully unaware of the truly shocking dimensions of the drug problem threatening to destroy America from within, their number must be exceedingly small in the aftermath of President and Nancy Reagan's dramatic Sunday night appeal to the American people to declare all-out "war" on drugs and drug pushers.

Granted, the President and Mrs. Reagan proposed no new ways of fighting the drug menace; that's probably because there are none. Rather, theirs was an unprecedented call by the nation's most prominent mother and father for a total commitment by every segment of our society to the anti-drug "war" in much the same manner that the entire nation rallied to defeat the menace of Nazism and Fascism during World War II.

But "war," of course, entails self-sacrifice and unrelenting commitment to victory. The cynics, therefore, will scoff. They will say sneeringly that "we've heard it all before," that words, even when spoken in dramatic fashion by the President and First Lady, are no substitute for action and that, in the "war" against drugs, most Americans are pacifists. They will contend that the problem is too big, that "everyone's doing it," that the past glorification of the drug culture (for which we can thank principally the news and entertainment media) is woven inextricably into the national fabric. They will cite the obvious: that at best our past response to the menace was weak, platitudinous and hypocritical. And time may well prove that the presidential call for an end to moral neutrality concerning this issue was foredoomed to have few practical results.

We should not have to wait long to see whether such cynics are right. If the nation's school and legal authorities do not demonstrate to the nation's youth that *they* accept the President's reminder that "drug abuse is a repudiation of everything America is," if they act as if they do not really believe that "the destructiveness and human wreckage" of drug abuse "mock our heritage," then young people, most of whom really do want strong corrective action consistently applied against drug and alcohol abuse, will not be convinced either.

"Drugs out of the schools" should mean precisely that. Let there be no temporizing with the costly (estimated at $60 billion annually) problem, no inconsistency in applying anti-drug policies, no discriminatory favoring of superior students over those less intellectually endowed, no legal gimmicks that allow convicted druggies to "beat the system" and continue to stroll the corridors of the nation's schools with impunity.

Here in New Hampshire, we believe there is one easy yardstick to apply to determine just how seriously school authorities view the drug problem beyond the bounds of mere rhetoric: Let us see how many communities across the state follow the example set by the Portsmouth School Board and mandate the suspension of students apprehended with illegal drugs and alcohol. Let us see whether Manchester, Concord, Nashua and other cities and towns will follow suit.

Then let us see whether effective follow-up programs are put into effect to rehabilitate the drug- and alcohol-crazed outcasts.

Only those who fail to comprehend the nature of the drug-alcohol problem, who refuse to face the fact that students have a *right* to function during school hours in a drug-free atmosphere conducive to serious education, a right that is being outrageously violated, only these head-in-the-sand types will regard the Portsmouth policy, put into effect on the first day of this month, as too harsh.

Oh yes. Did we fail to mention it? The biggest cynics of them all when it comes to viewing the practical effects of dramatic warnings against drug abuse are young people, the principal target of the drug pushers. And they are cynical with good cause: They are accustomed to adults promising much and delivering little.

The Burlington Free Press

Burlington, VT, September 18, 1986

As one of the hottest issues in an election year, drug abuse has drawn the frenetic attention of politicians from all points on the political spectrum.

Democrats and Republicans are trying to outdo each other in their efforts to introduce proposals for curbing drug usage in the country. At times, it indeed appears as if their zeal borders on hysteria.

Several politicians want to put the country on a war footing to combat drug trafficking. With President Reagan playing the role of the general and a bipartisan group of congressmen his lieutenants, the battle to eradicate the drug scourge in the country is being plotted.

An arsenal of weapons, including mandatory drug testing of federal workers in "sensitive" jobs, capital punishment for some drug-related crimes and more research and treatment programs, will be used as a means of curbing drug use.

The House passed a bill last week which would require Reagan to send U.S. military forces within 45 days to halt the drug traffic along the nation's borders. Secretary of Defense Caspar W. Weinberger was a vehement opponent of the proposal.

Yet all the grandiose and politically popular schemes, some of them questionable, will be meaningless if a massive grassroots educational effort is not launched to impress young people with the harmful consequences of drug abuse.

Drug dealers cannot flourish and foreign suppliers cannot survive if the demand for such substances is drastically reduced. However undramatic that it may seem to many politicians, the place to begin the war is in the nation's schools.

What is equally important is that people assume responsibility for their actions. If they choose to use drugs, no amount of Big Brotherism is going to change the fact that addiction is the inevitable outcome.

Treatment programs certainly could help many people but the amount of money allocated in the House bill is niggardly in comparison to the amount that will be spent on halting the drug traffic.

The dollars spent on education and treatment undoubtedly will be more effective than some of the other measures advocated by the White House and Congress.

To win the drug war, it will be necessary to use those measures which will cut down the demand for drugs to such a point that drug dealers will find it unprofitable to do business in this country.

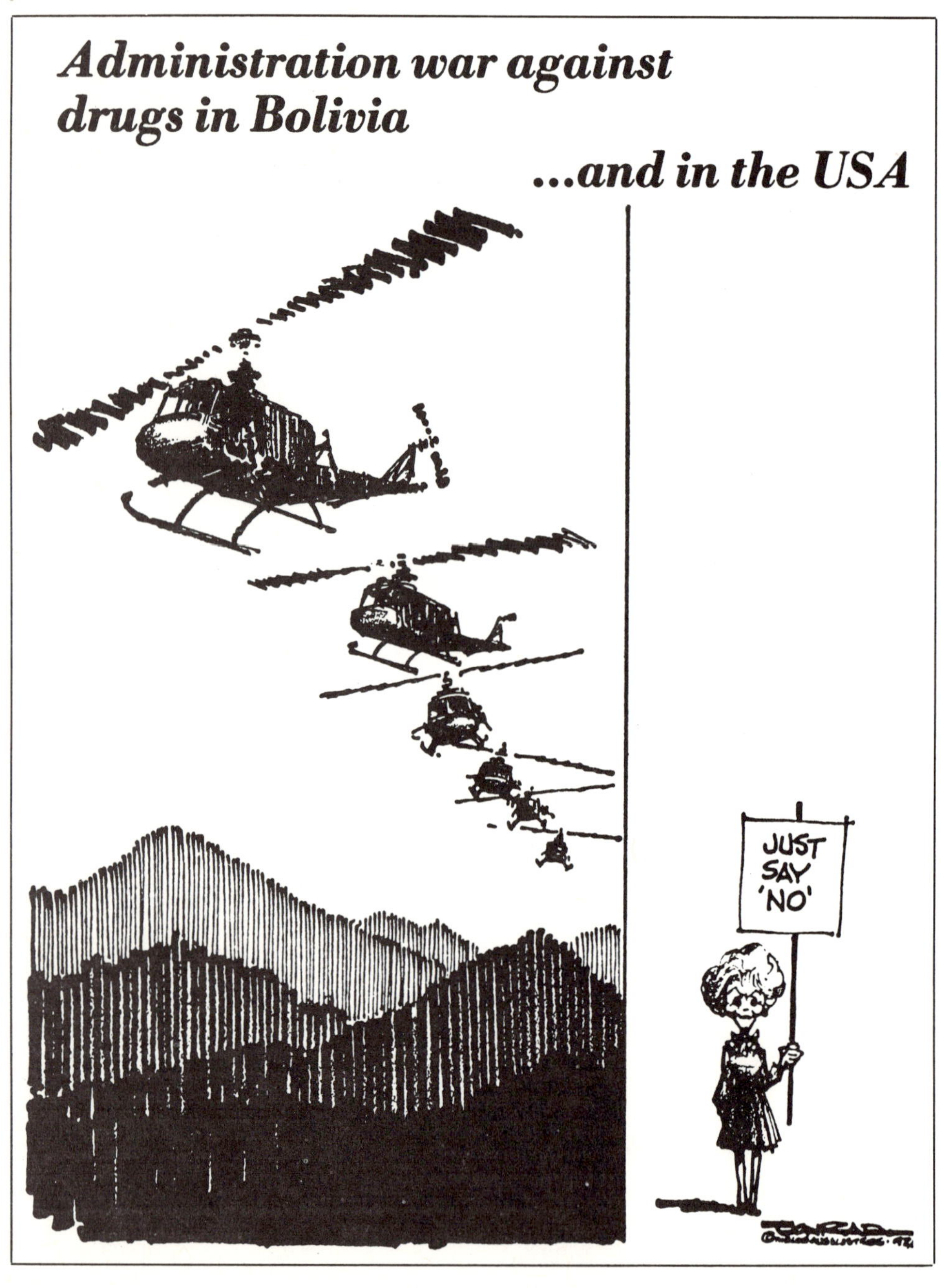

Administration war against
drugs in Bolivia
...and in the USA
JUST
SAY
'NO'

Part III: Smuggling

It has been estimated that over 90% of the illicit drugs consumed in the United States are produced in foreign countries. Supplies originate in diverse areas but basically they come from Latin America, Southeast Asia and Southwest Asia. Shipment to the U.S. is accomplished in a variety of ways. Large-scale professional smugglers use commercial planes and ships for trafficking, but they also tend to use small private aircraft. A private plane is often used on a one-time only basis to avoid detection, and landings are made at makeshift airfields in rural areas. Small boats are also used extensively for trafficking; often they are disguised as charter fishing craft. Drug-trafficking networks are not always this sophisticated, however, often employing amateur couriers who are relatively safe from arrest. The couriers are well paid and use every conceivable way of concealing drugs. Drugs have been found in suitcases with hollow bottoms; in toy dolls and animals; pressed thin and placed in books. Other innovative smugglers have been known to hide drugs in body cavities; soak their clothes in a drug solution; or swallow small pouches of a drug and later excrete them.

Drug cartels have recently appeared, such as Colombian groups known as "Cocaine Cowboys," and Southeast Asian groups. The common objective is money and the primary tactic is violence. Organized crime also engages in weapons trafficking, prostitution, gambling, pornography and other activities that directly or indirectly involve many innocent people and institutions. There are also reports of public officials at all levels who are being corrupted by drug money, particularly rural police officers who accept large sums to "look the other way" during smuggling operations.

Most illicit drugs are smuggled into the U.S. by way of New York City, Florida and California. The Drug Enforcement Administration is responsible for developing interdiction intelligence and participating in cooperative efforts with the U.S. Customs Service, the U.S. Coast Guard, and the U.S. Border Patrol (part of the Immigration and Naturalization Service), which provides the principle anti-smuggling operations at ports of entry and along land and water borders. But whether these efforts are having an effect is open to scrutiny. The South Florida Task Force, for example, which was established in 1982, claims to have reduced the flow into this key transshipment point. And while smugglers at least seem to have diversified their traffic lanes to Texas, the Carolinas and the Northeast, the Task Force has at least kept them off balance, and similar task forces have been established throughout the country as well.

Slaying of Drug Agent Adds to U.S.-Mexico Tension

Two decomposed bodies found on a ranch southeast of Guadaljara were firmly identified March 7, 1985 as those of an agent of the United States Drug Enforcement Administration (DEA) and a Mexican pilot who had sometimes flown missions for the agency. A few days earlier, Mexican federal police searching for the missing men had engaged in a gun battle with suspected drug traffickers at the ranch. The shootout resulted in the deaths of the couple who owned the ranch, their two sons and a federal police agent. Five suspects were arrested but were later released without being charged. Police reportedly confiscated weapons and two pounds of cocaine. Both the murdered men had been kidnapped in separate incidents a month before. Mexican federal officials March 14 confirmed that 13 people had been arrested in connection with the murders, including three top state police officials and at least four other policemen.

U.S. Secretary of State George Shultz met with Mexican Foreign Secretary Bernardo Sepulveda Amor March 11 in an effort to ease tensions between the two countries resulting from the murders and from an increase in crimes against Americans in Mexico. U.S. officials charged that Mexico had not acted vigorously enough in seeking to apprehend the U.S. agent's kidnappers and that police officials had aided those responsible. Mexican officials for their part, complained of U.S. searches of cars crossing the U.S.-Mexican border after the kidnapping. Those delays caused by the searches had damaged the economies of border towns.

The Washington Post

Washington, DC, March 9, 1985

The kidnapping and murder of American drug enforcement agent Enrique Camarena Salazar in Mexico must stiffen the nation's resolve to beat back the drug menace with whatever it takes.

And the lingering doubts about the way Mexican officials have handled the follow-up investigations on the case must not be brushed aside. There are indications the case could have been pursued much more vigorously.

By cold-bloodedly dispatching the agent and his pilot, the drug traffickers showed the kind of stakes they are playing for. They respect no boundaries; they will allow nothing to come between them and their massive shipments of drugs to this and other countries. Murder and the worst kinds of corruption are standard operating procedures for the narcotics traffickers.

Camarena will not have died in vain if our country commits more resources to drug interdiction — and tightens the screws on any country not fully cooperating in the effort to put the poppy, marijuana and coca fields out of business for good.

THE KANSAS CITY STAR

Kansas City, MO, March 7, 1985

Relations between the United States and Mexico have been festering slowly for some time over trade, immigration and Mexico's debt crisis. But now the pace of irritation has picked up in light of recent violence against American citizens in Mexico. This, more than the others, may be the issue that could send the fulcrum flying.

Already it has resulted in the sealing of nine border points and State Department warnings to American tourists who plan to visit certain Mexican cities.

Life can be dangerous in the United States, too. But Americans are getting the impression that not only is it risky to visit Mexico, particularly Guadalajara, but that Mexican authorities will do little to protect those who do. Although the fear of traveling to Mexico may be exaggerated, a concern for safety is valid.

While much government and media attention has been focused on the disappearance of U.S. Drug Enforcement Agent Enrique Camarena Salazar, whose body was believed to have been found Wednesday wrapped in a plastic bag, the plight of at least six missing Americans has received little notice.

Mr. Camarena and the six others disappeared in three separate incidents within a 10-week period. At least five of them were forced into cars by uniformed men in front of witnesses.

On Dec. 2, Dennis and Rose Carlsen, of California, and Ben and Patricia Mascarenas, of Nevada, vanished from a residential section of Guadalajara, where they had been distributing religious literature.

On Jan. 30, John Walker, who moved to Guadalajara from Minnesota, and Alberto Rabelat, a friend visiting from Texas, vanished after a night on the town. Mr. Camarena, possibly the most visible U.S. narcotics agent in Mexico, was lured into a car on Feb. 7.

About 27,000 Americans, mostly retirees, are believed to be living in Guadalajara without any problems. But U.S. officials have claimed the city is home to one of the largest and most powerful narcotics rings in Mexico. Narcotics was believed to have been the motive behind the Camarena kidnapping although no motive has been given for the other cases.

The Mexican government is considering establishing an office to investigate crimes against foreign visitors, but its citizens and the press have claimed such an office would discriminate against Mexicans.

A special office may not be the answer, but something has to be done pronto before the wounds become irreversibly gangrenous.

The Morning News

Wilmington, DE, March 11, 1985

IF WE truly are in a "war" against drug traffickers, use of sophisticated military equipment in the campaign seems appropriate.

Sen. Lloyd Bentsen reported Thursday that Air Force AWACS — planes equipped with very advanced radar and other detection devices — have been used on five missions in the search for airplanes being used to smuggle drugs across the U.S. border from Mexico.

The Texas Democrat said that Secretary of Defense Caspar Weinberger is "enthusiastic" about the use of the planes for this purpose and that more such missions are likely.

It really would be of great benefit to society if the drug traffic could be cut off. Just this past week the body of a U.S. agent and his pilot, presumably slain during investigations below the border, were discovered in Mexico.

The dealings in illegal drugs are staggering in the harm they do and also in the sums of money involved.

That latter is the factor which complicates the AWACS development.

Such stupendous sums change hands that the drug traffickers find it profitable to use very sophisticated equipment of their own. The stakes are such that boats and even aircraft can be abandoned after a single delivery.

It would surprise nobody, for example, if the criminals who are engaged in this body- and soul-destroying traffic could find and buy countermeasures against even these multi-million dollar flying radar installations.

Something even more fundamental than the use of military equipment — use of troops themselves apparently would be illegal — may be required for an effective crackdown.

Other observers have even suggested that the way to deal with the illegal drug traffic is to make the drugs legal — taking away from the traffickers the staggering profits which stem from their very illegality.

But if the AWACS don't do the job, something else must. Society cannot and must not bear the costs much longer.

BUFFALO EVENING NEWS
Buffalo, NY, March 13, 1985

THERE ARE big bucks involved in the international narcotics traffic, and the money attracts ruthless killers and corrupt officials. All these elements were apparently present in the kidnapping and brutal murder of an American drug agent and a Mexican pilot in Guadalajara, Mexico.

American officials have expressed justifiable anger at the inept Mexican investigation of the kidnappings and the indications of some police corruption, at least at the lower levels. The escape of one prime suspect appeared to have been aided by some police officials at a time when other Mexican police were moving in to arrest him.

Another indication of the sinister, corrupting influence of the narcotics traffic came recently with the arrest in Miami of Norman Saunders, the head of the government of the Turks and Caicos Islands, a British protectorate near the Bahamas. He is accused of accepting $50,000 from undercover agents as protection for a plot to use the islands as a transshipment point for narcotics.

The United States has major programs to assist the countries of origin in eradicating their illegal narcotic crops, but the results have been mixed at best. Colombia cooperated in the destruction of an estimated third of its illegal marijuana crop, but it is still a major source, and, in addition, Colombia is the largest source of refined cocaine.

Peru, the largest grower of coca leaf, the source of cocaine, is trying to destroy the crop with U.S. help, but the output continues to increase there and in Bolivia and Colombia. Major coca cultivations have just been discovered in Ecuador. Jamaica is the third-largest producer of marijuana and still has no agreement with the United States on eradicating or limiting the crops.

The magnitude of the problem is demonstrated by Mexico, where opium-poppy and marijuana crops increased last year despite crackdowns that included the largest narcotics raid in history. In that operation, 10,000 tons of marijuana plants were seized. The problem is aggravated by the highly organized nature of the trafficking in Mexico and the corrupting influence of Mafia-like organizations on law enforcement and political figures.

It was this sordid world of the international narcotics traffic that the slain American drug agent had penetrated at the cost of his life.

The State Department's annual report on the narcotics trade indicated that various aid programs were effective in encouraging cooperation by source countries. These programs should be continued and expanded, and, where the problem is ignored, the threat of cutbacks in aid can be a useful tool. Only by concentrated efforts on many fronts can this deadly drug trade be brought under control.

The Hartford Courant
Hartford, CT, March 15, 1985

There is shock, but no surprise, to be found in the news that an American drug enforcement agent and his Mexican pilot were found murdered on a ranch near Guadalajara.

There is shock in the singular brutality of the murders of the men, who were viciously beaten and perhaps buried alive after being kidnapped. But there is no surprise that the escalating war on drugs from Latin America should claim two more casualties.

Enrique Camarena Salazar, the U.S. Drug Enforcement Administration agent, was involved in an investigation of Guadalajara-based syndicates; his work had already cost the drug traffickers 3,600 pounds of cocaine, worth $20 million.

They were hurt and they struck back. They've got to be hurt more, until they can't or are too afraid to strike back.

The anger shown by Secretary of State George P. Shultz over the murders, and at growing suspicions of collusion by Mexican police to assist the drug traffickers in Guadalajara, should be expressed as sanctions unless the Mexican government provides hard evidence of a more aggressive crackdown on the drug trade.

The detention by Mexican authorities this week of three federal police commanders and 27 other people in connection with the murders is a hopeful sign that they are beginning to take the problem seriously.

The traffic in illegal drugs, after all, is not a harmless way for poor countries to bring in foreign currency. The stakes are so high that corruption of officials has become endemic in the countries where many of the drugs originate.

Indeed, some of the drug traffickers have become so rich and powerful that they can openly defy the government when it does try to bear down on them. Colombia, which has launched a war against cocaine, has seen some bloody battles as a result. In Peru, drug money is even being used to help finance anti-government guerrillas.

Last week five Mexican policemen were shot to death and three wounded by a group of drug traffickers.

The DEA, which has been pressing its fight to prevent drugs from reaching the United States with courage and persistence, deserves the continued support of the administration and Congress. It also deserves the support of the American people, who, it should be recalled, provide the market for the drugs.

The market includes not just addicts, but casual consumers, who ought to keep in mind the image of Mr. Camarena in a plastic body bag when they argue that cocaine or imported marijuana is a harmless indulgence.

The Times-Picayune
The States-Item
New Orleans, LA, March 9, 1985

It is no longer much of an exaggeration to describe U.S. efforts to reduce the smuggling of illegal drugs into this country as a war. The murder in Mexico of Enrique Camarena Salazar, an employee of the U.S. Drug Enforcement Administration, and his pilot, Alfredo Zavala Avelar, is tragic evidence of the deadly nature of the international drug conflict.

Mr. Camarena, a veteran drug enforcement agent and ex-Marine from Calexico, Calif., was abducted near the U.S. Consulate in Guadalajara, Mexico's second-largest city, Feb. 7. His body and that of Mr. Zavala, who also was abducted Feb. 7 by gunmen while he was on his way to the airport, were found Tuesday in plastic bags on a ranch 60 miles north of Guadalajara.

The way in which the two men were abducted and slain is worthy of the worst deeds of political terrorists, hence the similarity to the most insidious form of modern warfare. Mexico's illegal drug producers and merchants clearly wanted to send a message to the U.S. Drug Enforcement Administration and to the White House, for that matter.

The murders were not the first attempt by foreign drug dealers to discourage and demoralize U.S. drug enforcement officials. Seven DEA agents have died in the line of duty since the agency was formed in 1973. Two U.S. drug enforcement agents were lucky to survive after being kidnapped, shot repeatedly and left for dead in Colombia three years ago.

The calculated murders of Mr. Camarena and Mr. Zavala show what the U.S. government is up against as it attempts to cut off the foreign drug traffic at its source. The effort will undoubtedly be futile without the complete cooperation of foreign governments.

Unfortunately, the response of the Mexican government so far, unlike that of some other governments involved such as Colombia, has been disappointing. Secretary of State George Shultz and DEA officials have not bothered to hide their disgust over the sluggish reaction of Mexican authorities to illegal drug production in Mexico.

So what can the United States do? More diplomatic pressure is about all, it seems. For good reason, Mr. Shultz rules out economic sanctions against an otherwise friendly government of considerable importance to the United States that is struggling to strengthen its shaky economy.

Unintentionally, the murder of the U.S. drug enforcement agent and his pilot delivers another message to American society. That message is simply that the widespread demand for illegal drugs in this country played a major part in the deaths of the two men and puts the lives of other U.S. agents at risk. The drug war can't be won on the foreign front without major changes within the enormous U.S. market for which the drugs are produced.

The Miami Herald

Miami, FL, March 2, 1985

DRUG trafficking is not likely to be eliminated from the Western Hemisphere unless the human frailties that create both the demand and the temptation to profit from it are eliminated. Even so, the impossibility of actually ending drug trafficking is no excuse for exerting less than the nation's best efforts to combat it.

Containment *does* make a difference. Adolescents who never see pills don't get hooked on them. Young adults who aren't offered cocaine don't use it. People who don't have access to heroin don't buy it. Police officers who rarely see a dealer are not as likely to accept a bribe as are those who see them every day.

A staff report submitted on Tuesday to the House Foreign Affairs Committee urges an increased international effort against drug trafficking in the Americas. The committee, chaired by Rep. Dante Fascell of Miami, plans the report as the starting point for moving anti-drug efforts into the making of foreign policy. That welcome goal should be applauded throughout the nation and the hemisphere.

The committee staff highlighted corruption in Latin American police departments as a major problem, along with deficiencies in communication among various U.S. police and foreign-affairs agencies. Clearly the documenting of foreign-police complicity is a potential step toward tying economic-development and other U.S. aid to improvements in local drug enforcement. And certainly U.S. assistance to various Latin American military bureaucracies should be hinged on those commands' strict adherence to anti-drug efforts.

Ultimately illicit drugs endanger the providing nations as well as the receivers, as any Bahamian today could attest. Colombia lost a justice minister to drug-king assassins. Mexico today has its largest city's police chief awaiting extradition from California while authorities search for a U.S. drug agent kidnapped in Mexico by drug traffickers.

Fast, dirty money corrupts law enforcement and the judiciary even in societies with a long history of democracy and impartial justice. In nations steeped in oligarchy and feudal class privileges, the temptation is overwhelming. Further, widespread trafficking inevitably leads to broad local use. That makes victims of those same communities that once thought only to profit from the weakness of foreigners in the North.

Representative Fascell's committee staff has taken a crucial step toward moving this common threat onto the main agenda of the hemisphere's bargaining tables. Follow-through efforts deserve support from the entire Congress and the Administration.

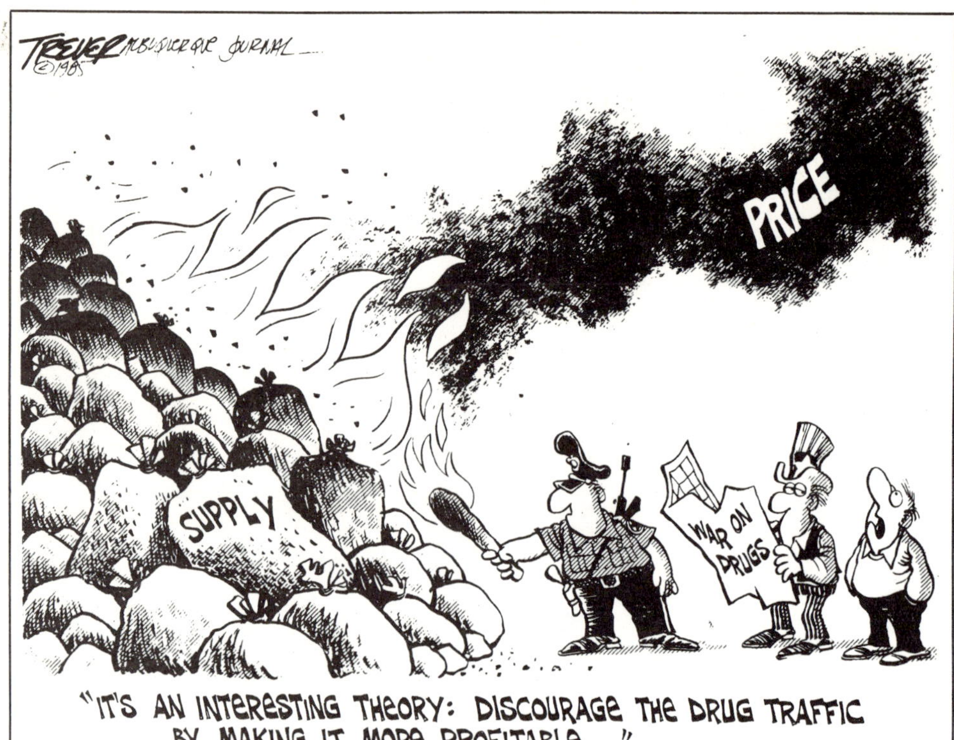

"IT'S AN INTERESTING THEORY: DISCOURAGE THE DRUG TRAFFIC BY MAKING IT MORE PROFITABLE...."

The San Diego Union

San Diego, CA, February 21, 1985

The United States is sending a message to Mexico with its intensified inspection of luggage and vehicles entering the United States. The message needs to be sent, even if it appears that the wrong people are suffering the greatest inconvenience.

Delays like those being experienced at San Ysidro are aggravating, but we trust there is no plan for a return to business as usual in the immediate future. That is the point of the message — that there can be no business as usual along our border so long as law enforcement officials in Mexico conduct business as usual with people producing illegal drugs.

U.S. officials are convinced that the Mexican federal police assigned to look for a U.S. drug enforcement agent kidnapped in Guadalajara are not really interested in finding him. A Mexican police official assigned to the case has been seen in the company of members of the drug ring believed responsible for the kidnapping. Money is said to have changed hands so the investigation will not go too far.

The *mordida* system of bribery which is known to make the wheels go round in many areas of Mexican life can be tolerated only up to a point. The point is exceeded when such corruption endangers the lives of U.S. citizens sent to Mexico to enforce the law in cooperation with Mexican police agencies. It is also exceeded when the law winks at the production and transportation of illicit drugs that are causing untold misery in the lives of citizens of this country and others.

The White House has indicated that putting a squeeze on border traffic is a tactic that would have been employed even if Enrique Camarena of the U.S. Drug Enforcement Agency had not been kidnapped Feb. 7. The administration has been growing more and more impatient with the failure of Mexico to be a more determined participant in efforts to stem the international narcotics traffic.

The State Department's annual review of the drug problem released last week praised Colombia and Peru for their programs to eradicate coca crops used to produce cocaine, but mentioned that Mexico continues to be a major source of both heroin and marijuana. A major impediment to law enforcement, according to the report, is the existence of a mafia-like organization in Mexico that wields both economic and political power to protect its drug operations.

Officials familiar with the international drug traffic say the key to success in enforcement efforts is to convince the governments of countries where drugs are produced that all the bad consequences are not being exported. Countries that once were indifferent if not hospitable toward illicit drug production have become enthusiastic partners in stamping it out when their own people, especially young people, begin turning up for treatment as addicts.

The United States is employing another device to get the attention of a reluctant government. Delays at the border affect the income that Mexico otherwise enjoys from the easy flow of commerce between our two countries. The people of Tijuana may suffer, but if they do, they should address their complaints to Mexico City. It is at the highest level of government where the power lies to replace corrupt drug enforcement officers with honest cops.

The 🌳 State

Columbia, SC, March 4, 1985

MEXICO'S suspect performance in investigating the kidnapping of an American drug enforcement agent raises anew the specter of rampant corruption in the government of the Latin American nation.

Meanwhile, the abduction of the victim, Enrique Camarema Salazar, outside the U.S. Consulate in Guadalajara, has sparked other disconcerting moves.

The United States has considered a "travel advisory" warning Americans who travel to Mexico might be unsafe. Mexico replied with a threat to limit travel of drug hunters in its territory. And Mexican President Miguel de la Madrid has complained to the White House about a border crackdown, during which U.S. Customs people have meticulously searched incoming vehicles, creating mammoth traffic jams.

What concerned Uncle Sam most was the possibility that a key suspect, a cocaine magnate, had some police protection in Mexico City. Washington charged the suspect was allowed to board an aircraft despite attempts by Mexican police to arrest him under a warrant.

As if in reply, Mexican officials arrested three former police officers Sunday and a pilot Monday in the kidnapping, but they apparently were not involved.

The American charges obviously stung the Latins, but corruption and graft are no strangers to Mexico. President de la Madrid has paid at least lip service to stopping extortion and payoffs that have permeated the government from top to bottom. From petty policemen to agency heads, officials have sought "favors," preying on a population that is dependent on the bureaucracy. The situation has helped spawn a major drug connection in Mexico.

Even though Mexican officials maintain publicly that their officials are no more corrupt than others, Mr. de la Madrid is certainly aware that scandals threaten to erode his government's credibility. Thus, he created the Federal Comptroller Secretariat to crack down on fraud.

But many suspect this agency is more show than substance. Francisco J. Rojas, who heads this newest ministry in the Mexican government, told 25 American editors who interviewed him earlier this winter that "the phenomenon of corruption is a universal one" and that cases in his country are isolated ones.

Nevertheless, the drug case, the disappearance of six other Americans in the Guadalajara area since December and the roughing up of tourists have sorely tested U.S.-Mexican links.

Mr. de la Madrid, a technocrat with noble aspirations for his nation, certainly has the right idea about reforming Mexican government. But he is now confronted with a case which will impact significantly on his country's relations with its most important neighbor. Mexico's effectiveness in dealing with the Salazar investigation will be closely watched from north of the border by a nation which is not only concerned about the safety of its agents but the further encroachment of the drug traffic.

Birmingham Post-Herald

Birmingham, AL, March 5, 1985

The kidnapping of a U.S. drug enforcement agent in Guadalajara Feb. 7 and the ineffective "investigation" by Mexican police into his disappearance have focused attention on how safe foreign visitors are in that country. The answer seems to be not very.

The State Department has been considering warning tourists of the dangers in visiting Mexico. But it has put the matter "on the shelf" for fear of roiling diplomatic relations with a country that needs a flow of tourist dollars.

Nevertheless, the U.S. Embassy in Mexico City confirms that 54 American citizens died violently in Mexico in 1984, and 1,475 assaults against Americans were reported in the Mexico City consular district alone. In Guadalajara seven U.S. citizens have disappeared in the past several months.

In response to U.S. complaints about laxness in investigating crimes against Americans, Mexico now plans to set up a new office to oversee the handling and prosecution of crimes committed against foreigners.

Prudent Americans may want to see how effective the new office will be before making a trip to Mexico. After all, when it is so easy to get mugged at home, why invest time and money to suffer the same treatment abroad?

ALBUQUERQUE JOURNAL

Albuquerque, NM, March 8, 1985

Drug smuggling has come a long way in the last decade.

In the mid 1970s, the stereotypical marijuana smuggler was a skilled pilot of a single-engine airplane, plying his trade largely as an individual entrepreneur. There was danger, but the danger came from landing on dirt roads, or flying close to the ground to evade radar. The whole thing had a certain air of derring-do and lawlessness on a lark. But violence between the chasers and the chased was rare.

Today, violence has become the lowest common denominator of the organized criminal activity related to drug smuggling. This was made chillingly apparent in the kidnap-slaying of an American Drug Enforcement Agency agent and his Mexican pilot, and in the shootout in which four Mexican drug agents died trying to stop a tank truck marijuana load.

In the case of the DEA agent's death, there were even indications that the drug lords had offered a bounty of $30,000 for the death of a senior member of the American anti-drug agency. In the drug underworld of the Americas, nothing is off limits; there is nothing without its price and the money is available to meet any price.

We recall a recent report from Colombia that drug lords offered to pay off the country's national debt in exchange for favors — or the recent drug smuggling arrests in Florida of high government officials from an obscure Caribbean island group.

Illegal drugs — marijuana, cocaine, heroin — and the astronomical sums of money they generate, have become a cancer on the societies of the countries which produce them. The debilitating effect of the illegal drug trade on the social mores of Colombia, or Mexico, is at least as serious as the effect of heroin in an American ghetto, or of cocaine in the U.S. sports and entertainment industries.

Additionally, the non-addicted, socially adjusted, productive member of American society who partakes of a little marijuana for purely social pleasure should examine his stash of crushed green leaves to make sure it isn't bloodstained.

The brutal deaths in Mexico are this violent underworld's ugly side bursting through the skin of government and society.

They should be the catalyst for a new era in the war on drugs and drug smugglers. The corruption and violent arrogance of the drug underworld have become too apparent. The recent body count should help convince the governments of the producing and exporting countries that their end of the drug problem is every bit as serious as ours.

Ending the power and corruption of the drug underground should be one of the primary focuses of hemispheric cooperation. This profit-fed guerrilla fifth column among us is as serious a threat to peaceful coexistence as any ideology-fed band of guerrillas in the hills of El Salvador — or Nicaragua.

Colombia Continues as a Top Source of Narcotics

Colombia has the dubious distinction of being the world's principal drug source, a fact which may be attributed to its strategic location on the South American continent and its geographical makeup, as well as to its experience as well-ordered trafficking community. The major processing and transshipment center for Peruvian and Bolivian coca, Colombia is allegedly responsible for 70% of the cocaine entering the United States and for 50% of the world's supply. U.S. drug enforcement officials estimate that 44 tons, with a street value of $29 billion, is annually smuggled into the U.S. from Colombia. The country also cultivates coca on some 7,200 acres that yield an estimated 4 tons of cocaine annually. Colombia is also a major exporter of marijuana to the U.S., allegedly supplying 75% of the market. An estimated 80% of other dangerous drugs entering the U.S., particularly methaqualone, are supplied through Colombia. Most of the illicit drug traffic passes through south Florida, the Gulf of Mexico and East Coast port areas. Trafficking in cocaine and marijuana, the top two money-producers, has a value to the Colombian economy of an estimated $1 to $1.5 billion, perhaps $500 million of which stays in the country and—untaxed and inflationary—undermines the legitimate economy.

Although the Colombian government has been charged with not perceiving drug abuse as a major problem, it has been suggested by outside observers that there has been an increase in the use of cocaine, marijuana and methaqualone among Colombian youth—not surprising when considering the availability of the drugs. The recent political unrest in Colombia has made it difficult to forsee what government efforts and actions will be effective. There have been reports that guerilla groups are trafficking drugs as a source of income to pay for arms shipments. Other charges have been levied against the U.S. and Colombian governments themselves alleging their tacit approval of the drug trade and the money it provides to facilitate payments of the huge International Monetary Fund (IMF) debt which Colombia owes. It is thought that even the threat of default by Colombia or any one of the drug-producing South American nations with outstanding IMF debts could send catastrophic ripples through the international economic community.

Houston Chronicle
*Houston, TX,
January 2, 1985*

More evidence of the insidious nature of the drug problem in Colombia surfaced last week, with the arrest of the second secretary of the Colombian Embassy in Madrid on drug trafficking charges.

The secretary, who had worked in the embassy for seven years, was charged with smuggling cocaine from Colombia to Spain in diplomatic packages that are exempt from customs checks. The packages were sent from the presidential press office in Bogota, still another black mark for the government.

Official corruption and the temptation of high profits have brought more and more Colombians into drug trafficking, making it one of the country's biggest industries. It is easy to see why the Colombian government is having such a tough anti-drug fight.

Because of threats connected with the crackdown on drug traffickers, dozens of American families have left Colombia, and last week U.S. Ambassador Lewis Tambs, a staunch defender of the get-tough policy, returned to the United States with his family.

Colombian President Belisario Betancur, who instigated the crackdown after the assassination of Justice Minister Rodrigo Lara last year, also has been threatened, primarily because of his insistence that Colombia extradite drug traffickers to the United States for trial. Six of the extradition requests have already been approved, although the prisoners are still in Colombian jails.

It is only a beginning, and a belated one, but the reports coming out of Colombia indicate the problem is getting the publicity and the serious attention it rightly deserves.

THE MILWAUKEE JOURNAL
Milwaukee, WI, February 25, 1985

The US State Department reported the other day that international drug trafficking is getting worse. Anybody surprised by that news must have been asleep in recent months, or smoking something weird.

In the same week that saw release of the report, Miami drug agents seized a Colombian 747 cargo jet loaded with more than a ton of cocaine. A few days earlier, drug merchants in Mexico kidnapped a US Drug Enforcement Administration agent. And terrorists reportedly have embarked from Colombia to attack DEA agents and buildings in this country.

Although the State Department cautioned that it was hard to be precise about such figures, its report indicated that in most of the world's drug-producing countries, drug-producing crops (like marijuana) were more plentiful in 1984 than in 1983. The production of coca (used to make cocaine) grew by more than one-third in Bolivia, Peru and Colombia. Clearly, much of the end product ends up in the US market.

What can be done? Under a new law, the president must cut off US aid to countries that don't cooperate in the war against international drug trade. Not surprisingly, some members of Congress want those sanctions invoked, and one State Department official says he wouldn't hesitate to recommend such aid reductions.

That might backfire. In Bolivia and certain other countries, traffic in drug-producing crops has become a major source of foreign exchange. A cutoff or reduction of US aid to those countries might make them even more dependent on illicit drug commerce. In Burma, the government report noted, another problem exists: Most of the opium-growing regions are controlled by anti-government militias.

Well, if aid reduction is a less-than-promising weapon against drug merchants, what can the United States do?

For one thing, it can recognize that international drug commerce is a national security issue rather than mainly a problem in state and regional law-enforcement. In a real sense, this country is under attack. Several southern governors have appealed for (and deserve) help from the Defense Department in intercepting drug-laden ships and planes that are bound for the US. That needs to be done in accord with international law, of course, but it seems to us that ways can be found to bolster US barriers against such poisonous cargo.

US technical help in the specific task of eradicating drug-producing crops ought to be offered to countries that demonstrate a will to fight illegal drugs. Some governments are up to the task. Despite political violence (including at least one assassination) and an increase in coca production, Colombia destroyed as much as one-third of its marijuana crop last year. If Colombia can do that, so can other countries.

US officials should make it plain to those countries, such as Bolivia and Jamaica, that unless they get moving to follow Colombia's lead, an aroused Congress is likely to cut off aid or maybe take even more drastic action. Those countries also should be reminded that rampant drug crime threatens the stability of their own regimes.

The choices are difficult. The worst choice, though, would be to do nothing more than is already being done about the growing drug threat to the nation's security.

The Evening Gazette

Worcester, MA, July 13, 1985

If, as reported, the major Colombian cocaine producers have called a truce and formed a production cartel, cocaine trafficking may become even harder to control than it is now.

Investigators say that three major Colombian distribution networks have reached an understanding, pooling resources to convert cocaine base into cocaine power in rural "factories" in the United States. Officials say the laboratories used to produce the drug represent a "major change" in the distribution of cocaine in the United States.

Formerly, processed cocaine was smuggled into this country. Raids on Long Island, upstate New York and Virginia Wednesday netted enough base and chemicals to produce 7,000 pounds of the cocaine. Each network has its own supplies of cocaine base but has agreed to share the facilities and equipment needed to process it for the illicit drug market, investigators claim.

Ten Colombians were arrested during the raids, but authorities failed to net Jaime Orjuela, the reputed and long-sought top U.S. agent of Colombia's cocaine "families."

The raids slowed down the operation, but cooperation among drug traffickers is bad news for U.S. enforcement officials. The trend toward drug-production factories in the United States will further complicate the daunting job of controlling the drug traffic from South America.

The Washington Post

Washington, DC, March 20, 1985

AN IMPORTANT conviction was obtained in a trial that ended last weekend in federal court here. Marcos Cadavid, a major figure in the Colombian drug trade, was found guilty of conspiracy to distribute cocaine in the Washington area between 1976 and 1983. In a series of transactions, he had been paid more than $20 million in cash.

The prosecution is significant as the first in what is expected to be a series of trials made possible by a new extradition treaty signed between the United States and Colombia. Until recently, the powerful and dangerous narcotics kingpins in Colombia were not only hard to prosecute in that country, they were also safe from prosecution for crimes committed here. But now, President Belisario Betancur's drive against drug dealers has produced dramatic results, in his own country and here.

Four Colombian traffickers have already been extradited and a number of sealed indictments have been handed up that will result in additional American prosecutions of Colombians. There has been some backlash from criminals in Colombia. The State Department, fearful of reprisals against Americans visiting that country, advised travelers to be particularly careful. But the crackdown continued. With the help of the armed forces, Colombian law enforcement officers moved in, seizing drugs, burning marijuana fields and making arrests. Some large producers have already moved their operations to neighboring countries.

This assault on the drug trade is important for its connection to crime in this country, and for what it means for the Colombian government. According to U.S. Ambassador Lewis Tambs, the growth of the narcotics trade has caused widespread addiction in Colombia and has handsomely financed armed revolutionaries operating in the rural regions.

Mr. Cadavid's six-day trial was conducted under tight security, for threats had been received that were taken very seriously. The jurors were sequestered; steps were taken to protect the judge and prosecutors; armed guards were even stationed on the roof of the courthouse when the defendant was moved to and from the building. It was all worthwhile. A major criminal will be sent to prison here for many years, and the Colombians have been reassured that American courts are a valuable ally in the effort to stem this vicious trade between the two countries.

THE SUN

Baltimore, MD, August 2, 1985

Those concerned about drug abuse should be cheered by recent events in Latin America. In one operation, Colombian and Peruvian police, aided by U.S. drug agents, used helicopters to storm four cocaine processing centers 700 miles northeast of Peru's capital, Lima.

One laboratory, in a complex of buildings valued at $500 million, had its own 2,000-foot long, concrete airstrip; five planes with computerized navigation; six dormitories holding 100 people each; and equipment to handle 500 pounds of cocaine a week.

Under pressure from U.S. agencies, the Colombian government cracked down on drug traffickers last year, chasing them into Peru, Brazil and Ecuador. Now authorities are tracking the drug kings to their jungle hideouts.

There is progress here as well:

☐ In Philadelphia, FBI agents broke up a multi-million-dollar cocaine ring allegedly run by dentists who began dealing drugs in professional school. Agents in Miami and other cities arrested most other members of a ring that was alleged to be national in scope.

☐ In June, Maryland State Police arrested three airline passengers from Florida and confiscated a kilogram of cocaine. Troopers then raided six residences, netting $800,000 worth of cocaine, autos and records.

☐ Police stopped a 60-year-old man in a 1980 Malibu on the Harbor Tunnel Thruway recently and found 17.6 pounds of cocaine, sealed in plastic bags and stashed in the trunk. A raid in Waverly turned up 26 more pounds. Officers said a "ring of middle-aged men" had been importing $18 million in drugs a year.

☐ A *New York Times* series detailed drug use among professional baseball players. Records show that a photographer and a telecommunications salesman in Pittsburgh and a Philadelphia caterer are charged with selling drugs to players on several teams, the *Times* said. A Pittsburgh heating manufacturer pled guilty to similar charges, and a Kansas City man was sentenced in 1982 to six years in prison.

Many think the amount of cocaine available and the wide demand for it mean that the epidemic can never be stemmed. But law-enforcement officials say the big seizures are proof they are penetrating the "circles of friends" supplying middle-class customers.

If they are right, if people who have careers, businesses and reputations to lose continue to go to prison, cocaine will lose its respectability. The higher probability of prosecution would then put a damper on open drug use at parties and casual trading in middle-class circles. The drug epidemic may not be so unstoppable after all.

THE LINCOLN STAR

Lincoln, NE, February 20, 1985

News reports tell of a disturbing offer by narcotics traffickers in Colombia of up to $350,000 for the kidnapping of Drug Enforcement Administration chief Francis M. Mullen. From the streets of Mexico, four suspected drug dealers recently captured DEA agent Enrique Salazar Camarena and he has not been heard from since.

But the drug dealers are in for a surprise. The billions that are a part of the total illegal drug business in this country will not be enough to sustain the traffickers in their entry into the field of terrorism.

This country has faced well organized, well financed and ruthless crime in its past and will continue to do so. But crime and criminals have invariably come out the losers.

Just this past week, several of the more famed Mafia families of this country were decimated with a series of arrests by the FBI, including the arrest of family patriarchs.

But while the barons of illegal drug dealings ultimately will fail, they present a challenge that is highly threatening. It is reported that hit squads from South America are being sent into this country to capture, torture and kill DEA agents.

The drug business has become an international matter of high importance. If the threat posed by this business is to be successfully met, it will require the understanding and support of the American people. It will take a substantial investment to curtail a movement that has millions of dollars to throw around as rewards for acts of violence against law enforcement officials.

Intimidation has long been a tool of the lawless, and today's drug dealers use it with a vengeance. There is no alternative for this country but to appropriate the funds and enlist and train the personnel who are essential to bring this dirty business to its knees.

DAILY☰NEWS

New York, NY, February 17, 1985

A new law bans U.S. aid to countries that don't cut production of dangerous drugs. Last year there were bumper crops, and the culprits include seven that receive aid. Among them are Bolivia, Belize and Jamaica, and if they don't shape up, all aid should be cut off. They need American support desperately. There's a price, and they must pay it.

Others are making an effort, notably Colombia. Peru is fighting terrorism and has abandoned the war on cocaine. It's not good enough: The U.S. must insist there is nothing more corrupting than to let the drug dealers take over.

Even if all these countries stamped out coca, marijuana and opium, others would replace them. Production is rising rapidly in Brazil, for instance. The war on drugs can only be won by an international effort, and it's hard for the U.S. to organize because the worst culprits are the American customers, yuppies from Suffolk to Marin County who get their thrills sniffing coke through a $20 bill.

The Kansas City Times

Kansas City, MO, February 19, 1985

Reports that Colombian drug traffickers are offering up to $350,000 for the kidnapping of Francis M. Mullen, chief of the U.S. Drug Enforcement Administration, show that the enforcement methods of the two governments are working.

Colombia's Justice Minister Rodrigo Lara Bonilla was assassinated last April as a warning to President Belisario Betancur to cease the anti-drug campaign. Now this threat against the American.

There also have been bombings outside the American Embassy in Bogata where many U.S. personnel and their families have been evacuated. Others may leave as the situation worsens.

Colombia is believed to be the primary source of illegal drugs for the U.S., and both governments are trying to combat the problem which continues through this symbiotic relationship. Last May Colombian authorities destroyed a cocaine-processing center believed to be capable of producing 13,000 pounds a month.

U.S. helicopters were sent to Colombia in September to spray thousands of acres of marijuana with herbicide and strip coca leaves used to make cocaine. These important deterrents only temporarily disturb the cycle. Extradition of traffickers is proving to be the more effective method. It is what the drug dealers warned the two governments not to do.

At least three extradited Colombians are to stand trial in Miami and another in Washington. They have hired some American lawyers. While the extradition process has been slowed by Mr. Betancur's reluctance to send his drug-smuggler citizens to be tried in a foreign land, this important campaign by the two governments should not stop.

Those extradited can reveal far more about the problem than a naked coca tree or dead marijuana forest. And that's what has Colombian smugglers and their American customers worried the most.

The Miami Herald

Miami, FL, January 10, 1985

THE FIRST four Colombians ever extradited to the United States to face drug-trafficking charges have arrived amid much-deserved praise for Colombia's President Belasario Betancur. Despite mounting violence directed at American diplomats, Colombian officials, and U.S.-financed drug-eradication programs in his country, President Betancur has been steadfast in his heroic commitment to rid his country of its infamous drug industry. Colombia is the world's largest supplier of illicit drugs.

The four Colombians extradited are not the kingpins that authorities have been trying to apprehend. However, they are "important cases," according to a U.S. Justice Department spokesman.

The four are Hernan Botero Moreno, president of the *Atletico Nacional* soccer team in Medellin, Colombia, wanted on money-laundering charges involving a Broward County bank; Said and Ricardo Pavon Jatter, sought in the 1982 Operation Swordfish money-laundering investigation involving a Miami business set up by Federal agents and charged with several counts of conspiracy to import and distribute cocaine; and Marco Cadavid, a businessman facing charges in connection with a nationwide cocaine ring that allegedly laundered its profits through a Washington bank.

Although the U.S. and Colombian governments had signed an extradition treaty in 1982, it lay fallow until the assassination of Colombian Justice Minister Rodrigo Lara Bonilla in May 1984. That killing, believed to have been ordered by drug traffickers, convinced President Betancur finally to allow Colombian nationals to be extradited for prosecution. Mr. Lara Bonilla had become a threat by making impressive hits on drug-processing laboratories, at one time seizing 13.8 tons of cocaine, the largest seizure ever.

Colombian officials have agreed to extradite 18 people accused of drug-trafficking. However, the United States has asked the Colombians to extradite 70 of their nationals, most of them wanted on drug charges in this country.

These four initial extraditions are an encouraging step. May President Betancur now take the next one by extraditing all those Colombians against whom U.S. authorities have brought drug charges.

Miami, FL, February 21, 1985

U.S. CUSTOMS officials had every right to impound the Avianca Airlines Boeing 747 cargo plane in which inspectors found 1.25 tons of smuggled cocaine worth $600 million on the street. The seizure caused ill will between Customs and the Drug Enforcement Agency, however, and it also brought strenuous protests from Colombia's ambassador to the United States and from lawyers for Avianca, the Colombian government's airline.

Now the plane — Avianca's only all-cargo 747 — is back in Avianca's hands in a negotiated settlement that preserves equity all around. The airline will put up cash and notes totaling $1.98 million against possible civil penalties should Avianca be deemed at fault for the smuggled cargo, the 34th seizure made from its aircraft since April 1980. Moreover, Avianca will forfeit the 747 should a U.S. court so order. Refusal could cost Avianca its authorization to operate in the United States. That's a penalty that Colombia wouldn't dare risk.

It would have been self-defeating U.S. diplomacy to prolong the plane's impoundment. After all, Colombia has made enormous efforts to curb its pervasive drug industry since the assassination last year of its justice minister. Colombia's continued crackdown is essential if the flow of cocaine and marijuana from there to Florida is ever to be stemmed.

The plane's release doesn't solve the larger problem involving Avianca and smuggled drugs, however. The U.S. Government must insist that Avianca be more diligent in preventing illegal drugs from being smuggled aboard its aircraft in Colombia. If nothing else, the seizure of this key aircraft should persuade Colombian authorities that, absent that diligence, Avianca's planes will be impounded and sitting idle instead of flying legitimate cargo and earning legitimate profits.

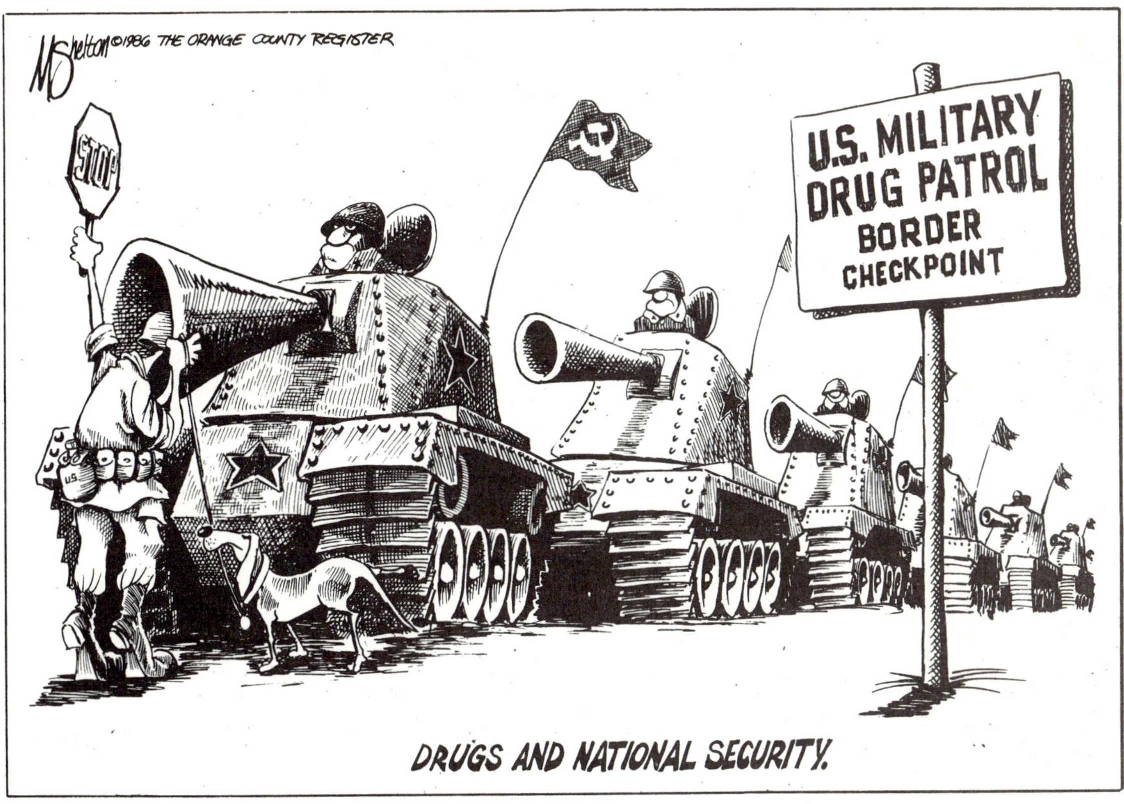

THE LINCOLN STAR

Lincoln, NE, June 26, 1986

Judging from news reports on the extensive influence of illegal drug trafficking in South America, the threat of political upheaval may be a minor issue. The Associated Press reported trafficking families offered to pay Colombia's $12.5 billion foreign debt and bring home their enormous fortune if the government would give them immunity from extradition to the United States.

Similar reports of massive use of illegal drug gains were reported in many other nations of South America. The money from criminal drug activity has infiltrated and corrupted many levels of government throughout the region.

Officials have noted that those who traffic in illegal drugs are able to pay more for the services of public officials than the governments for whom such officials work. A Bahamian official spoke of the great difficulty for society when one night of drug trafficking can earn you $10,000 as opposed to a legitimate wage of $3 an hour.

A U.S. official has referred to the sumptuously rich traffickers in cocaine, marijuana and heroin. Most of these drugs are coming into the United States.

That means, of course, that the billions being paid for the drugs are coming from the United States. The sale of illegal drugs, therefore, is even of major economic concern in this country's balance of trade. Those sales are a total loss of wealth from the United States.

The many other consequences of this traffic in illegal drugs are devastating to both the United States and South America. Use of such drugs in this country feeds crime at all levels and creates endless social problems. The human loss from the situation is absolute disaster.

In South America, the destruction of the moral fiber of society and of government presents far more of a political threat than the ideology of communism. What communism could not win in any free exchange of ideas it might well win in the ebb and flow of laundered dirty drug money.

With all its other problems, billions of dollars in tainted funds is not what the nations of South America need. It is exactly the opposite of the kind of discipline that might otherwise build a productive and satisfied society.

Legal action against this drug traffic does not come easily or inexpensively. But given the nature of the threat and its economic liability, far more financial resources and manpower than exist at present are justified in the fight against this insidious criminal activity.

The Seattle Times

Seattle, WA, September 21, 1986

IT'S EASY for North Americans, from a comfortable distance, to decry the power of the Colombian cocaine kings. People who challenge those underworld lords in their own country are singularly brave.

Raul Echevarria Barrios, a newsman in the Colombian city of Cali, wrote an editorial last week supporting a bill in the U.S. House of Representatives that calls for the execution of drug dealers.

"Those that produce cocaine and its derivatives," Echevarria wrote, "those that sow marijuana, those that introduce those toxic substances in their countries and put them within reach of the public, are executioners."

The brave journalist was proved precisely right the very next day, when he was shot to death by a man who sped away on a motorcycle.

Seattle, WA, January 6, 1985

THE power of Colombia's cocaine kings has seldom been more disturbingly evident than in recent days, when they in effect drove the U.S. ambassador out of their country.

Lewis Tambs and his family, who have received telephoned threats from drug traffickers, packed up and left for home.

Because of the threats, some nine other U.S. diplomats and their families also have left Colombia. Many U.S. business executives working in Colombia have said they were leaving or at least sending their families out of the country.

Being in the Foreign Service these days, particularly in some Third World countries, is more dangerous than most forms of military service. Most of the danger is related to politics rather than drugs, of course.

The troubles in Colombia center on a U.S. request for the extradition of 70 Colombians on drug charges. Showing great personal courage, President Belisario Betancur has approved at least six of the requests. It remains to be seen how much compliance actually will occur.

The Reagan administration should resort to a policy, briefly followed in the Carter administration, of relating the degree of economic aid to certain Latin countries to the degree of their cooperation in battling the illegal narcotics trade.

Panama's Army Chief Tied to Drugs, Murder by U.S.

Panama's army commander, who is effectively the leader of the country, was deeply involved in a number of illegal activities, including drug trafficking and the supply of arms to Colombian rebels, according to information gathered by United States intelligence sources. The officer, Gen. Manuel Antonio Noriega, was also involved in the 1985 murder of a political opponent, Dr. Hugo Spadafora, senior U.S. State Department, Pentagon and intelligence sources said. The charges were published in the June 12, 1986 edition of the *New York Times*. The *Times* said senior White House officials were aware of the charges against Noriega but initially refused to discuss them for fear of damaging relations with Panama. Panama is vital to U.S. interests in Latin America. The U.S. has a vast intelligence-gathering network there to monitor all of Central America and most of South America. It was through this network that the extensive file on Noriega's illegal activities was said to have been gathered. Noriega's activities were said to have caused a dilemma for successive U.S. administrations, which had to weigh Panama's strategic value to the U.S. against denouncing illegal operations by its top officers. The *Times* said officials in the Reagan and past administrations had decided to overlook Noriega's various illegal operations because he had cooperated with U.S. intelligence agencies and permitted the U.S. military to operate in Panama.

The *Times* cited a recent classified report by the Defense Intelligence Agency that said Noriega tightly controlled drug trafficiking and money laundering by associates in the Panama Defense Force. According to a White House official, Noriega directed the most significant drug trade in Panama, which had been described in a 1985 assessment by the U.S. House Foreign Affairs Committee as a "drug and chemical transshipment point and money-laundering center for drug money." U.S. intelligence sources were quoted as saying Noriega played the role of "facilitator." As such, he was paid a percentage of drug profits for "protection of the traffic." He provided facilities to traffickers through his secret investments in Panamanian companies and his involvement in a number of trading concerns. Noriega and Panamanian President Eric Arturo Delvalle denied the charges June 12, 1986 after an emergency meeting of top Panamanian government officials.

THE SACRAMENTO BEE

Sacramento, CA, June 26, 1986

Officially, the Reagan administration is treating accusations of political murder, election fraud, drug smuggling and gunrunning by the military strongman of Panama as "basically a Panamanian affair." That's as it should be. At the same time, key administration officials are letting it be known that they consider the allegations to be true. That, too, is as it should be.

If even half the charges in the intelligence dossier on Gen. Manuel Antonio Noriega — officially the armed forces chief but in fact Panama's dictator — are true, the calculated risk Washington is taking in confirming press reports of his misdeeds is one worth taking. There's strong popular opposition to Noriega, so that making known U.S. displeasure with his behavior is less likely to be seen, as it would elsewhere, as unwelcome Yanqui meddling. It's important, though, for the U.S. response to remain a low-key one. This country has 10,000 troops and a strategic interest in Panama, which by treaty will take full sovereignty over the Panama Canal in just 14 years.

For years U.S. officials found it expedient to deal with Noriega, who supplied intelligence information about Cuban activities in Panama (all the while keeping Havana posted about U.S. operations there). But since becoming Panama's kingmaker, Noriega apparently has committed the sin of excess. He is charged with subverting Panama's return to democratic rule, first by rigging the 1984 presidential election for his handpicked candidate, Nicolas Ardito Barletta, then, in 1985, by forcing Barletta to quit after he dared to call for an investigation of a political murder that opponents say Noriega ordered. At the same time, the general is accused of supplying leftist Colombian guerrillas with weapons in return for narcotics whose final destination is this country.

Narcotics production for export, mostly to the United States, has become a major industry in a number of Latin American countries. Poverty, corruption and intimidation of officials make eradication of large-scale drug trafficking all but impossible. Given the unsavory history of its ruling military clique, that may be the case in Panama. It's just possible, though, that the spotlight now focused on Noriega will persuade his colleagues that such egregious behavior mandates a change. Whether that happens or not, it's important that this country dissociate itself from a dictator's ugly abuse.

Detroit Free Press

Detroit, MI, June 22, 1986

U.S. RELATIONS with the military strongmen of Latin America have long been problematic. Often, our policy has been to close our eyes to their human rights abuses because they have brought stability to a part of the world where it is often lacking. Yet sometimes their excesses become too great to ignore.

The activities of Gen. Manuel Noriega, head of Panama's armed forces and the power behind the Panamanian president, appear to be just such a case. And, according to recent news reports, U.S. self-interest and Gen. Noriega were on a collision course in 1972 when his alleged involvement in drug trafficking prompted the suggestion that he be assassinated. Cooler heads in the Nixon administration wisely rejected that notion.

Recent news reports have alleged the general's continuing involvement in the drug trade, as well as in gun-running and money-laundering activities. They also claimed that he has close links to Libya, Cuba, the Palestine Liberation Organization, and leftist insurgents in Colombia and El Salvador, and, citing U.S. intelligence officials' secret testimony before Congress, that he planned and supervised the murder last year of a political opponent.

Understandably, as Secretary of State George Shultz said last week, the reports about Gen. Noriega are "of importance and concern" to those responsible for formulating U.S. foreign policy, particularly as they look ahead to the year 2000, when Panama is to take over defense of the Panama Canal.

In anticipation of the transfer of responsibility for that strategic waterway, the Panama Defense Force has already swelled to 15,000 members and is expected to reach 20,000. Its budget is approximately $90 million. Panama is nominally a civilian-run country, but few deny that Gen. Noriega is the boss.

Though the allegations against him should not be used as an excuse for heavy-handed U.S. meddling, they must be taken seriously, and the situation closely monitored.

THE PLAIN DEALER
Cleveland, OH, June 28, 1986

The disclosure that Panama's military leader stole his country's 1984 presidential election for a comrade was leaked to the press by the Reagan administration for a reason. The public should keep that in mind the next time the president or CIA Director William Casey denounces government leaks.

In this case, the leak was orchestrated by the administration to counter Sen. Jesse Helms' efforts to undercut the treaty that returned the Panama Canal to Panama. To save the pact and neutralize Helms, who has been hammering away at Gen. Manuel Antonio Noriega, the administration has been forced to acknowledge the sordid details of the stolen election.

Noriega is said by administration officials to be involved in drug dealing and in feeding sensitive information to Cuba. They say he is responsible for stealing the 1984 Panamian presidential election from Arnulfo Arias Madrid, a popular nationalist the United States considered anti-American and a threat to U.S. interests in Panama.

The White House instead supported Nicolas Ardito Barletta, whose candidacy also was supported by Noriega. When it became apparent that Barletta was losing the election—Panama's first for a president since 1968—Noriega halted the vote count. National guard troops seized ballot boxes and the count was rigged in Barletta's favor.

In blowing the whistle on Noriega, who among his other misdeeds forced Barletta from office in 1985 when the president insisted on probing the murder of a Noriega critic, the administration now admits:

• That it knew before the election that Noriega was prepared to steal it for Barletta.

• That Noriega did steal it and the United States had massive evidence of the fraud at the time it was being committed.

• That the administration adopted a policy to ignore the vote theft and to support Barletta because it was in the United States' interests to do so. Thus, in response to widespread charges of fraud after Barletta was declared the winner, the United States claimed it had received no evidence of fraud. Yet, before the election, the administration had warned that any attempt to steal votes could result in a cut off of U.S. aid to Panama.

Only the naive would consider that threat genuine, given the strategic value of Panama and its canal to the United States. That warning, however, in light of what the administration now admits happened, places the United States in an awkward situation. Does the United States stand four-square behind the democratic process or doesn't it?

Noriega undoubtably is a bad egg. He has only been exposed now by the administration, in a rare airing of dirty linen, because of Helms' use of previously classified information to undermine the canal treaties.

The affair reveals much about the struggle for influence over foreign policy in Washington. It also points to the historical weak link in America's policy toward Latin America.

Gratitude is only temporary for foreign political or military leaders whom Washington buys politically. The administration's policy in Panama was to look the other way while the Panamanian people were being deprived of the right to elect the person a majority wanted to be their president. Neither they nor the interests of the United States have been served well by that bit of double-dealing.

St. Petersburg Times
St. Petersburg, FL, June 26

It's common knowledge that Gen. Manuel Antonio Noriega is the true power behind the presidency in Panamanian politics. Authoritative U.S. intelligence reports show that Noriega, commander of the Panamanian army, worked to rig Panama's 1984 presidential election in favor of Nicolas Ardito Barletta — and then forced Barletta out of office last year because of a fear that the new president would pursue charges that Noriega was involved in the torture and murder of a political opponent.

And unless the Reagan administration and Congress act quickly to determine the facts surrounding the 1984 Panamanian election — including the American role in its staging and outcome — it will appear that Noriega also is capable of wielding inordinate power behind the closed doors of our own government.

Administration officials acknowledge that Barletta was chosen as a figurehead presidential candidate equally acceptable to Washington and Noriega. Among other assets on Barletta's resume was a stint as an economics student under George Shultz at the University of Chicago. Still unexplained, however, is the logic behind the Reagan administration's apparent decision to do business with Noriega, who was already known to be a corrupt and unreliable ally.

Panama had had no presidential election since 1968; in the meantime, the country was led by a government controlled by a succession of military strongmen. Noriega's predecessor, Brig. Gen. Omar Torrijos Herrera, was generally considered a dependable friend of the United States. But questions of Noriega's character and ultimate loyalties have been unresolved for more than a decade.

Documents show that officials of the Nixon administration were so concerned with Noriega's involvement in illegal drug trafficking that they considered several proposals, including assassination, to remove the general from power. Beyond that, U.S. officials accuse Noriega of having provided vital intelligence information to Cuba and other governments (as well as our own) for at least 15 years.

The United States' connection, however tenuous, to Noriega's strongman rule makes a mockery of the Reagan administration's general policy of promoting democratic reform in Latin America. Of more immediate importance to our own security, Noriega's erratic leadership threatens the future of the agreement under which the United States gradually turns control of the Panama Canal over to Panama.

The United States obviously has a vital long-term interest in the maintenance of a friendly, reliable government in Panama. But that interest will not be served by a marriage of convenience with a tyrant whose loyalty is constantly on sale to the highest bidder.

Noriega was warned prior to the 1984 elections that any attempt to subvert the political process would result in a cutoff of U.S. aid. Despite evidence of fraud at the time, aid continued unabated. A similar threat, with real meaning behind it, is needed to convince Noriega and his associates that Panama must join the democratic movement that has swept most of its Latin American neighbors.

THE KANSAS CITY STAR
Kansas City, MO, June 17, 1986

Panama's armed forces chief, Gen. Manuel Noriega, received a most unpleasant welcome while in the U.S. last week. The general, who has made certain his path is unobstructed in pseudo-democratic Panama, walked right smack into a real democracy and its free press. While in the U.S., Gen. Noriega was treated to a front-page story in *The New York Times* in which intelligence sources accused him of drug trafficking and other corruption, running guns to terrorists, murder, and supplying information to the Cubans and the U.S. simultaneously. What was not in the newspaper was broadcast on NBC television.

As the general is the true head of state in Panama, not President Eric Arturo Delvalle, it is safe to assume that Panamanian newspapers would not have carried such stories. The general runs the country and things have a way of happening to uncooperative media people and dissidents. The decapitated body of one outspoken critic, Hugo Spadefora, was found last year at the Panama-Costa Rica border.

The charges against the general, if true, could have adverse affects on U.S.-Panamanian relations. Regional peace plans would also be imperiled. Gen. Noriega has been accused of supplying Colombia's leftist M-19 guerrillas with guns to overthrow the Colombian government. Panama and Colombia are half the Contadora Group.

Gen. Noriega seems to be loyal only to himself. He has supplied the U.S. with intelligence information about Cuba and the Nicaraguan Sandinistas and offered the same to Cuba on American activities in Panama, the media reported. Panama is a training ground for numerous military exercises and other national security activities. For this reason, the administration must step lightly in solving what is not only a domestic problem for Panamanians, but a bilateral one, requiring U.S. action.

The Washington Post
Times Herald

Washington, DC, June 24, 1986

Suddenly in parts of the press and television there is a retelling of the more or less familiar story of Panama's strongman, Gen. Manuel Noriega, accused drug trafficker, weapons peddler, murderer, double agent (spying for both the United States and Cuba), election fixer and coup maker. Interesting details have come to light, but what is even more intriguing are the possible explanations of why the rerun is occurring and of whose interest it serves.

The more innocent explanation is that the information on Gen. Noriega took on a shape so ominous and undeniable that the American intelligence agencies collecting it and the political bureaus receiving it simply could not keep it to themselves. The administration was caught between an American habit of winking at local foibles in order to enjoy the strategic comforts of close association with Panama, and its growing apprehension that Gen. Noriega's misrule was threatening to undermine the American interest in the stability of the country and its great canal.

A darker explanation is that elements on the American right who have never reconciled themselves to the Panama Canal treaties are pumping out damaging information about Gen. Noriega in order to make a case for going back on the American treaty commitment to turn over the canal to Panama in the year 2000. Sen. Jesse Helms (R-N.C.), who has used his Senate Foreign Relations subcommittee to air some of the charges, allows that "it may be entirely necessary down the road" for the United States to try to assume power over the Panama Canal again. An odd political matchup is taking place in Washington: conservatives whose interest is to demonstrate Panamanian frailty, liberals appalled by Gen. Noriega's human rights record.

In this murky scene, two things are clear. Gen. Noriega, who presides over a system that does not permit a fair judgment of the shocking charges against him, does not have a mandate from the Panamanian people and must allow the country's admittedly frail and uncertain democratic process to get back on its feet. Meanwhile, the United States—and this means Congress, too—cannot afford to give the slightest sustenance to the notion of revising the canal treaties. That way lies a cynical cultivation of instability in Panama and a threat to the strategic assets that the United States removed from risk precisely by the treaties some would now casually reopen.

Birmingham Post-Herald
Birmingham, AL, June 16, 1986

As if the United States did not have enough headaches in Central America, it now must decide what to do, if anything, about a Panamanian businessman whose business is, well, Panama.

The amigo in question is Gen. Manuel Antonio Noriega, head of the Panama Defense Force, who rules the strategically placed nation through a dummy civilian president, Eric Arturo Delvalle.

According to U.S. intelligence sources, quoted by The New York Times and NBC News, Noreiga is a busy beaver who intends to get as rich as such world-class crooks as Baby Doc Duvalier and Fredinand Marcos.

Noriega and his cronies in the Panamanian military run money-laundering activities for drug dealers. They protect drug shipments in and out of the country for a price. And they provide weapons to M-19, pro-Cuban guerrillas who are fighting to overthrow the democratically elected government of neighboring Colombia.

In addition, the good general is a secret investor in a Panamanian company that sells embargoed American technology to Cuba and the communist bloc in Europe. And for 15 years he has provided valuable information to the CIA, while evenhandedly furnishing Havana with intelligence on the United States.

Noriega presents a dilemma to Washington policymakers. He clearly is an asset to international drug traffickers who are ravaging this nation's youth. He also permits American actions that a successor might not: He allows the National Security Agency to eavesdrop on much of Latin America and the U.S. Army to conduct clandestine missions from Panama.

For this newspaper, the choice is easier than for the CIA and NSA. When you stay too close to a corrupt dictator for too long, as with Cuba's Batista, Nicaragua's Somoza and Iran's shah, you end up with virulently anti-American successor regimes.

Thus, if the Reagan administration can figure out how, it ought to facilitate Noriega's departure and his replacement by an honest democrat. He already has a vast fortune hidden in European banks and a house in southern France, not far from Baby Doc's, and the French economy needs all the help it can get.

Lexington Herald-Leader
Lexington, KY, June 24, 1986

Don't look now, but there's a crisis to the south. A Central American nation located near a vital U.S. strategic interest has been selling secrets to the Cubans. Its leaders are involved in smuggling drugs into this country. The military helped rig the country's last elections.

Clearly, it's time to send the Marines in to clean up this mess in Nicaragua, right?

Wrong.

The country in question is Panama, not Nicaragua. And the Reagan administration seems perfectly tolerant of this state of affairs.

This is a peculiar state of affairs. The Reagan administration has repeatedly denounced Nicaragua's government for its ties to Cuba and the Soviet Union, alleged that the Nicaraguans are involved in drug smuggling, and dismissed Nicaragua's 1984 elections as a sham.

The administration has known about the situation in Panama for some time, and has begun to tell reporters about it. But officials remain curiously silent about it in public. Although the government had extensive knowledge of the election irregularities, Secretary of State George Shultz congratulated the Panamanians on their 1984 elections, which he described as offering "Panamanians of all political persuasions a new opportunity for progress and national development." Our government recently sent the Panamanian government a note assuring them that we would keep quiet on the topic.

From one perspective, our desire not to stir up trouble with Panama is understandable. The Panama Canal remains a key strategic concern. The United States military's southern command center is in Panama, and overall the government remains friendly to us.

This policy is nothing new, of course. It is precisely the same kind of tack we took with the Somoza regime in Nicaragua and with scores of preceding military dictatorships in other countries in the region. So long as a government remains ostensibly friendly toward us, we will ignore its shortcomings.

This short-sighted attitude has gotten us into trouble before, and it will get us into trouble again. In fact, it is likely to cause trouble for the Reagan administration in short order.

The administration is trying again to push through Congress $100 million in aid to Nicaraguan rebels. Revelations about the rebel leaders' misuse of funds have made the administration's job harder. The news concerning Panama is apt to make it even more difficult.

This sort of double standard is at the heart of the administration's problems with its Central American policies. If Panama and the Nicaraguan contras are the best we can do for friends in that part of the world, maybe it's time to try embracing our enemies.

The Houston Post

Houston, TX, June 24, 1986

Panama's Gen. Manuel Antonio Noriega has been the target of allegations that he was involved in illicit activities ranging from narcotics-smuggling and money-laundering to assassination and election-rigging. U.S. officials have privately corroborated many of these disclosures, and Sen. Jesse Helms, R-N.C., has charged the Panamanian military chief with running "the biggest drug-trafficking operation in the Western Hemisphere."

Now a State Department spokesman says the reports that Noriega is connected with drug-smuggling are hearsay, circumstantial or speculative. That raises questions about other claims. Did the general, for instance, order the military to intervene in Panama's 1984 presidential election?

Political opponents of the Panamanian government have also attempted to tie Noriega to the death of a political dissident. Is this, too, hearsay? If we have hard evidence that Noriega is involved in corruption, that he has acted against U.S. interests, we shouldn't leak it and then issue a qualified repudiation of it. Such contradictory behavior damages our position in a strategically crucial region and our relations with the country that will control the Panama Canal in another 15 years.

The Providence Journal

Providence, RI, June 25, 1986

General Manuel Antonio Noriega, the strongman of Panama for the past five years, poses an interesting problem for the United States.

On the one hand, he is a strategic player in the broad scheme of Central American events: He is now, and has been for some time, a useful source of intelligence information for the region. He has granted the United States considerable latitude for military operations within Panama. And of course, he is the most important Panamanian with whom this country deals in the proposed transfer of authority over the Panama Canal. The canal treaties, ratified in 1977, take effect at the end of the century.

But General Noriega is also "head of the biggest drug trafficking operation in the Western Hemisphere," according to Sen. Jesse Helms (R-N.C.), and "a business partner with (Fidel) Castro."

Senator Helms is the first public official to confirm details of two-week-old news reports that accuse General Noriega of drug trafficking, money laundering and the murder of a political opponent. It also claims that he has been systematically providing intelligence data to Havana, as well as Washington, and sold restricted American technology to Cuba and various Eastern bloc governments. He is also alleged to be supplying arms to pro-Cuban rebels in democratic Colombia.

Such revelations put the United States in a quandary. Of course, in his day, Senator Helms was the most vocal opponent of the Canal treaties, and is no friend of the regime in Panama City. But as a senior member of the Foreign Relations Committee, he speaks with considerable authority, and his assertions have been met with a disconcerting silence in the two capitals.

After all, as armed forces chief, General Noriega is the real power in a country where his hand-picked prime minister is the nominal administrator. And for many strategic, military and diplomatic reasons, the United States must reckon with whomever or whatever governs Panama.

General Noriega has many friends in Washington. His predecessor, General Omar Torrijos, had many friends, too — and even some exotic admirers, such as the British novelist Graham Greene. But General Torrijos died in a mysterious helicopter crash in 1981, and his successor seems to have wormed his way into the confidence of military, intelligence and political circles in a variety of hemispheric capitals.

Senator Helms was asked over the weekend whether the United States should intervene in Panama, to oppose the government, as we have sought to exercise influence in Nicaragua, for the same reason. He declined to answer, partly because he does not wish to speculate about hypothetical matters, but largely because President Reagan is the Commander-in-Chief "and I am not."

Accordingly, President Reagan should take a hard look at the Panamanian in charge, and ask some pointed questions of his own: Are these allegations true, or can General Noriega prove that they are false? And if they are true, is this the sort of person with whom the United States can do business as we divest ourselves of the strategic waterway between the Atlantic and Pacific oceans?

These questions should be asked in Panama, by General Noriega's military associates and fellow countrymen. Perhaps they can furnish some answers about which Washington can only speculate.

Chicago Tribune

Chicago, IL, June 27, 1986

Even hardshell cynics might concede that Gen. Manuel Antonio Noriega of Panama has compiled for himself a fairly impressive resume as all-around villain and menace.

The military strongman, ostensibly an American ally who currently runs a country in which vital U.S. interests are at stake, is accused, on what appears to be substantial evidence, of: ordering up the assassination of at least one political opponent, who was, in especially grisly style, decapitated and deposited in a U.S. mailbag; possibly arranging the helicopter crash which killed his predecessor; providing intelligence information and American technology to Cuba; running guns to a pro-Cuban guerrilla organization in Colombia; and stealing the 1984 Panamanian presidential election for his candidate (whom he subsequently and unceremoniously dumped).

When not occupied with such delicate affairs of state the general, whose official title is commander of the army, also is accused of dabbling in a major-league money laundering operation and presiding over what Sen. Jesse Helms (R., N.C.) calls the "biggest drug trafficking operation in the Western hemisphere."

Sen. Helms, ardent conservative and achingly disappointed leader of the fight against the Panama Canal Treaty, which provides for the U.S. to turn the canal over to Panama in the year 2000, is floating another option.

Asked on a TV interview program if he thought the U.S. should move to reassert authority over the canal, Sen. Helms responded, "Well, I think it may be entirely necessary down the road. That depends on how the present situation involving Mr. Noriega is handled."

No, it doesn't. Even to suggest reopening the canal treaty question, to threaten now to take back and reclaim sovereignty over part of of another people's country, is as dumb and as extreme an idea as was the suggestion by law enforcement officials in the 1970s that the general be assassinated.

What the U.S. might do, for a start, is quit turning a blind eye to Gen. Noriega in return for his willingness to permit extensive American military and intelligence operations in Panama. For the State Department spokesman to declare only that "we find these allegations to be disturbing," which is approximately all the administration has done so far, is hardly an adequately robust response.

U.S. Troops Aid Attack on Cocaine Targets in Bolivia

United States Administration officials July 15, 1986 said U.S. Army personnel and equipment had been sent to Bolivia to help in the war on drug traffickers. Six U.S. Black Hawk helicopters and some of the roughly 160 pilots, officers and support personnel to be involved in the operation had arrived in Santa Cruz, Bolivia July 14 from their U.S. Southern Command bases in Panama, the officials said. They would assist the Bolivian military in raids in the Beni region in north-central Bolivia, where a large part of the world's cocaine is produced. The helicopters, equipped with M-60 machine guns, would transport Bolivian troops to drug installations, according to the officials. A U.S. Drug Enforcement Administration (DEA) officer would be aboard each helicopter. U.S. Army personnel would not be involved in the raids but would be permitted to return fire if shot at. The 60 day-operation would be directed at 35 targets.

The U.S. had wanted to keep the operation a secret until Bolivian troops could be trained, but news of the arrival in Santa Cruz of a U.S. C-5A transport plane carrying the U.S. troops and helicopters quickly appeared in the local press. The leak was expected to allow drug traffickers time to flee along with their equipment and drugs. The raids, due to start July 16, had to be delayed because of "logistical problems," according to the Bolivian embassy in Washington, D.C.

Bolivian President Victor Paz Estenssoro reportedly had been prompted to request U.S. aid in part because of the growing political influence of drug traffickers, who had financed candidates for local and national office. In addition, drug abuse among Bolivian young people was increasing, and legitimate business operations were being threatened by the growth of illegitimate businesses to launder drug money.

The Bolivian operation was the first under an April 8, 1986 national security directive approved by U.S. President Ronald Reagan. The directive described the international drug trade as a threat to U.S. security and permitted U.S. military personnel to aid American agencies in planning raids on narcotics traffickers and equipping police forces and transporting them to the sites of the raids. Critics questioned the Administration's assertion that the involvement of the military in law enforcement was not covered by the War Powers Act of 1973. Under the War Powers Resolution, the President must to consult Congress whenever U.S. troops are to be introduced into hostilities or "situations where imminent involvement in hostilities is clearly indicated by the circumstances."

The Washington Times

Washington, DC, July 17, 1986

At first glance, the six helicopters and 140 Army pilots and support personnel the U.S. sent to Bolivia to help stamp out illicit drug production look mighty impressive. The huge profits that are part and parcel of the drug trade may lose their appeal when drug makers look up to see the working end of a M60 machine gun. But as Confederate Gen. Nathan Bedford Forrest is reputed to have said, the fellow who wins is the one who "gits thar fustest with the mostest."

Let's face it. A handful of Army choppers is hardly enough to turn the tide in a war against an enormous drug trade that reaches to every nook and cranny in America. Anyone who has read the stats knows the dimensions of the struggle, knows that America is fighting for her life. The age at which youngsters begin experimenting with drugs continues to drop each year. We're talking hard drugs here, poisons such as cocaine and its sinister derivative, crack. News items about teen-agers overdosing are so common that they hardly get a paragraph back among the swimsuit ads.

In April President Reagan signed an executive order declaring the drug traffic a threat to national security. If that is the case, and no one denies it, something a lot tougher than the Bolivian operation is required. It's one thing to pop in unannounced on a couple of drug processing labs, quite another to deal the drug trade a blow from which it cannot recover. To do that, Bolivia — and Colombia and Peru and Mexico — will have to clean house at the top while we go to work at home.

Corrupt politicians and police officials, without whose help the drug trade would not have become the empire it is, will have to go. They, as well as the producers and growers, ought to be right up there on the "target acquisition list." The Reagan administration is going to have to put a lot more muscle where its mouth is. As William Tecumseh Sherman observed, war is hell. It's time for the United States to give drug pushers, at home and abroad, a whole new definition of the term.

WORCESTER TELEGRAM.

Worcester, MA, July 21, 1986

The use of U.S. troops in Bolivia to help that nation move against clandestine cocaine factories presents contradictory faces.

If this nation is in a declared war on drugs, then we must be prepared to use military force, just as we have in the war on terrorism, which has claimed far fewer American victims than drugs have. But we are a nation of democratic and constitutional principles. One of the most sacred is the segregation of police and military powers. The use of soldiers to do civilian police work in far off lands raises the specter of encroaching martial law.

Congress has already passed measures that allow the military to come to the aid of law enforcement agencies in combatting drugs. And President Reagan in April issued a directive that made curbing the international drug traffic a matter of national security.

Here at home, many Americans are worried that drugs are sapping the country of its moral fiber. They see drug dependency as crippling the American will to meet its responsibilities. The international drug trade is the subversion from without destined to make our nation fall. In those terms, drugs are indeed a threat to the national security, and the flow of drugs is an invasion.

Opponents of drug enforcement efforts by the armed forces worry about the casualness with which the military might be called into police affairs. This is not a nation accustomed to seeing military personnel patrolling on street corners. That image is reserved for dire emergencies. Military commanders are concerned, too. They worry that police exercises might rob their troops of combat readiness.

Congress generally supports the Bolivian operation. But the road to military deterrence in the drug war is not a clear one. We must stand ready to assist in the fight on all fronts, here and elsewhere, but our role in Bolivia must be maintained as that of a limited helper.

The Detroit News

Detroit, MI, July 17, 1986

The Reagan administration has joined the war against "crack" by dispatching six helicopters and 100 pilots and support troops to Bolivia to help that country conduct raids against drug traffickers. Much of the world's cocaine allegedly is grown in that area of South America. While we agree that drugs are one of the most serious problems the United States faces, we're not at all persuaded that using soldiers as "narcs" is a very wise idea.

Not the least of the ironies in the Bolivia deployment is that if 100 soldiers and some helicopters had been deployed to, say, "help" the government of El Salvador, Congress and the liberal isolationists would be going bonkers.

President Reagan recently declared drugs to be a serious threat to the national security. But when he declared Communist insurgency in Central America to be a threat to the national security, Congress used every means at its disposal to prevent or limit the use of military forces for military purposes. The danger of a quagmire was too great, the critics said.

If it's quagmires we fear, sending troops into the front lines against the drug trade, a mission for which they are neither trained nor equipped, has the makings of a doozy.

The United States should be using its influence with its friends to get them to crack down on their own drug smugglers. Indeed, the United States currently is withholding nearly half of its $40 million in economic aid to Bolivia as punishment for Bolivia's failure to eradicate more coca fields itself. Why not cut off all aid? Bolivia exports an estimated $450 million of cocaine a year. (Neighboring Peru is the other big exporter, making the area the "Kansas of cocaine.")

If the military is going to be seriously involved in the anti-drug trade, it might make more sense to employ it in a more traditional way: replacing governments that either can't or won't put a stop to massive, prolonged drug production within their borders. This, at least, would have the benefit of "encouraging" other countries to get serious about their own efforts.

Our laws have wisely tended to limit the use of the military for nonmilitary police purposes, lest the armed forces become politicized and corrupted. We have a feeling that the Bolivian caper is the international equivalent of the stunt by New York Sen. Al D'Amato the other day in dressing up in a leather jacket and going to Harlem to purchase some crack. These sorts of showy gestures may only be cover-ups for lack of a real strategy for dealing with the drug problem.

We can't offer any instant solutions ourselves. Stiffer penalties for drug trafficking, combined with a serious effort to educate our children to the dangers of drug use, are probably the most effective combination. But nobody should expect miracles. The effort to enforce the prohibition on alcohol earlier in this century should be a cautionary experience. The more resources we put into trying to catch drug smugglers and sealing off our borders to drugs, the worse the problem seems to get — as the continued decline in street prices of heroin, marijuana, and cocaine attests.

The Reagan administration's action in Bolivia may prove popular. The conventional wisdom is that drug use has become an epidemic, and the spread of such dangerous substances as "crack" into the middle class has congressmen rushing to get aboard the get-tough bandwagon. But if the Reagan administration is going to commit the military to expeditions around the world on random search-and-destroy missions against drugs, it may be getting us into a true quagmire. Other countries will be only too happy to let us take on a task that they themselves should be performing much more effectively. And U.S. forces will be distracted from their primary mission, the military security of our country.

THE BLADE

Toledo, OH, July 21, 1986

SENDING six helicopters and 100 U.S. personnel to help Bolivia wage war against the booming illegal drug-production business has a certain Rambo-like flourish to it. But it will take more than firepower to make a dent in the international drug problem.

Questions can be raised about the mission, which is designed to help Bolivian forces smash suspected cocaine-processing laboratories and other installations in an area where most of the coca leaves are grown.

The landing of U.S. troops outside this nation's borders could be misinterpreted. The mission also may be misdirected in that the task of eradicating drug production should be first and foremost a Bolivian responsibility.

Several South American countries have likewise failed in trying to stamp out the source of drug supplies. As long as Bolivia invites U.S. troops, perhaps they can help get a small part of the job done. But raids have been conducted in recent years in both South and North America, and the flow of illegal drugs just keeps growing.

And what if the impossible happens and all the coca crops south of the Rio Grande River are eradicated and the border closed to smugglers? Domestic marijuana production in the United States would still assure users in this country of a substitute for cocaine.

There is no magic solution to be found in the Bolivian raids, just as no other single strategy works. Stiffer penalties against drug traffickers, education programs aimed at children, sharp reductions in foreign aid to offending countries, and similar approaches may have a cumulative effect. No overnight miracles should be expected.

Wisconsin State Journal

Madison, WI,
July 22, 1986

Like a mischievous child who's always looking to point the finger of blame at someone else, the United States has fallen into a pattern of blaming other nations for our drug problems.

In May, U.S. Customs Service Commissioner William von Raab, speaking of the drug trade in Mexico, alleged there was "massive" corruption by Mexican officials and "ingrained corruption in the Mexican law enforcement establishment up and down the ladder."

The fact that von Raab was probably correct didn't change the basic problem: the *demand* for illegal drugs exists in this country, not south of the border.

Now the Reagan adminstration has deployed U.S. Army helicopters and troops in Bolivia, home to a cottage industry of cocaine processors and traffickers, for a much-publicized series of "raids" on suspected laboratories.

To date, the Bolivian-U.S. raids have turned up only one processing center, a small airplane, some cocaine-refining chemicals and a lone suspect. But even if the continuing raids turn up tons of cocaine and hundreds of suspects, a much larger point is still being missed.

How much good is accomplished by trying to cut off a "supply" that can almost certainly be duplicated elsewhere when so little is being done to limit the "demand" at home?

Major drug dealers in this country, when they are sentenced to prison terms, aren't put away for very long. Few drug users or small-time peddlers are even arrested. It seems the legal system puts drug abuse near the bottom of its list of priorities, perhaps because of the myth that it's a "victimless" crime, perhaps because the political pressure is so misdirected — as has been the case with the Bolivian excursion.

Public education efforts, while vastly improved over a decade or two ago, still have a long way to go toward dispelling the notion of "recreational" drug use. About the time people are convinced of the dangers of one drug (LSD, heroin, etc.) another pops up to take its place (cocaine, "crack," etc.).

Of course, Bolivia and Mexico are major sources of illegal and harmful drugs. But so are Thailand, Pakistan, Colombia and a half-dozen other nations. Will the United States dispatch Black Hawk helicopters there, too?

Our drug problems begin at home. Bolivian peasants would not be growing coca leaf if they weren't guaranteed a willing and lucrative market.

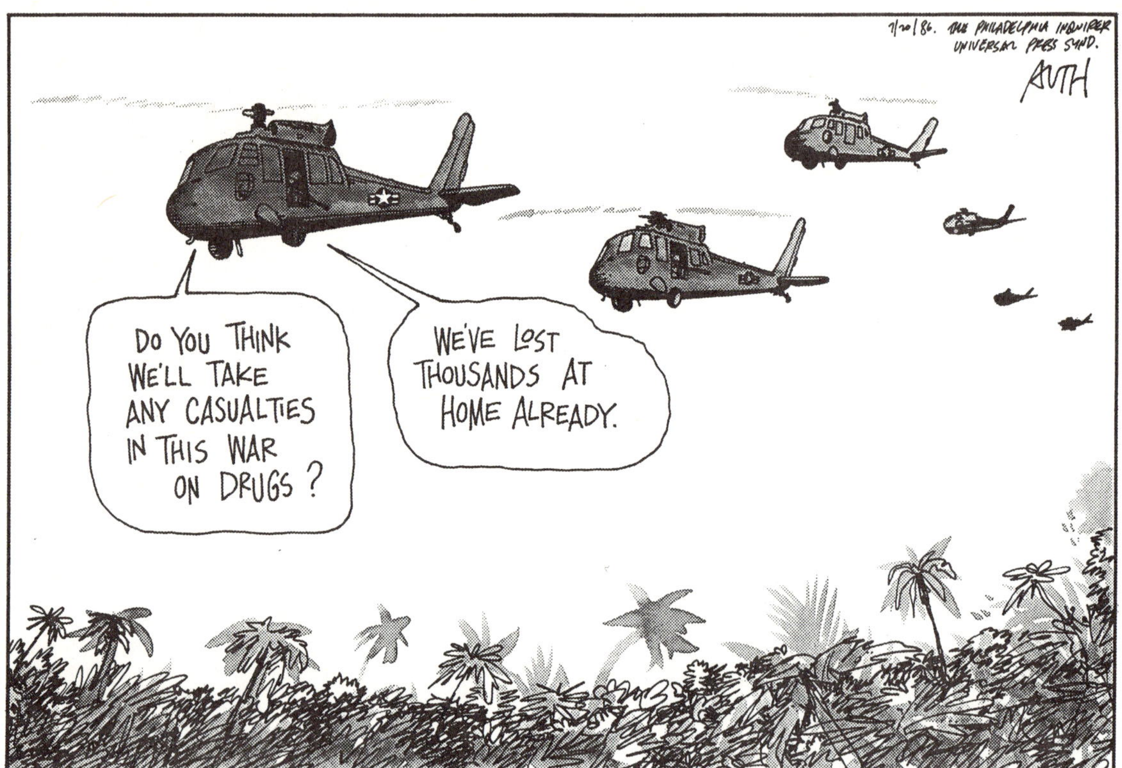

ST. LOUIS POST-DISPATCH

*St. Louis, MO,
July 29, 1986*

American soldiers and helicopters have been in Bolivia for about two weeks to help in operations against drug traffickers, and the only demonstrable conclusion is that they face a difficult task. Indeed, the question remains what it was when President Reagan announced the mission: Is this unusual use of U.S. military personnel justified?

A day before the Americans landed, men working in one major cocaine laboratory in the northwest of Bolivia flew out from their landing strip. Later, Bolivian police carried on U.S. helicopters raided two cattle ranches and found them to be cattle ranches. The Bolivian agents then found an empty complex of cocaine laboratories. They have arrested 18 suspects.

U.S. spokesmen contend that the operation has stopped cocaine production for about six months; they also hope that it will create a glut of coca leaves, forcing down prices and encouraging poor farmers to grow something else. Yet the immediate effect has been the opposite. Coca prices have risen since the raids began. Coca has replaced tin as the major Bolivian export and, as the Bolivian ambassador to Washington noted, poor peasants would be hurt most by destroying coca plants.

A few days ago President Reagan himself conceded that there was no way to turn off the flow of illegal drugs to the United States and said that the real answer has to be, "Let's turn the customers off." The customers in this market are Americans. No doubt it will prove as difficult to curtail the buyers as it is to block the sellers, but the emphasis in drug control has to be in this country, and it will not require the use of troops. The soldiers in Bolivia ought to be brought home.

The San Diego Union

San Diego, CA, July 19, 1986

The Reagan administration's campaign to stem the flow of illegal drugs from Latin America began in earnest yesterday as six U.S. Army Black Hawk helicopters swept into the jungles of eastern Bolivia. The aircraft, flown by U.S. pilots, carried Bolivian anti-drug forces that are raiding 50 of that nation's clandestine cocaine labs.

The bold joint operation, which is expected to last two months, is designed to destroy the facilities in Bolivia that produce most of the 100 tons of cocaine that are shipped abroad each year by Bolivian drug barons. This staggering figure accounts for 25 percent of the world supply and nearly 30 percent of the cocaine coming into the United States each year.

Although cocaine is the largest single component of Bolivia's $3 billion economy, the new Bolivian government seems determined to put an end to this deadly trade. Last April, President Victor Paz Estenssoro requested U.S. assistance in the drug raids. That request, it should be noted, was prompted by a recent U.S. decision to cut off a large share of American aid to Bolivia so long as that government refused to eradicate a significant portion of the country's coca crop.

The timely strike is the first to be carried out under a directive signed April 8 by President Reagan that declared drug trafficking to be a national-security threat. But this is not the first time U.S.-manned helicopters have assisted an anti-drug effort by another country. Operation Bahamas has seen American pilots transport Bahamian troops throughout that Caribbean country during the last three years.

More encouraging still, U.S.-supported assaults against cocaine facilities in Peru and Colombia are under consideration. These operations, which could begin as early as next month, would be more limited than the Bolivian strike. Agents from the U.S. Drug Enforcement Administration would assist local troops and police in raids against cocaine-producing areas.

Taken together, these joint operations represent a dramatic step in the Reagan administration's campaign to staunch the flood of drugs that menace the United States. Granted, the use of U.S. personnel in these raids presumes the possibility of American casualties. Indeed, the soldiers have the green light to defend themselves if fired upon. But the attendant risk seems completely justified, given the grim toll of death and suffering that cocaine causes each year in this country.

That sentiment was generally reflected on Capitol Hill, where the operation received strong bipartisan support. Such support began to surface six years ago, when it became apparent that the United States ought to use its military resources to supplement law-enforcement efforts in the war against international drug dealers.

This strategy has already paid dividends off the coast of South Florida, where the illicit drug traffic was dramatically reduced by the use of Navy patrol boats and surveillance aircraft. President Reagan's recent executive order allows the military freer rein to undertake drug-enforcement missions for their own sake without working them into existing missions.

Which isn't to suggest that American paratroopers will be dropping into Panama in the near future to disrupt Gen. Noriega's drug deals. Or that the U.S. Air Force will be conducting surgical strikes against Colombia's cocaine factories. But it does increase the risks to the international drug traffickers as they ply their deadly trade. And that bodes well for the United States to gain some ground in this dirty war.

The Des Moines Register

Des Moines, IA, October 17, 1986

Officials of the U.S. Drug Enforcement Agency had a bad trip last week when they tried to raid a Bolivian town in search of cocaine traffickers and had to flee during a protest by hundreds of angry residents shouting "Kill the Yankees" and "Yankee go home."

The raid by 110 U.S. and Bolivian drug-enforcement officials was prompted by reports that several major cocaine traffickers were hiding in Santa Ana, a town of 5,000 people. After drug agents had searched homes and cars and questioned residents, a crowd gathered in the town square and chased the officials to an airfield 3 miles away, where helicopters were used to scatter protesters while the plane took off.

Not surprisingly, no drugs were seized and no arrests were made. But the incident casts doubt on whether using U.S. troops overseas is the most effective way to stop drugs. In any case, fighting drugs and still maintaining good relations with neighboring nations may require more Yankee ingenuity, not to mention sensitivity, than was shown last week.

THE INDIANAPOLIS NEWS

Indianapolis, IN, July 29, 1986

After nearly a week in the jungles of Bolivia, U.S. soldiers and drug agents, along with Bolivia's elite police unit, the leopards, have arrested a few dozen suspected drug traffickers, captured two large cocaine labs and mistakenly raided three cattle ranches.

The most optimistic view is that the joint Bolivian-U.S. cocaine raids have forced Bolivia's top drug lords into hiding and shut down the bulk of Bolivia's cocaine manufacturing operations until after the November-to-March rainy season. Bolivia, according to experts in drug trafficking, supplies about one-fourth of the cocaine sold on international drug markets.

That is the most optimistic view.

By all accounts, the highly publicized operation, tagged Operation Blast Furnace, has been a fiasco.

For starters, the operation was scheduled to begin on July 4, but delays prevented the U.S. Army helicopters and 160 support personnel from arriving until July 14. Then, a petroleum workers strike prevented planes and helicopters from getting fuel.

By the time the planes got off the ground, press reports — many of them irresponsibly stemming from the American media — had already publicized the raids. Other sources, however, say Operation Blast Furnace had already been infiltrated by the Bolivian drug mafia. Jorge Roca, a top cocaine trafficker, had reportedly been tipped off a month before the operation began by corrupt Bolivian officials.

Then, what bad weather and public disclosure of the raids didn't hamper, outdated intelligence, poor coordination and maintenance problems did. On two days mechanical problems with a DC-3 airplane used to refuel helicopters at more remote sites kept aircraft grounded.

Maj. Carlos Vizcarra, deputy commander of the Bolivian antinarcotic police unit, complained that U.S. Drug Enforcement Administration agents had picked the sites to raid without consulting Bolivian police. "They don't trust us Bolivians," he said.

On the first Sunday, three helicopters loaded with more than 30 Bolivian police went to a site based on coordinates given by the DEA agents. No laboratory was found.

The failure of the raids to capture Bolivia's major drug traffickers and to destroy more than two of the nation's 60 cocaine processing plants may have been the least of its shortcomings.

Failure connected with the mission resulted in ridicule or intensified local anger about U.S. troop presence in Bolivia. It also reinforced the image that many Bolivian drug traffickers enjoy — an image of being Robin Hoods.

Although Bolivia requested U.S. assistance, in part out of fear that the drug mafia was totally corrupting the government and to some degree because of growing drug problems among its own youth, it also had a gun at its head. The United States is withholding nearly half of its $40 million in economic aid to Bolivia as punishment for the country's failure to eradicate more coca fields itself.

One Western diplomat noted that U.S. presence in the raids risks offending members of Bolivia's armed forces, who see it as highlighting their inability to handle a military operation. "The Bolivian military noses have been really put out of joint by this."

As for the average Bolivian peasant farmer, there is ambivalence. It must be remembered that cocaine sales pump an estimated $600 million a year into Bolivia's economy — about one-fifth its gross national product.

Nestor Sanchez, a dry goods salesman in the Beni region — the heart of Bolivia's cocaine growing area, shrugs and says, "I would guess that about half of our economy is based on coca. It's not a good thing, but what can one do?"

Many Bolivians believe that if the United States is so concerned about its drug problem, it should concentrate on dealing with the problem within its own borders.

LAS VEGAS SUN

Las Vegas, NV, July 22, 1986

The Bolivian government's invitation to have U.S. soldiers come into that nation to help fight the world-wide narcotics dilemma is a bold move that could have resulted in the most effective strike ever at the heart of the growing problem — if it had been kept secret and run properly by both countries.

For years, the hands of U.S. police officers and federal agents have been tied because most action had to be taken against drug smugglers as the narcotics were entering our shores or already here, and not at the source of manufacturing.

The decision to call for U.S. help shows a great deal of courage and foresight on the part of Bolivia President Victor Paz Estenssoro, whose country rates second behind neighbor Peru in the production of cocoa leaves (used to make cocaine).

By inviting a foreign power into his land to battle a problem that most countries choose to handle with their own forces, Estenssora risks not only his political career in the face of failure, but also his life.

For we're sure Estenssora is aware that Bolivia's cocaine industry brings in $2 billion a year and that 100,000 of the nation's 6 million inhabitants are involved in it.

And it is an industry that has left a trail of addiction and death in this nation and others.

Earlier this month, in separate incidents days apart, the drug was partially, if not totally, responsible for taking the lives of a collegiate basketball standout who had great NBA potential and a pro football player on the verge of stardom.

Last week, in a Mexican border town across from Brownsville, Texas, a newspaper publisher and his 24-year-old star reporter, who had taken strong stands against narcotics smuggling, were gunned down in a wave of machine gun bullets.

The list of drug-related tragedies is almost endless.

But now, a military force from a nation that has the manpower and financial resources equal to or greater than the drug dealers has the opportunity to fight the problem at its source.

Some have argued that sending in 160 U.S. soldiers and six helicopters is a violation of the constitution of the South American nation, which is the size of Texas and California combined.

But this isn't really a question of whether one nation did the wrong thing for good reasons. Our troops went in at the invitation of that nation's leaders.

It's the old question of which is more important, preserving the rights of criminals who profit off an illegal and deadly trade or the rights of citizens who don't want drugs or the shifty characters who deal in them running rampant in their country.

Las Vegas has long had a problem fighting drug trafficking from all over the world. One Metro police officer was sent thousands of miles to the Orient to break up the source of a major ring operating in Las Vegas.

Local police deal daily with the problems of drugs and youth gangs who finance other criminal activities with the sale of rock cocaine to the most affluent individuals who have money to throw away on so-called coke parties.

And the starting point of the problem can be traced to nations like Bolivia, where the drug rates among the top cash crops.

One U.S. official has been quoted as saying that U.S. soldiers "are not going in there in a military operation. They are carrying Bolivian police and U.S. drug agents. We're not sending guys who shoot up the fields where the stuff is grown."

Just as we're not so naive to believe that the world's drug problem can be eradicated overnight — or in an eternity for that matter — we also are not so naive to believe that soldiers, if being shot at, won't return fire.

The fact is, this is a war — the bitter and long war on drugs.

The use of U.S. soldiers to back up another nation's forces is an idea whose time has come. And it's time that others take note and not thumb their white powder-stained noses at the operation.

U.S. DEA Agent Tortured by Police; Mexico Denies Mistreatment

An agent of the United States Drug Enforcement Administration (DEA) and a Mexican informant were detained and allegedly tortured by Jalisco state police August 13, 1986. Mexican officials denied that the agent, Victor Cortez, Jr., had been mistreated. At the time of the incident, Mexican President Miguel de la Madrid Hurtado was in Washington on a visit intended to improve relations between the two nations. The disputed incident began in Guadalajara, the capital of Jalisco state, on the afternoon of Aug. 13. Cortez and the unidentified informant were stopped by three police officers after residents reported suspicious behavior by the two men, who apparently had been watching a house for several days. Five more officers in three cars soon appeared at the scene, and Cortez and the informant were taken to the Jalisco state police headquarters after weapons were found in the trunk of the informant's car. Cortez claimed he was a DEA agent and said he carried no identification because he was working under- cover. The incident was witnessed by a U.S. embassy officer, who followed the police, traced the number of their car and then went to Mexican authorities to seek the agent's release. Cortez and the informant were allegedly held for six hours and were freed only after DEA agents urged representatives of the Mexican attorney general to intercede on Cortez's behalf. The two men were flown to the U.S. the next day.

Details later emerged that Cortez and the informant had been stripped, bound and interrogated. Cortez was reportedly tortured with electric shocks and "severely beaten—and worse," according to one U.S. official. According to DEA chief John C. Lawn Aug. 15, the Jalisco police had sought to learn details of the agency's investigations and personnel in Mexico. The DEA Aug. 21 in Washington began meetings with agents stationed in Mexico to determine the future of the agency's involvement there.

Mexican federal officials Aug. 15 contended that Cortez had been detained only for about two hours and denied that he had been tortured. However, in a news conference Aug. 15, U.S. Attorney General Edwin Meese 3rd said, "There's no question that our agent was badly mistreated, and we're not going to stand for this kind of conduct." In a separate statement, the White House accused Mexican police of vigilantism that harmed the ability of the two countries to work together to fight drug trafficking.

Fort Worth Star-Telegram

Fort Worth, TX, August 21, 1986

The arrest and torture of an American under- cover drug agent in Mexico last week is yet another chapter in the exposure of corruptness that grips certain segments of officialdom in our neighbor to the south.

The Mexican police at the Jalisco headquar- ters in Guadalajara obviously knew that the agent, Victor Cortez Jr., worked for the U.S. Drug Enforcement Administration. There was even one report that his arrest was ordered by a known underworld drug pusher in that area.

Cortez and another person, identified as an informant, were held at the Mexican police head- quarters for six hours. They were released only after the intervention of the Mexican attorney general and other U.S. officials, who went to the jail to rescue them.

Cortez reportedly was stripped, bound and interrogated in a jail cell during the six hours, being questioned specifically about the opera- tions of the Drug Enforcement Administration in Mexico.

That tends to authenticate the report that the arrest was ordered by drug pushers, who obvi- ously would have some sort of control over the Jalisco police in such a case. Information about U.S. drug agents in Mexico certainly would be of enormous benefit to drug pushers and dealers there.

The United States has about 30 DEA officers working in Mexico. As in other countries, they work with the full knowledge of the government there. They have no arrest or direct police pow- ers, and any such action is carried out by Mexican police.

Mexican authorities originally denied that Cortez was tortured. They also have denied that there is widespread corruption in that land, but events keep popping up that tend to show other- wise. An example is a statement that appeared recently in a Mexico quarterly, *Voices of Mexico.* It was made by Sergio Aguayo, a senior research- er at the Center for International Studies of El Colegio de Mexico. Speaking of the differences between the United States and Mexico, Aguayo said one reason many U.S. journalists do not understand how business is done in Mexico is because they "don't realize we are speaking of different species of animals.

"They take the U.S. private sector as the model, but it in no way resembles the Mexican private sector, which is as corrupt and inefficient as is the state, and this can be supported with exam- ples."

We are the first to acknowledge that the cur- rent drug problem is as much our fault as it is the fault of drug pushers and dealers in other coun- tries. Mexico says she wants to cooperate with the United States in fighting the drug problem. But we suggest that Mexico will never be able to conquer any of her problems until several layers of corruption are removed from her govern- mental structure.

The Cincinnati Post

August 20, 1986
Cincinnati, OH

The fine words about Mexi- can-American cooperation in the war against narcotics al- ready sound false. Even as Pres- idents Reagan and Miguel de la Madrid were meeting in the White House last week, a U.S. narcotics agent was being ab- ducted and tortured by police in Guadalajara.

The incident is the latest proof of the staggering resis- tance the anti-drug campaign faces from Mexican narcotics bosses and corrupt officials. It brings to mind the torture and murder of another Drug En- forcement Administration agent, also based in Guadalaja- ra, in February 1985.

Victor Cortez Jr. was luckier: Two fellow agents witnessed his abduction Aug. 13. Then DEA officers surrounded the police detention center where they suspected he was being held and demanded his release. More than six hours later, Cortez was finally freed.

Some reports say de la Madrid himself ordered the American released. But the Mexican gov- ernment, unmoved by medical evidence of torture by electric shock, flatly denies that Cortez was mistreated.

Such outrageous non-cooper- ation from the central govern- ment is one obstacle U.S. anti-drug efforts meet in Mexi- co. Another is the drug lords' power over local police. U.S. of- ficials believe the same police unit that abducted Cortez was involved in the slaying of DEA agent Enrique Camarena Sala- zar 18 months ago.

Mexico has failed to prose- cute a major drug dealer in more than 10 years. Meanwhile, it remains the world's third- largest producer of marijuana and the main supplier of am- phetamines and barbiturates to the United States. American of- ficials estimate 30 percent of the cocaine coming into this coun- try passes through Mexico.

During his visit to Washing- ton President de la Madrid called drug trafficking a "can- cer of modern society." But in the affair of Victor Cortez, his country again has shown a will- ingness to tolerate that cancer.

The Birmingham News
Birmingham, AL, August 16, 1986

Neighbors must work together to solve neighborhood problems, and that is exactly what the United States and Mexico have pledged to do in fighting illict drug trafficking and improving the region's economy.

President Reagan and Mexican President Miguel de la Madrid this week issued a "joint declaration of war on drug trafficking" and moved to expand cross-border trade and investments.

Relations between the United States and Mexico have been strained for a number of reasons, including U.S. allegations of fraud in recent elections in Chihuahua state, which were won by de la Madrid's ruling party, and charges by Reagan administration officials that widespread corruption that included Mexican government officials has promoted flourishing traffic in illegal drugs. The illegal arrest and torture of a U.S. drug agent, Victor Cortez Jr., has added to that perception.

But the meeting by the two heads of state should bring constructive results. One international irritant was taken care of immediately, as Mr. Reagan also announced that a 6-year ban on imports of tuna from Mexico, imposed after the Mexican government seized U.S. fishing boats off the Mexican coast, has been lifted.

De la Madrid promised to cooperate in combating drug trafficking but said the problem must be attacked "simultaneously at all links of the chain — production distribution and consumption." Included in that pledge of support was a reminder of Mexico's contention that the United States is not doing enough to discourage the demand for drugs.

On the economic front, Mr. Reagan praised Mexico's "courageous efforts" to come to grips with its economic crisis. Those efforts include sharp budget cuts over the next three years and the sale or closure of money-losing state enterprises. In return, the International Monetary Fund has agreed to provide Mexico with $1.6 billion over the next 18 months and the World Bank has pledged an additional $2 billion.

Mr. Reagan and de la Madrid announced their governments will open negotiations on a new agreement aimed at expanding trade and investment, with a target date of 1987 for reaching an agreement.

We hope the combination of austerity at home and new trade opportunities abroad will help to restore Mexico's economy, since our neighbor's problems so quickly become our own when workers cross the border to escape a depressed economy.

Mr. Reagan's personal relationship with de la Madrid, which has sustained our neighborly relations through difficult times, apparently is paying dividends in the areas of law enforcement and economic development.

Newsday
Long Island, NY, August 22, 1986

If the Reagan administration hopes to develop a credible antidrug program, it must figure out a way to protect its enforcement agents from the Mexican police. It had better make sure the torture of an American agent in the city of Guadalajara by Jalisco state police is the last incident of its kind.

Agent Victor Cortez of the Drug Enforcement Administration says he was seized, beaten and tortured for six hours last week while the Mexican police tried to learn the identities of informants, the addresses of other American drug agents in Guadalajara, the types of weapons and cars they use and the nature of current drug investigations.

Under a 20-year-old agreement, DEA agents collaborate with Mexican police to investigate and hinder narcotics traffic to the United States. There's reason to think that Cortez, one of 30 DEA agents working in Mexico, was singled out because he had a role in the recent seizure of 2,200 pounds of cocaine.

Mexican officials denied any mistreatment even though Cortez' injuries were severe enough to be photographed and further verified by medical examination. The torturers belong to the same unit that was implicated 18 months ago in the kidnaping and killing of another DEA agent, Enrique Camarena. It takes no imagination to think that Cortez might have met the same fate if DEA colleagues hadn't witnessed his arrest and brought pressure for his release.

The incident couldn't have come at a worse moment for Mexico's President Miguel de la Madrid. He was in Washington to talk to President Ronald Reagan about stepping up a joint war against drug trafficking. Mexico has become this country's leading supplier of heroin and marijuana, and it serves as a transshipment point for 30 percent of the cocaine flown in from Colombia and points farther south.

The handling of the Cortez incident provides an early test of de la Madrid's good intentions. Washington can't accept the kind of foot-dragging that has left the Camarena murder still an open case with no arrest or trial. And the corruption of police and public officials by drug traffickers should concern Mexico's government even more than our own.

The Houston Post
Houston, TX, August 31, 1986

Mexico has a funny way of waging a war on drugs. And it makes one wonder about the recently declared increase in cooperation between the two countries in combating drug trafficking.

Last week Mexico sent a harshly worded message to Washington warning that henceforth U.S. Drug Enforcement Administration agents would be "restricted to exchange of information."

First reports were that Mexico was ordering the agents out of the country. That would have eliminated problems like the killing of one DEA agent by Mexican drug lords and the torture of another by Jalisco state police. But apparently Mexico never wanted the agents to leave. The bellicosity of the note might have been more for internal Mexican consumption than for U.S. consideration.

The gist of the Mexican message seems to be that DEA agents have to conduct their activity "within the limits of the law." It is hard to object to that. Those agents are there to help enforce the laws of both the United States and Mexico.

The real problem seems to be not with violations by United States officials, but with corrupt Mexican law enforcement officers. It is a long-standing problem that Mexico's administration acknowledges and is trying to solve. Until it succeeds better than it has in the past, there is little hope of stemming the drug tide from Mexico.

The Seattle Times
Seattle, WA, August 25, 1986

THE Mexican government's initial reaction to the kidnapping and torture of U.S. drug-enforcement agent Victor Cortez Jr. was to deny that the crime took place. Now that government is questioning whether such agents even have a legal right to work in Mexico. If this artful dodging continues, Mexico will pay a heavy price in lost credibility, lost tourist business, and lost good will where it is needed most.

The foreign ministry in Mexico City says there is no accord permitting Drug Enforcement Administration agents to work in Mexico. A U.S. spokesman says that there is a verbal agreement to that effect, and that DEA agents have been operating in Mexico for 20 years.

The brutalization of Cortez by the same Jalisco state police unit that has been implicated in the killing of another DEA agent, Enrique Camarena Salazar, 18 months ago — and the central government's woefully inadequate reaction to both crimes — makes a mockery of grandiloquent promises of drug-enforcement cooperation made by Mexican President Miguel de la Madrid in Washington the other day.

Although a number of people have been implicated in Camarena's murder, none has been brought to trial. In fact, Mexico has failed to prosecute a major drug dealer in more than a decade.

Much of Mexican officialdom and press loves to indulge in a little gringo-baiting. But De la Madrid's government ought to know that the Camarena and Cortez cases are far too serious for that.

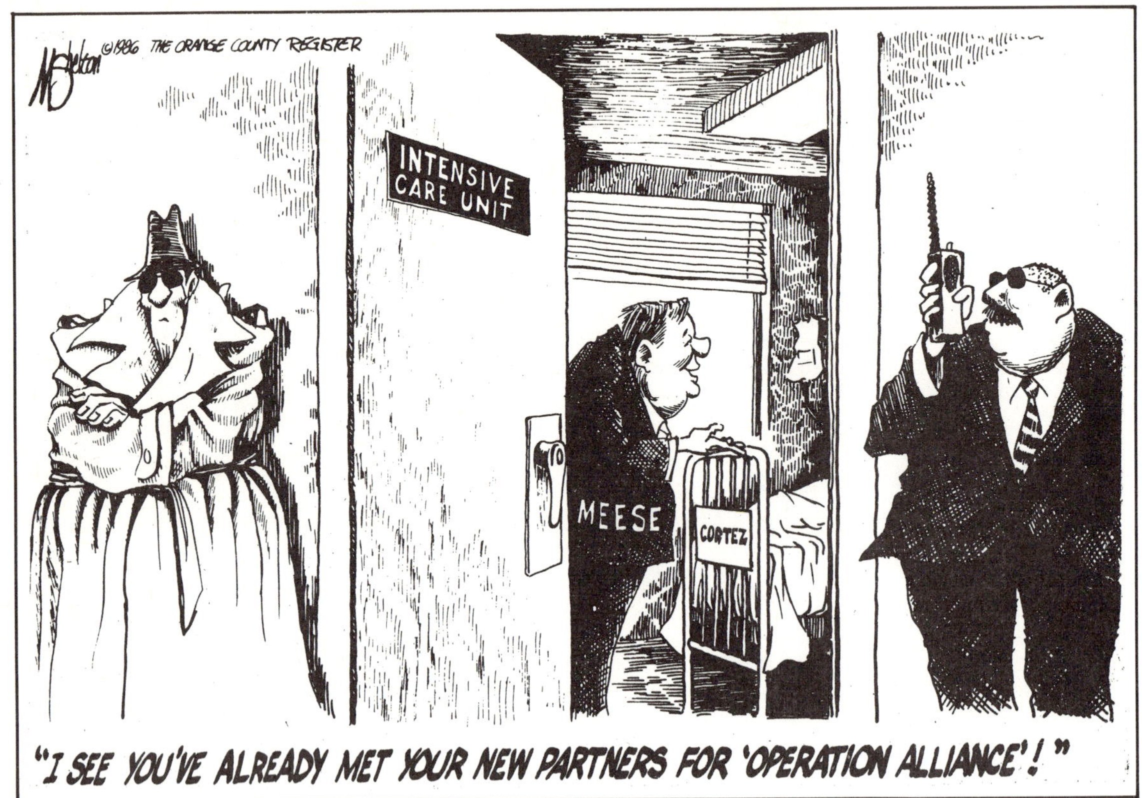

CHARLESTON EVENING POST

Charleston, SC, August 25, 1986

The Reagan administration's announcement of a massive campaign to halt the flow of drugs across the Mexican border was accompanied by a new vow of cooperation from Mexico. The vow immediately took on a hollow ring in light of the reported detention and torture of an American drug agent by police in Guadalajara. The implications of such base actions are far-reaching.

Officials of this country's Drug Enforcement Administration contend that agent Victor Cortez Jr. was literally kidnapped, beaten and tortured with a cattle prod. They suspect he was tortured to make him divulge information the DEA has on drug traffickers and their protectors. They suspect he was tortured, too, in retaliation for recent seizures of drug shipments by U.S. agents — seizures which deprived Mexican police of their accustomed payoffs and of other money they could have made by selling confiscated drugs to other smugglers.

They suspect also a link between the kidnapping of Mr. Cortez and the torture and slaying of DEA Agent Enrique Camarena Salazar and his Mexican pilot last year, also in Guadalajara. DEA sources said at the time they believed the agent was snatched off the street and murdered because he was "doing his job too well."

Washington's not blaming Mexico's president or attorney general for the two incidents, but it is no secret that anti-drug efforts in Mexico are so corrupt that the big-name traffickers operate with impunity. The circumstances surrounding the abduction and torture of an American drug agent, like the earlier slaying of a fellow agent, has raised the question of who is running things in Guadalajara — the central government, or the provincial police and the drug smugglers? It is a question President de la Madrid must answer. How he responds will determine whether — in the eyes of neighbors — Mexico passes Cortez test. And whether the anti-drug campaign works.

Rockford Register Star

Rockford, IL, August 21, 1986

Mexican President Miguel de la Madrid's "declaration of war on drug trafficking" into the United States can be applauded only when it's backed up by action.

Given the Mexican government's poor performance on drug enforcement in the past, it is difficult to give much credence to the Mexican president's promise.

Recent revelations that U.S. drug enforcement agents have been tortured and abused by Mexican police makes a mockery of de la Madrid's formal statement. DEA agent Victor Cortez of Tucson, Ariz., was abducted and tortured by Mexican police in Guadalajara last week. The United States has lodged a formal protest with the Mexican government.

Cortez is not the first agent to receive such treatment from so-called law enforcement officers within the corruption-riddled Mexican ranks. There are dozens of similar cases of American agents being detained and tortured so that Mexican police can learn more about the scope of U.S. anti-drug operations in Mexico.

In addition, the U.S. State Department's Bureau of International Narcotics Matters said earlier this year that Mexico's performance toward drug eradication was the "principal disappointment" of 1985.

Mexico produced more marijuana and opium poppies (used for heroin) in 1985 than in 1984. The bureau believes Mexico is the leading exporter of both illegal products to the United States.

Only Burma and Jamaica, of 14 countries with drug-eradication programs, met crop reduction targets set in agreements with the U.S.

Mexico didn't come close.

With the Mexican government in the grips of a crippling economic crisis, there are many measures President Reagan has at his disposal to encourage President de la Madrid to live up to his declaration against drugs.

Our president should use them.

The Washington Times

Washington, DC, August 22, 1986

A lot of people owe Customs Commissioner William von Raab an apology. It was Mr. von Raab, it will be recalled, who blew the whistle in May on the flagrant corruption that exists at all levels of the Mexican government. When he did so, U.S. officials, state and federal, outdid themselves denouncing the commissioner and heaping praise on their political brethren south of the border.

Last week it was revealed that Mexican police, knowing his identity full well, nearly tortured to death a U.S. Drug Enforcement Administration agent, Victor Cortez Jr. Mr. Cortez was picked up on a street in Guadalajara and taken to the local jail, where Mexican cops worked him over with electric cattle prods and forced carbonated water laced with jalapeno peppers up his nose.

Previously, Mexican dealers gunned down DEA agent Glenn Miles as he returned from a drop in Arizona, and more Mexican drug traffickers kidnapped, tortured, and murdered Enrique Camarena, another DEA agent. In the Camarena murder, a number of Mexican policemen have been indicted.

When, testifying before the House Select Committee on Narcotics, Mr. von Raab charged that corruption was widespread among Mexican officials, the Reagan administration hurriedly apologized. No less an eminence than Attorney General Edwin Meese assured his Mexican counterpart that Mr. von Raab's remarks by no means reflected the thinking of the administration. Other prominent officials, including Gov. Bruce Babbitt of Arizona, also moved with unbecoming alacrity to distance themselves from the truth.

It was a humiliating performance. One would have to live on the far side of the moon to believe that Mexican officials are not deeply involved in the drug trade. John Gavin, a former U.S. ambassador to Mexico, told a Senate subcommittee in June that "at least two" Mexican governors were "up to their elbows in the drug trade," and in February the State Department's Bureau of International Narcotics Matters called Mexico's anti-drug efforts the "principal disappointment" of 1985 and warned that Mexico had become the largest exporter of heroin to the United States.

In addition to supplying untold tons of heroin and marijuana, Mexico also is our largest supplier of black market amphetamine pills. And although Colombia remains the world's foremost producer of cocaine, in the past 18 months Mexican dealers have become the major wholesale brokers of American-bound coke. This is a snowstorm of immense proportions, and it has made countless Mexican politicians and police officials big rich.

No one — at least no honest person — will deny any of this. The niceties of U.S.-Mexican relations may prevent top U.S. officials from speaking with the candor of Mr. von Raab, but need they have compounded their cravenness by denouncing him? Someone in the administration should have the decency and courage to apologize to the gentleman now that he has been proved so right.

The News and Courier

Charleston, SC, August 29, 1986

Mexico's greatest problem is not so much corruption as the fact that it has become institutionalized. Because "la mordida" ("the bite" or kickback, as it would be called in English) is an accepted, unquestioned indecency of everyday life, along with many other abuses inflicted by authority on the long-suffering ordinary Mexican citizen, it is not surprising that moral standards are not considered to be a suitable subject for public debate.

When Mexicans are forced to consider the behavior of their police, for example, — usually because some unfortunate foreigner has fallen afoul of the Mexican authorities — they usually respond by expressing nationalistic outrage at outside meddling in their affairs. Such has been the predictable reaction in Mexico to American outrage over the allegations made by Victor Cortez Jr., a U.S. drug enforcement agent, that he was kidnapped and tortured by Jalisco state police. That is the same unit that detained Enrique Camarena Salazar, another American narcotics sleuth who was found murdered, with signs of torture, in Guadalajara a year ago.

Under U.S. pressure, Mexican authorities went through the motions of investigating the murder of Mr. Camarena. But the appalling treatment that Mr. Cortez says he was subjected to bears witness to the fact that nothing has changed. Although 11 Jalisco police officers have been charged with mistreating Mr. Cortez, the official government position, as outlined in a note from the foreign ministry, is that the police were in the right and Mr. Cortez was in the wrong.

Nothing will change until Mexicans stop trying to evade self-examination by arguing that they are "different" and do not have to live up to what they call "gringo" moral standards. Torture and murder are not ethnic foibles that can be overlooked. Unfortunately, although President Miguel de la Madrid is a distinct improvement on his shamelessly corrupt predecessors, he does not appear to have the moral fiber to come to grips with institutionalized corruption. The following statement (published in The Wall Street Journal on Sept. 10, 1984) explains why there is no action from the top to crack down on Mexico's institutionalized crooks: "I think that attempts are often made to analyze us with the same criteria and parameters used to analyze the American situation. The analysis does not come out right because we are different. Different as to our origins, evolution and as to the current configuration of our societies."

As long as Mexicans, from the president downward, go on claiming that they are not subject to "gringo standards," Mexico cannot change. Corruption will remain institutionalized, and even torture and murder, if committed in the Mexican way, will not be looked upon as crimes.

The Miami Herald

Miami, FL, August 17, 1986

WHILE champagne still bubbled in Washington in celebration of the jointly declared war against drugs by the United States and Mexico, the first American wounded in that war was flown in from Guadalajara, Mexico, to a Tucson, Ariz., hospital.

U.S. Drug Enforcement Administration (DEA) agent Victor Cortez, Jr. was abducted in Guadalajara by the Jalisco State Police. He was interrogated for about eight hours and was beaten and savagely tortured with electric cattle prods and with soda water forced through his nostrils. This is outrageous.

After his release, Mr. Cortez was brought to a U.S. hospital for checkup and treatment. A Mexican citizen tortured with Mr. Cortez is now in U.S. protective custody.

Cops can go crooked when ensnared by drugs. It has happened in Miami, where several officers face drug-related charges. In Mexico, however, existing government corruption grants a certain degree of impunity to such actions. Indictments of police officers are difficult and infrequent.

"The United States protests the unprovoked and totally unjustified detention and torture of one of its officials," said White House spokesman Larry Speakes. "Vigilantism by a state authority causes serious harm to the relationship necessary for our two countries to be able to combat drug trafficking and production."

A connection has been found in the torture of Mr. Cortez and the beating and murder last year of DEA agent Enrique Camarena Salazar. Mr. Camarena was killed by drug lords in collusion with the police of Guadalajara, the capital of Jalisco. It is this same police department that now has tortured Mr. Cortez and interrogated him about DEA investigations in Guadalajara.

Although several arrests were made in the case of Mr. Camarena, some people involved in the murder are still at large.

The Reagan Administration should exert all necessary pressure to get to the bottom of such acts against U.S. officials in a supposedly friendly country. The culpable Mexican authorities — regardless of how high they may rank — must be brought to justice for their intolerable conduct.

Malaysia Hangs 2 Australians Convicted of Heroin Trafficking

Two Australians convicted of heroin trafficking were hanged July 6, 1986 in Kuala Lumpur amid international protests. The executions, the first of non-Asians under the country's stringent drug laws, followed a string of legal appeals by the defendants as well as personal pleas on the part of Australian Prime Minister Bob Hawke and Prime Minister Margaret Thatcher of Great Britain. The two men were Brian Chambers and British-born Kevin Barlow, both 28. They had been arrested in 1983 for possession of 180 grams of heroin. In Malaysia, trafficking in more than 15 grams of the substance is a mandatory capital offense.

Thirty foreigners have been arrested in Malaysia for drug offenses since 1983 and faced death sentences if convicted. No one has yet been executed under the new law, but 31 drug traffickers have been executed under noncompulsory legislation in recent years, and another 50 people have received commutations of death sentences.

Roanoke Times & World-News

Roanoke, VA, July 8, 1986

TWO YOUNG American athletes recently paid with their lives for indulging in drug use. Two young Australian men recently paid with their lives for trafficking in drugs. They were hanged in Malaysia under that country's get-tough anti-drug laws.

The hanging of Brian Chambers Jr. and John Barlow brought outcries from the Western world. Australian Prime Minister Bob Hawke said his government did all it could do to "persuade the Malaysian authorities that whatever view they had about the guilt of these two young men, it was barbaric to take their lives."

British Prime Minister Margaret Thatcher also appealed on behalf of Barlow, who held dual Australian-British citizenship.

Chambers, a building contractor from Sydney, and Barlow, a welder from Perth, were arrested in November 1983 at Penang International Airport at Kuala Lumpur, Malaysia's capital, on charges of possessing 6.2 ounces of heroin. They were convicted of drug trafficking and sentenced to death in August 1985.

It remains for each society to determine what crimes merit that extreme measure. While we cannot recommend Malaysia's remedy for American society, we can sympathize with the small country's reasons for adopting such drastic measures. Prime Minister Mahathir Mohamad cited drug abuse as Malaysia's biggest problem, with about 500,000 addicts — one out of every 30 citizens. If that same ratio applied in this country, we would have 8 million addicts in our population.

"Anybody who violates Malaysia's anti-drug law will have to face the consequence," Mahathir said. "We cannot consider the color of the skin, philosophy or any other matter in our fight against this evil."

It is well to remember that Malaysia is in a part of the world that long has felt the drug scourge. The Chinese fought a war with Britain in 1840-42 over the opium trade, which was ruining China's economy, corrupting its society and sapping its national energy. China lost the war and still suffers from the effects of economic and technological backwardness, which the loss helped perpetuate.

The Chinese case was presented then in a letter to Queen Victoria from Lin Zexu, a commissioner appointed by the Chinese government to stop the opium trade. He wrote:

"You do not allow your own people to smoke [opium] or severe penalties for disobedience, evidently [. . .] a curse it is and therefore strictly prohibit-ing the practice. But better still than forbidding people to smoke, would it not be to forbid the sale and also the preparation of opium? . . . Not to smoke yourselves, but yet to dare to prepare and sell to and beguile the foolish masses of the Inner Land — this is to protect one's own life while leading others to death, to gather profit for oneself while bringing injury upon others. Such behavior is repugnant to the feelings of human beings and is not tolerated by the ways of God . . .

Malaysia's government sees the drug problem as serious enough to require draconian measures. It has therefore imposed the death penalty. It will be interesting to see whether this measure actually proves to be a deterrent.

The conventional wisdom is that capital punishment does not deter. But Dr. Philip J. Cook, a Duke University authority on criminal justice, notes that "the death penalty might serve as a deterrent . . . but not if we apply it half-heartedly. The Nazis used it effectively in the occupied territories during World War II."

The key to the death penalty's effectiveness as a deterrent therefore seems to lie in the ruthlessness with which it is applied. In American society, that degree of ruthlessness would be unacceptable. Americans would fear that they might execute the innocent. And they would wonder about the possibility of rehabilitating the pusher; selling heroin or cocaine is not considered quite as heinous as, say, shooting a cashier in an armed robbery.

We are a humane people and we pay for our humanity by exposing our children and ourselves to the dangers of drug addiction and the violent crime that supports it. Ernest van den Haag, in his book, "Punishing Criminals" (Basic Books, 1975), observed that "No matter what can be said for abolition of the death penalty, it will be perceived symbolically as a loss of nerve: social authority no longer is willing to pass an irrevocable judgment on anyone."

We have seen repeated evidence that drug addiction can sentence young people to lives of living hell. And we have seen how a drug as ubiquitous as cocaine can be deadly when ingested by certain people. The sellers of these substances are killers, whether they intend to be or not. The penalties should be tough and consistent.

While we cannot take pleasure in the deaths of the two young Australians, nor recommend the Malaysian approach to American states, we contemplate the deaths and ruined lives brought on by drug abuse and we cannot find it within us to call the Malaysian remedy barbaric.

The Honolulu Advertiser

Honolulu, HI, July 14, 1986

The hanging of two Australians for drug trafficking by the Malaysian government is a case expected to have political and emotional echoes. The death sentences were carried out despite mercy pleas from Australia, Britain and Amnesty International.

Anyone who opposes the death penalty is likely to find the dual hanging draconian. But whether it was unfair in any other sense is far from certain.

IT IS HARD to argue for special treatment because these were the first Westerners hanged under Malaysia's tough drug law, which requires the death penalty.

Since 1975, 36 others have been hanged under the law, including six non-Malaysians from neighboring Singapore. Some 120 more drug traffickers are in death row there, including 18 other foreigners.

Some fear reprisals against Malaysians in Australia, and other public relations problems in the West. However, some who deplore the death penalty feel this case could also have a deterrent effect on other Westerners who might be tempted to get involved in the Asian drug trade.

CONTROVERSY is going to continue, but the New Straits Times in Kuala Lumpur says there is at least some hope that this celebrated case will lead Malaysians to ask some questions. It said they include:

"Is capital punishment a civilized concept? Is mandatory death an effective deterrent? Should the judiciary be left with no choice but to dispense death with no facility to temper justice with mercy? Should the process of legal defense be reduced to a desperate quest for delaying tactics leading up to the prospect of a royal pardon?"

Good questions for any society. But Malaysia has an especially difficult drug problem, and it seems unlikely the tough law will be changed soon now that this traumatic point has been passed.

The Houston Post
Houston, TX, July 8, 1986

Two Australians died in Malaysia on Monday. The cause: drugs. Again.

Kevin Barlow, 28, and Brian Chambers, 29, didn't die of drug overdoses. They were hanged. Malaysia's harsh drug laws demand a mandatory death sentence for anyone caught trafficking in more than 3.3 ounces of heroin. Malaysian courts convicted the men of being in possession of 6.3 ounces of heroin in July 1985. Since the death penalty was imposed there in 1975, 36 convicted drug smugglers had been hanged. On Monday, the number rose to 38.

Whether Malaysia acted in a humanitarian way is beside the point. In that part of the world, most people, especially drug dealers, know the penalty for drug trafficking in Malaysia. Barlow and Chambers knew and took the risks. They paid a horrible price for a few ounces of heroin. More and more, drugs and death are becoming inseparable.

Richmond Times-Dispatch
Richmond, VA, July 12, 1986

Despite the growing public furor following the cocaine-related deaths of athletes Len Bias and Don Rogers, U.S. concern about drug abuse is nothing compared with that of Malaysia. There an estimated 500,000 people out of a total population of 15 million are considered drug addicts, and officials consider drug use — not the budget or the economy or joblessness — the No. 1 problem. Moreover, they are in deadly earnest about addressing that problem. The death penalty is mandatory for those convicted of drug trafficking there.

This week the Malaysian government put to death two Australians convicted of trafficking in heroin — despite the protests of Australian Prime Minister Bob Hawke and British Prime Minister Margaret Thatcher. Both referred to the hangings as barbaric. But Malaysian officials show no sign of relenting in their fight against this "evil," as Prime Minister Mahathir Mohamad refers to drug use. Shortly after the two men were hanged, the high court in Malaysia imposed the same sentence on a 69-year-old woman convicted of trafficking 46 ounces of raw opium.

Critics of the Malaysian government might be more sympathetic to capital punishment for drug trafficking if their countries suffered drug abuse to the same degree as Malaysia. New York state, for example, has a greater population than that country but is now treating some 43,000 drug addicts, which is far less than Malaysia's estimated 500,000.

We, however, are not advocating the death penalty for drug trafficking, heinous though the act is. Pushers, for example, didn't kill Len Bias or Don Rogers. They contributed to the deaths, to be sure, and may be subject to charges of manslaughter. But the evidence so far indicates that the two victims voluntarily took the cocaine that took their lives. No one held a gun to their heads and forced them to use it.

Stiffer penalties, short of hangings, for traffickers is an approach to drug abuse with which more and more people will likely agree, particularly as public awareness of the problem grows. But sooner or later the United States will have to realize that getting serious about drugs also means getting serious about the demand for them. That might mean kicking out of school any pupils found with drugs, improved drug education programs and more: in short, acknowledging that the trafficker alone is not to blame for drug abuse.

The Washington Times
Washington, DC, July 8, 1986

Indifferent to entreaties from Prime Ministers Margaret Thatcher of Britain and Bob Hawke of Australia, Malaysia on Monday strung up two men — both Australian, both 28 years old — convicted of trafficking in heroin. Malaysia has sent 38 persons to the gallows since it enacted no-nonsense drug laws in 1975, though until Monday only Asians had been hanged.

"Death to Traffickers!" posters are plastered everywhere. An explicit warning is printed on the landing card that every traveler must fill out. Only an imbecile — or a drug dealer — would try to pull one on the Malay cops. The law makes possession of more than 15 grams of heroin a capital crime; Monday's hangees were nabbed trying to leave the country with nearly 180 grams. You figure it out.

What is curious is the strenuous attempts by Mrs. Thatcher and Mr. Hawke to win a reprieve on humanitarian grounds. To be sure, politics and lingering jingoism probably dictated some sort of expression of concern. But to seek clemency on "humanitarian" grounds sort of bends the word out of shape.

When you come down to it, one might argue that, if anything, non-addicted drug pushers, since they deal in misery and death on an enormous scale, should be *executed* on humanitarian grounds.

Most of them think that, the profits being what they are, trafficking in drugs is worth the risk. In its own small way, Malaysia has set out to prove them wrong.

San Francisco Chronicle
San Francisco, CA, July 9, 1986

MALAYSIA'S EXECUTION by hanging of two Australian heroin dealers, punishment in the extreme by western standards, reflects that nation's deep and sincere concern for the tragic consequences of drug addiction.

The executions were the first carried out on non-Asians under a law mandating the death sentence for anyone found guilty of trafficking in more than 15 grams of heroin. The two Australians were found to have nearly 180 grams when they tried to leave the country at the international airport on Penang Island.

A number of countries in the region have enacted stringent narcotics legislation, both in response to growing addiction problems at home and to pressure from the United States to curb the flow of drugs from Southeast Asia. Malaysia Prime Minister Mahathir Mohamad said just this week that, "Anybody who violates Malaysia's anti-drug law will have to face the consequences. We cannot consider the color of the skin, philosophy or any other matter in our fight against this evil."

VISITORS TO MALAYSIA have ample warning that the penalties for drug smuggling are severe. Announcements are made on planes arriving in the country and immigration landing cards carry notices. Posters in the airports proclaim "Death To Traffickers."

The Kuala Lumpur government, concerned that some 500,000 people out of a population of 15 million are addicts, is fully justified in administering its uncompromising narcotics laws as it sees fit. Smugglers from abroad can hardly expect a double standard to apply.

Reputed Top Colombian Drug Trafficker Extradited to U.S.

Colombian police and military personnel February 4, 1987 captured a reputed leader of the world's largest drug trafficking ring and immediately extradited him to the United States. The trafficker, billionaire Carlos Enrique Lehder Rivas, 37, considered one of the world's most violent and successful drug traffickers and had long been sought by the U.S. Lehder and 14 bodyguards were captured in a predawn raid at a mansion in the Rionegro area near Medelin after a brief exchange of gunfire. Lehder was flown later that day to Tampa, Florida, arriving amid heavy security early Feb. 5. He appeared the same day in U.S. District Court in Tampa on drug- trafficking charges. Lehder was wanted in Jacksonville, Fla. in connection with a 1981 indictment charging him with importing 3,000 kilograms of cocaine. An August 1986 indictment returned in U.S. District Court in Miami charged him with a further 13 counts of drug smuggling and racketeering. Lehder became the 10th Colombian national and the 14th person overall to be extradited to the U.S. under a 1979 extradition treaty signed with Colombia. An order for his extradition to the U.S. had been signed in 1984.

Lehder was said to have begun his trafficking career selling marijuana in New York. In time he became a leader of the so-called Medilin Cartel, which was said to be responsible for 80% of the cocaine entering the U.S. In the late 1970s, Lehder bought a Bahamian isalnd, which was reportedly used as a base for his drug-trafficking activities before moving his operations to Colombia in 1981. In 1982, Lehder, who was a former senator, reportedly formed the Latino Nacionel political party, which sought to end the U.S. extradition treaty. The Colombian was said to be a political theorist who admired Adolf Hitler and the political philosophy of Friedrich Nietzche. In a 1985 television interview, he had called cocaine Latin America's "atom bomb," capable of destroying the U.S. He called on army officers and leftist revolutionaries to join the "cocaine bonanza," which he described as an "arm of the struggle against America" and the "Achilles heel of American imperialism."

U.S. Drug Enforcement Administration (DEA) chief John C. Lawn Feb. 5 said security at DEA offices worldwide had been intensified after Lehder's arrest. In 1985, Lehder had offered a payment of $350,000 to anyone who killed or captured the DEA chief and had also issued death threats against other law enforcement officials. He reportedly had threatened that if arrested, he would kill a judge a week until he was freed.

The Kansas City Times

Kansas City, MO, February 10, 1987

Colombia and the United States do not trade insults the way this country does with Mexico. There are no U.S. troops burning coca plantations in Colombia, as in Bolivia, where their presence has raised a domestic furor. America's misguided narcotrafficking policies in Bolivia and Mexico waste more time and money than results can justify. They mostly serve to scatter traffickers from parts of the country where enforcement assumes a high profile to parts where this presence is next to nil.

The arrest and extradition of Colombian Carlos Lehder Rivas, a reputed cocaine kingpin, is a good example of how a bilateral anti-drug policy should work. Colombian and American officials negotiate a way to net the big fish and rid their countries of a common plague. Negotiation would be ineffective were it not for conscience-minded officials who cannot be baited by traffickers' lavish offerings. That seems to be a key to Colombia's success.

Lehder is a very big fish. This former parking lot attendant with a fifth-grade education is believed to be one of the wealthiest drug barons in Colombia. He is a gangster with many low-life high-placed friends in the U.S.

Allowing Lehder to face the American judicial system was perhaps the bravest thing that a president could have done. Colombia President Virgilio Barco is now the most wanted man in Colombia because he has abided by legislation passed three years ago by Colombia's Conservative Party and which legalized deportation of drug fugitives to the U.S.

There are many who want Barco dead, just as they wished death for former President Betancur, who also netted big fish for the American courts. Betancur lives. The same cannot be said of his friends, relatives and those who assisted his anti-drug campaign. Elected officials, judges and journalists are among those hit by paid assassins or drug-financed leftist rebels. Since Lehder's extradition, more than a dozen Colombian notables, including Bogota Councilman Jorge Guzman, have been killed.

The Reagan administration must give Colombia more than a supply of funeral wreaths and kudos for its troubles. When Colombians "Just say 'No,' " they often sign their death warrants.

LEXINGTON HERALD-LEADER
Lexington, KY
February 8, 1987

The United States has managed, with the help of Colombian president Virgilio Barco Vargas, to extradite the man federal officials think is one of the world's biggest drug traffickers, a king of cocaine. What's important now is that Colombia be encouraged to stand firm with the United States in rounding up the rest of Colombia's cocaine royalty.

Carlos Lehder Rivas, a political disciple of Adolf Hitler, makes a fine trophy for the U.S. Justice Department and Drug Enforcement Administration: Serving up an alleged top dog in the world cocaine trade will stress to those who would follow in Lehder's footsteps that the United States and Colombia are serious about their drug-busting. But even more important is that Lehder can provide information about his friends in the drug business. Without a comprehensive, well-informed effort to rout the Colombian drug trade, it would be all too simple for another cocaine distributor to fill the gap left by Lehder.

Rounding up such men is not a tidy or safe business. Already death threats have apparently been made against law enforcement officials in connection with Lehder's capture. There are rumors that Lehder threatened to kill a federal judge a week if arrested. The DEA is tightening security at its field offices in response to the Lehder arrest.

With luck and the continued cooperation of Colombia, the arrest of Lehder will serve as a prelude to the arrest of Colombia's other top three drug dealers. Leon Kellner, the U.S. attorney in Miami, noted that the Lehder arrest means, "One down, three to go."

With continued help from Columbian officials, the other kingpins of the international cocaine trade may yet be brought to justice.

𝕷𝖔𝖘 𝕬𝖓𝖌𝖊𝖑𝖊𝖘 𝕿𝖎𝖒𝖊𝖘

Los Angeles, CA, February 2, 1987

Colombia is losing its war against illegal drug traffickers, and losing it badly. A poor but proud nation of 28 million people is literally under siege by a relative handful of powerful and violent criminals.

In a world plagued by illicit drugs, and the corruption and other social problems that they cause, no other nation has suffered the way Colombia has in recent years. Judges there are being murdered at the rate of one a month, according to a recent dispatch from Bogota by Times correspondent William Montalbano, and even a Supreme Court justice was killed by assassins. Three newspaper editors who crusaded against drug traffickers have been murdered, as have several top police officials —including one sitting attorney general. Even a former attorney general who was given an ambassadorial post behind the Iron Curtain to help protect him from restribution was tracked down in Hungary and killed by a hired gunman. And those are only the most extreme examples of the arrogant lawlessness of the Colombian drug gangs.

So rich and powerful have Colombia's drug lords become (they control an estimated 80% of the cocaine sold in the United States) that they have even begun spending their ill-gotten gains to try to win support from Colombia's poor. They have built social centers, funded food programs and tried to run for public office, portraying themselves as modern-day Robin Hoods. Some have gone so far as to suggest that they might repatriate the money that they have hidden in foreign banks to help bolster the Colombian economy—if the government of President Virgilio Barco lets up on the legal pressure that it has put on them.

To their credit, Barco and many other honest Colombian officials have resisted all efforts by the drug lords to intimidate them or to seduce them with the fantastic wealth that their filthy trade produces. Last month, in a particularly courageous act, Barco signed into law a new extradition treaty with the United States under which any arrested drug kingpins can be sent to this country for trial. It is the legal system in the United States, still largely beyond their corrupt and violent reach, that the Colombian drug lords fear most.

But the Colombians will not win their war on drugs by themselves. They need more help than they are getting from their allies, especially the United States. How sad and ironic that, as Colombia's president was exposing himself to physical danger by signing an extradition treaty with the United States, President Reagan was submitting to Congress a budget that would reduce the Administration's spending on drug-education and drug-eradication programs.

It should come as no surprise that, as in Mexico and Peru, prominent Colombian politicians are starting to ask why their nation should bear the pain of the drug war when the rich nation that consumes most of those illegal drugs is not doing enough to control the problem within its own borders. Until the United States is willing to do more to fight the war on drugs in this country, such as spending more to educate potential consumers about the dangers of drug use and to help police crack down on drug traffickers here, smaller and poorer nations like Colombia will fight a bloody but losing battle against the brutal drug kingpins of this world.

THE SACRAMENTO BEE

Sacramento, CA, February 7, 1987

Carlos Lehder, allegedly the biggest drug dealer in the world, is in U.S. custody at a secret location in Florida after being arrested in Colombia and quickly extradited. If he is convicted, it would be the first time a kingpin of one of the boldest and most violent outlaw organizations of modern times — one that's believed to control the flow of 80 percent of the cocaine and marijuana that reach American streets — has been brought to justice.

Yet Lehder's arrest, important as it is, also is cause for apprehension. Other big Colombian drug dealers remain at large and, in the violent and intimidating atmosphere that pervades Colombia, virtually a law unto themselves. They have made and kept threats to kill anyone who tried to shut down their operations: Two Colombian justice ministers, a supreme court justice, 20 judges, hundreds of policemen, a newspaper editor and two informants for the U.S. Drug Enforcement Administration are among the victims of the cocaine cartel's savagery. One Colombian official was even tracked down and murdered in Communist Hungary.

Paradoxically, the same thugs who now threaten to avenge Lehder's arrest may be the ones who turned him in because of the high profile he had assumed as a crackpot politician and admirer of Hitler who also supports some left-wing causes and describes illicit cocaine trafficking as an arm of "the struggle against America." Whether his fellow gangsters betrayed him or not, their threat to exact reprisals cannot be ignored, either in Colombia or in this country.

Colombian President Virgilio Barco has shown great courage in extraditing Lehder after his arrest last week in a shootout with police. U.S. officials must follow that example in prosecuting him and in standing firm against all attempts to thwart the course of justice by threats of reprisal. The joint Colombian-U.S. campaign against Colombian drug merchants has had little to show for the $70 million spent over five years. The arrest of Lehder thus is an important psychological breakthrough. Now it's vital to stand firm by refusing to let gangsters cow civilized society into backing down against this lawless threat.

𝕿𝖍𝖊 𝖁𝖎𝖗𝖌𝖎𝖓𝖎𝖆𝖓-𝕻𝖎𝖑𝖔𝖙

Norfolk, VA
February 10, 1987

The capture in Colombia and extradition to the United States of a man alleged to be among the world's biggest, richest and most vicious cocaine tycoons represents a major victory on a strategically important front in the war on drugs. Carlos Lehder Rivas, 37, former Colombian senator, admirer of Adolf Hitler and reputed billionaire kingpin of 80 percent of the U.S. cocaine trade, now sits in a Florida jail, awaiting federal prosecution on multiple counts of drug smuggling and racketeering. If convicted, he could be sentenced to life in prison.

Mr. Lehder's *modus operandi* makes him an especially choice war prize. When not combining their peculiar form of business and pleasure on Mr. Lehder's privately owned island in the Bahamas or at his estate in the Colombian resort city of Medellin, Mr. Lehder and his cohorts in the "Medellin cartel" — the OPEC of the drug trade — are busy intimidating and murdering Colombian government officials and private citizens who stand in their way.

Among those gunned down in the nation's streets since last July were a Colombian supreme court justice; a district-court judge who has ruled against Medellin traffickers; a police colonel who was head of the country's anti-narcotics unit, and two newspaper editors who opposed the cartel in print. The cartel's hired killers have roamed as far as Budapest, where a former Colombian justice minister was the target of an assassination attempt last month. Mr. Lehder also has placed bounties on the heads of top U.S. Drug Enforcement Administration officials.

Though Mr. Lehder is safely in custody, his countrymen remain at risk. Before his capture, Mr. Lehder warned that his minions would kill a judge a week until he is freed. The six-month-old government of drug-fighting President Virgilio Barco Vargas concedes that it is no match for the cocaine cartel's armed caravans.

Vice President George Bush, chairman of a federal anti-drug project, has sent a message to Colombian President Barco praising his courage. But words are not enough. Colombia deserves no less than Bolivia has received in its war on cocaine traffickers: U.S. military equipment, technicians and pilots last year assisted Bolivian officials in a major drug-eradication assault on cocaine fields and laboratories.

Such assistance has not yet saved Bolivia from narco-terrorists. Colombia cannot expect a quick blitz to victory, either. But of the Reagan administration's many fronts in its war on drugs, none has produced results so spectacular as the capture of Mr. Lehder.

Such advances may never vanquish foreign drug traffickers. But if Colombia seeks U.S. reinforcements, the Reagan administration should be prepared to shift resources from its overemphasized domestic drug-testing front to fight the war on drugs — and terrorism — at its source in places such as Colombia.

The Washington Post

Washington, DC, February9, 1987

IN THE WAR against drugs, Colombia has just set a very brave example. It arrested and extradited to the United States a man named Carlos Lehder Rivas, who is accused of being one of the great cocaine traffickers in his country. Drug dealers there have used their immense riches and their command of armed men to practice an arrogance unheard of in more fortunate places. Of the police, officials, judges, editors and others who have resisted their vast criminality, those they cannot buy they have sought to murder or intimidate, reaching out even to attack a conscientious justice minister who had been sent off for his safety as ambassador to Hungary.

Americans know the menace of drugs at home, but in such a country as Colombia, where the institutions of law enforcement and administration are weaker, the very integrity of the nation comes to be at stake. There is actually a proposal that the leading drug dealers, in exchange for a presumably friendly prosecution in Colombia, pay off the country's $13 billion foreign debt.

The extradition process in Colombia is infinitely delicate. It provides Colombians with a way to bring to justice and to send out of the country suspects who may be more dangerous when they are in official hands—because of the violence their thugs take to reclaim or avenge them—than when they are at large. Yet retaliation against those who take part in extradition is always a threat—see what happened to the ambassador in Hungary. There also seems to be a feeling, halfway between shame and nationalism, that makes Colombians hesitate to hand off these desperadoes to others, especially to the United States. The newly arrested Mr. Lehder had been known to characterize cocaine as a weapon against "American imperialism." He is only the first of the accused kingpins to be extradited. Florida has him now.

Cooperation in law enforcement with Colombia and other source countries is increasingly central to American drug policy. Colombians who look at the comparative costs to the two countries, however, can be forgiven for asking whether the United States yet does its full share. American diplomacy stresses the idea that drugs are a shared hemispheric concern; this is the basis for common action. This is so, but it is also so that many Latins see the United States, with its huge demand for drugs, as the principal cause of their terrible drug costs, including increasing rates of addiction among their young. The readiness of such a country as Colombia to take the risks of cracking down on the biggest traffickers deserves appreciation in this country—and matching seriousness.

The Miami Herald

Miami, FL, February 6, 1987

ONE DOWN, three to go." U.S. Attorney Leon Kellner applied these words to report the capture of drug lord Carlos Lehder Rivas, one of four leaders of the "Medellin Cartel." The Colombia-based organization is reputed to supply 80 percent of the cocaine consumed in the United States. Mr. Lehder was captured this week at a ranch near Medellin and immediately extradited to the United States, where he faces multiple drug-trafficking charges.

Only a few weeks ago the U.S.-Colombia extradition treaty was virtually nonexistent. A legal technicality — the document did not bear the actual signature of a Colombian president — had reduced the treaty to wet paper. Showing his commitment to the bitter anti-drug war, President Virgilio del Barco rescued the accord with his immediate signature.

Equal swiftness characterized the capture and extradition of Mr. Lehder. Colombian National Police moved fast on an informant's tip and made the arrest after a 15-minute gun battle. Once Mr. Lehder was under the custody of the Colombian government, President del Barco lost no time in handing him over to the U.S. Justice Department.

President del Barco and the Colombian police deserve praise for an excellent job done under strenuous and dangerous circumstances. The cooperation of American authorities is also to be commended. The U.S. Justice Department has been persistent in activating the extradition treaty. Also, Drug Enforcement Administration agents have stood behind Colombian agents in their difficult drug war.

Now it is up to U.S. authorities to carry this victory all the way. While Mr. Lehder is processed for trial, extreme security measures must be taken to avoid an escape attempt. This man counts his fortune in billions gleaned from street-corner drug sales, quite enough to buy his way out of most situations. Further, the U.S. Embassy in Bogotá should take special security measures, lest the cocaine king's vassals seek hostages or threaten other violence in pursuit of their boss's release.

It has taken a long time to bring Mr. Lehder in. Now the United States must keep him.

Miami, FL, February 13, 1987

THE CAPTURE of Carlos Lehder Rivas, one of four co-leaders of the Medellin cocaine cartel, brought justifiable exultation both here and in Colombia. One down, three to go? Yes — and no. For the cartel's reach is so broad, its ruthlessness so bestial, its illicit wealth so staggering that even this law-enforcement coup is unlikely to deter it much or for long.

That may sound pessimistic, but it isn't. It's simple realism.

Cocaine is a scourge. It's as deadly as the plague for Colombians who dare oppose it, as endemic as the sniffles among all strata of American society.

American demand drives the Colombian supply. American users lie, cheat, steal, and sacrifice family, career, and health to obtain cocaine. The Medellin Cartel viciously kills anyone — police officer, judge, cabinet minister, journalist — who attempts to loosen its pernicious grip on Colombian life.

So yes, it is exhilarating to have one of the Medellin Cartel's principals at last in the embrace of the American justice system. Yet whatever the result of Mr. Lehder's trial on multiple cocaine-trafficking charges, it will lessen neither the demand at South Florida's squalid "crack" houses nor the cartel's resolve to fill the demand.

Mr. Lehder's arrest *is* significant in another respect that could be — pray that it is — both telling and enduring. It came scant days before *The Herald* began to publish an exhaustive investigative report on the cartel on Sunday.

That was indeed a serendipitous confluence of events. It prompted the two national newspapers, *El Tiempo* and *El Espectador*, and the five regional newspapers in Colombia to request permission to reprint simultaneously the entire series — text, photos, charts, everything. Request promptly granted.

That request took great courage, because the cartel reputedly has assassinated 15 Colombian journalists since 1984 — most recently Guillermo Cano, editor of *El Espectador*, last Dec. 17. These newspapers' presentation *en masse* of *The Herald*'s wealth of information, supplemented with their own reporting on the cartel, will blanket Colombia with facts on the menace emanating from Medellin.

Thus Mr. Lehder's arrest already has galvanized the Colombian press. Perhaps that effect will suffuse itself throughout Colombia and create nationwide revulsion against the cartel. Revulsion — against suppliers in Colombia, against cocaine use in America — is the only true antidote to this scourge.

The Seattle Times

Seattle, WA, February 6, 1987

THE capture of cocaine king Carlos Lehder Rivas in a shootout at one of his luxurious Colombian hideouts and his immediate extradition to the United States provide a deeply satisfying example of the kind of cooperation this country has long sought with Latin American authorities in the war on illegal narcotics.

That sort of cooperation has often been hard to come by. Latin governments at times have taken the attitude that the drug problem is strictly a U.S. concern. Some Latin authorities have been bought off or scared off by the powerful drug racketeers, who can offer fortunes in bribes and do not hesitate to use assassination and torture as tools of intimidation.

Nowhere has the power of the narcotics barons been more brazenly on display than in Colombia, whose most lucrative export is not to be found among international-trade statistics, because it happens to be cocaine.

Former President Belisario Betancur showed great courage in signing Lehder's extradition order in May 1984. Lehder, described by U.S. officials as "the most violent of the Medellin Cartel," has thumbed his nose at U.S. and Colombian justice. The Medellin Cartel, a group of billionaire drug lords, is believed responsible for processing, shipping and distributing more than 80 percent of the cocaine consumed in the United States.

During the past year it appeared that Colombia had backed away from Betancur's resolve. But the killing of a fearless anti-racketeering editor, Guillermo Cano, last Nov. 17 prompted Colombia's current president, Virgilio Barco Vargas, to open a new offensive against the cocaine kings. The result was the capture of Lehder and 15 bodyguards.

Lehder is indeed a big prize. But final victory in the war on the international illegal drug trade will never be achieved as long as North American users continue to show contempt for the law and their own physical well-being.

The Saginaw News

Saginaw, MI, February 11, 1987

The arrest and extradition of alleged Colombian drug kingpin Carlos Lehder Rivas is extraordinary, as columnist Georgie Anne Geyer explains in her commentary today. Her fear — and ours — is that, for quite different reasons, this reputed controller of 75 percent of the cocaine traffic may escape justice in the United States as he has in Colombia.

Consider that drug dealers have tried to make a deal with the Colombian government: In exchange for lenient legal treatment, they would pay off the entire $13 billion foreign debt.

The drug trade is that lucrative. It is that dangerous. The dealers, and not only in Colombia, threaten to take over the country. Whom they cannot bribe, they kill.

Colombia's lightning transfer of Lehder to answer a U.S. indictment was a desperate, courageous bid for both self-preservation and self-respect. Its legitimate institutions are in jeopardy. No modern nation truly wishes to live off the suffering of others.

But now the American system of justice is under scrutiny, not because it is being bought off, but because of its traditional regard for the niceties of proper procedure. Already one attorney has questioned the manner in which Lehder was extradited.

That respect for the rights of the accused is a matter of pride in a civilized society. But Lehder, by all accounts, thinks and acts by other rules: He recognizes none that apply to him. How does society handle such a man?

Very carefully. Marshals ringed the Florida courtroom. Sharpshooters were posted atop nearby buildings. And the judge denied bail pending the scheduled March 23 trial.

If he did not, there almost certainly would be no trial. To men with incomes of $300 million a year and up, what does bail mean?

The further danger is that life also means little. In Colombia, the drug cartel has murdered dozens of policemen, judges, even ministers — and, yes, the journalists who expose their activities. What is its influence in the U.S.? This case may tell who holds the true balance of power.

It needs to be said once more that Americans are not entirely innocent in this matter. This country's appetite for illicit drugs engorges the dealers and undermines neighboring nations.

But the Lehder case goes to the source of the problem, and to the heart of justice. The U.S. alleges that he is one of the greatest drug dealers in the world. "Prove it," says his lawyer. It will be a trial that will allow, in many ways, no room for error.

San Francisco Chronicle

San Fransisco, CA, February 9, 1987

WITH THE ARREST and extradition of billionaire Carlos Lehder, believed to be one of the world's biggest cocaine dealers, the government of Colombia seems at last to have seized the initiative against a widespread narcotics traffic that tears at the country's vitals.

Recently, those who spoke out and acted against the drug business — journalists, judges and prosecutors — were threatened and often murdered. Traffickers made good their appalling boast: "We can kill whom we want." Fear did its work and the drug dealers went about their trade with arrogant openness.

By seizing Lehder, Colombian authorities have taken one of the reputed leaders of the so-called Medellin cartel, which U.S. Justice Department officials say is responsible for 75 per cent of all cocaine smuggled into America.

In mid-January, every newspaper in Colombia published on its front page a declaration of principles. Coming after assassination of the respected editor of El Espectador, this stated that the country was in danger of falling under "complete control" of traffickers. The government, political parties and Colombian society were urged to unify behind effective action against the criminals.

COLOMBIAN OFFICIALS and the American community in that country naturally fear reprisals now that this big fish is behind bars in Florida. But it took courage to grab him, and it will take continued courage and perseverance to turn the tide in this desperately-important battle.

Contra Drug Smuggling Charged

Two alleged drug traffickers had claimed that the Nicaraguan contras had smuggled drugs into the United States from Colombia via remote air strips in Costa Rica, according to *Newsweek* magazine in its January 26, 1987 issue. *Newsweek* had interviewed the two men who were being held in federal prison in Miami. They were Gary Betzner, 45, who said he had flown planes used in the operation, and George Morales, who said he had provided the aircraft. Betzner and Morales claimed that U.S. Central Intelligence Agency operatives and other U.S. officials had helped in an operation in which drugs were shipped out of Costa Rica and guns were were shipped in. Betzner claimed that the U.S. Drug Enforcement Administration (DEA) also knew of and assisted in the drug flights. Both men charged that contra leaders pocketed the money, which did not reach the contras in the field. *Newsweek* said a third alleged smuggler claimed to have seen planes belonging to Southern Air Transport Co. loaded with cocaine in Colombia in 1985. Southern Air had been linked to the El Salvador-based contra supply network set up by former National Security Council aide Lt. Col. Oliver North.

The *Washington Post* reported Jan. 20 that Jorge Ochoa Vasquez, reputedly a leader of the Medelin Cartel, said to be the world's largest drug ring, was in charge of a contra drug operation using Southern Air.

Separately, U.S. officials said Jan. 19 that DEA agents in 1986 had discovered evidence that the crews of the private contra supply network based in El Salvador were ferrying arms to El Salvador and then stopping in Panama on the return trip to pick up cocaine and marijuana. Officials were said to believe the Americans were motivated purely by personal profit and that a claim that they were protected by Lt. Col. North was a bluff.

St. Petersburg Times

St. Petersburg, FL, August 28, 1986

The Reagan administration's get-tough policy on drugs is by no means universal or consistent. While some officials go forward with plans to force millions of presumably innocent Americans to submit to the indignity of individual drug testing, another side of the administration is proving itself remarkably tolerant of well-documented drug smuggling activity on the part of its favorite "freedom fighters."

The White House's attitude seems to be that a little cocaine trafficking is okay, as long as the profits go to a good cause — such as an undeclared war on the government of Nicaragua.

It was reported last December that Nicaraguan rebels operating out of Costa Rica had become involved in a scheme to smuggle drugs into the United States. The profits of that operation helped to pay for their guerrilla war against the Sandinista government of Nicaragua.

White House officials didn't want to hear the story. Not long before the Costa Rican operation was exposed, the administration had made similar — but unsubstantiated — charges of drug smuggling on the part of the Sandinistas. When U.S. intelligence confirmed the *contras'* involvement in cocaine trafficking, the State Department publicly repudiated the charges.

In the meantime, Nicaraguans who said they were acting on behalf of the *contras* have been convicted in connection with two cocaine smuggling operations broken up by San Francisco authorities. Investigations showed that the profits from those operations also helped to finance the *contra* war.

At long last, a new report compiled by the State Department admits that "the available evidence points to involvement with drug traffickers by a limited number of persons having various kinds of affiliations with or political sympathies for resistance groups." The report says, however, that it is "inevitable that there will be some who have had drug connections" among the 20,000 or so active *contras.*

Incredibly, even the evidence included in this report — lamely worded and at least eight months late — is more than some administration officials want to admit to. A cover letter accompanying the report says "the administration believes these allegations are false."

A *contra* leader reading the language of the administration report must feel that he has been given official approval to continue to raise money by fair means or foul. After all, the number of rebels involved in trafficking, whether 10 or 1,000, will always be "limited." If such connections are considered "inevitable," there isn't much reason to bother trying to eliminate them. And some members of the administration will continue to question the validity of the accusations even after *contras* are convicted of criminal charges.

The administration's single-minded crusade against the Sandinistas has blinded many people to the troubling moral problems raised by our proxy army in Central America. The obvious unwillingness to crack down on the *contras'* drug trafficking is just another obvious example of that moral blind spot.

The Register

Santa Ana, CA,
April 14, 1986

As debate in the House of Representatives over supplying $100 million from U.S. taxpayers to anti-government forces in Nicaragua heats up, the charge has predictably been renewed that the so-called *contras* have been dealing in drugs to finance their insurrection. Rep. Michael Barnes, D-Md., says he thinks Americans will be outraged by this perfidy, while Rep. Bob Dornan, R-Garden Grove, suggests that it's understandable that the *contras* have turned to drug dealing since the United States cut off funds some time ago.

These allegations of drug-dealing by governments and political movements surface constantly, and it's likely that there is some plausibility to most of them. As long as the United States continues to try to outlaw certain substances for which there is a strong demand, thus driving up prices and potential profits, drug-dealing will be attractive to those who think they need lots of money (preferably not too traceable) quickly. Governments and political movements certainly fit this category.

Governments and insurrectionists are also well situated to deal drugs. Governments may be able to use diplomatic pouches and other prerogatives to move contraband. Insofar as governments and rebel movements effectively control territory and have weapons, trucks, airplanes and helicopters, they can be useful to drug dealers. And the government or political movement doesn't exist that doesn't think it can use more money.

Drug trafficking is no respecter of ideology. In recent years Bulgarian customs guards have resold seized heroin and both Colombian colonels and left-wing insurrectionists in Colombia have protected or dabbled in cocaine and marijuana. There is good evidence that some Nicaraguan government officials have trafficked in drugs. It is almost certain that the North Korean diplomatic service has smuggled heroin in diplomatic pouches and that the anti-communist, CIA-backed Hmong irregulars financed operations during the Vietnam war with opium and heroin.

Those facts are not pleasant, but they are facts. Drug dealing by political movements and governments is likely to continue unless the United States decides to decriminalize the possession and use of certain drugs. Having junkies indirectly finance political movements of varying degrees of unsavoriness is simply one more predictable result of U.S. laws against drugs.

The Courier-Journal & TIMES
Louisville, KY, February 15, 1987

IN MIAMI, prosecutors are having trouble getting drug convictions because alleged smugglers have begun resorting to what might be called the coke-and-*contra* defense. Instead of denying that they were dealing, the accused claim they worked secretly for the U. S. government, raising money for Nicaraguan "freedom fighters."

These claims may often be lies, but it's tough for law enforcement officials to disprove them. Prosecutors also worry that such stories may have emotional appeal to Miami juries that include Cuban Americans, many of whom favor U. S. support for the *contras.*

This is a sorry state of affairs. It's no worse, however, than the fog of lies and half-truths generated by the Reagan administration to obscure its arms trafficking with Iran and its efforts to skirt congressional restrictions on funding for the anti-Sandinista guerrillas.

According to *The Washington Post,* this willingness to resort to lies led some administration officials to work out a plan for misleading Congress — a plan that countenanced perjury.

William Casey, who has since resigned as head of the Central Intelligence Agency, was scheduled to submit testimony to a Senate committee last November on arms sales to Iran. In a story concocted by the CIA and the National Security Council, Mr. Casey was to allege that U. S. officials believed a shipment a year earlier from Israel to Iran had contained oil drilling equipment. In fact, as Mr. Casey, President Reagan and Secretary of State George Shultz evidently knew at the time, U. S.-made Hawk missiles were being shipped to Iran.

Mr. Shultz, according to *The Post,* got wind of the lie Mr. Casey planned to tell. The secretary of state then had what *Post* reporter Don Oberdorfer called "a tense showdown" with the President.

As a result of the Shultz protest, Mr. Casey's testimony was revised — though he still claimed that, "to the CIA's knowledge," the November 1985 shipment had contained drilling equipment, not missiles.

Four days after Mr. Casey told this tale to the committee, Attorney General Edwin Meese announced he had found evidence that proceeds from the Iran arms sales had been diverted to the *contras.*

Since then, congressional investigators have been trying to untangle a much larger skein of lies, and a special prosecutor is also looking into the Iran-*contra* connections.

Getting to the truth promises to be a daunting task. Compared to some high-level officials and former officials in Washington, those alleged drug smugglers in Miami sound like small-time fibbers.

The Philadelphia Inquirer
Philadelphia, PA, February 24, 1987

President Reagan wasn't content in his anti-Sandinista speeches last winter to paint Nicaragua as "a second Cuba, a second Libya," "a mortal threat to the entire New World." He liked to save up a kidney punch for the peroration. The punch was something called "narco-terrorism" and it focused on a Sandinista drug connection.

There was one photograph that would show up in State Department booklets and one — the same one — that the President would use on nationally televised appeals for contra funding. It purported to show a Sandinista official loading cocaine at a government-owned airfield. "I know every American parent concerned about the drug problem will be outraged to learn that top Nicaraguan government officials are deeply involved in drug trafficking," the President would say.

Exactly *how* deeply has remained something of a question, although the larger question in recent months has been not the Sandinista drug connection, but allegations that the contras' hands are pretty dirty themselves. The House subcommittee on crime, chaired by Rep. William J. Hughes (D., N.J.), has been investigating and now the Senate Foreign Relations Committee is about to take a look at both sides of the question, especially the contra side.

Given the state of affairs in Washington and the disarray over Central America policy in particular, the Nicaraguan drug connection (Colombia, let's face it, is the *real* connection) might seem like a sidelight. But it's time the administration's assertions were put to the test on issue after issue where official disinformation has obscured reality.

If the contentions of contra drug-running are substantiated, Mr. Reagan should explain why parents shouldn't be equally outraged at the administration's mercenaries. If there's a serious Sandinista connection, the White House can have satisfaction that it beat Senate investigators to the punch.

ST. LOUIS POST-DISPATCH
St. Louis, MO, February 28, 1987

For years, rumors have linked the Miami-based Contras with another group that has its unofficial headquarters in that city: cocaine smugglers. Now there's growing evidence that those sordid rumors may be based in sordid fact.

The FBI, which is investigating drug-running out of Miami, has a witness who swears he saw Southern Air Transport planes being loaded with cocaine in Barranquilla, Colombia. Southern Air Transport, you will recall, was the carrier of choice in the Contra arms supply scheme orchestrated by Lt. Col. Oliver North. Investigators suspect the planes would drop off a load of weapons to the Contras and fly on to Colombia before returning to Miami, where the drugs would be exchanged for more weapons and the trade triangle begun again.

Supporting testimony comes from two admitted drug smugglers, Gary Betzner and George Morales, in federal prison in Miami. The Contras weren't interested solely in buying weapons, Mr. Morales told *Newsweek.* The ringleaders pocketed the proceeds, he said, leaving the Contras in the field without even enough beans to eat.

More disturbing yet are these witnesses' accounts of complicity by CIA agents and officials of the U.S. Drug Enforcement Agency, who, the witnesses say, not only knew what was going on, but participated in the drugs-for-weapons exchange.

It's an unholy, implausible alliance, if it exists at all. At one point it would have been unthinkable — a radical, mind-bending suggestion entertained only by political enemies of the Reagan administration. In the wake of the Iran-Contra scandal, though, barriers to the unthinkable have come tumbling down. And that, more than evidence that may have been around for years, has made the start of congressional investigations of these rumors not simply justified but urgent as well.

Part IV: Education, Schools and Teenagers

Of major concern in the U.S. today is the early age at which drug users begin to experiment. The casualness which many parents have shown to the taking of drugs has extended to young people. A drug is often no further away than the family medicine cabinet. The adolescent is perhaps the most vulnerable individual confronting the growing social acceptance of drug use in the United States. But recent studies have indicated that drug abuse is even increasing among younger children. This is particularly disturbing becuase studies have shown that the younger a person begins to experiment with drugs, the more likely he is to progress to heavier drug use and stronger drugs. There are any number of theories why a child first experiments with drugs: questions of status, peer pleasure, thrills, boredom, stimulation, sophistication, difficulty coping with problems, and so on. Whatever the reasons, they have much to do with adolescence in general, a time when a child is developing physically and emotionally and is caught up in an identity crisis. When an adolescent has difficulty meeting society's demands, as well as his own internal demands, the result can be extreme anxiety and a feeling of powerlessness. The need to relieve these tensions can result in drug experimentation and give the adolescent a temporary high feeling and an exaggerated sense of competence and power. Instant gratification and the feeling of euphoria can dampen the fear of developing independence and decisionmaking. However, because every adolescent is a unique individual with his or her own physical and psychological problems, there can be no definitive cause of drug use.

While the treatment of drug dependence is extremely important, the greatest hope for combating the problem lies in preventing drug abuse from starting in the first place, or interfering with its use during the early experimentation stage. There are four generally recognized prevention stages:

1. *Information.* This includes providing accurate and objective information about all types of drugs and their effects on the body.

2. *Intervention.* This includes providing assistance and support to adolescents during critical periods of their life through counseling, the use of hotlines, etc.

3. *Education.* This includes clarifying values and improving problem-solving skills within a structured setting. Group discussion and role playing are common techniques in helping young people improve their ability to cope.

4. *Alternatives.* This includes promoting confidence and self-reliance through new, challenging experiences in school and providing positive alternatives to drug-taking behavior. Such alternatives include restoration projects, volunteer services in the community and helping such causes as environmental preservation.

Various parent groups have been organized in the last ten years to combat the drug blight among the young. Perhaps one of the driving forces behind the organization of parent groups stems from the feeling of helplessness parents feel when they realize their child has been experimenting with drugs. Many parents have no idea what actions to take, what questions to ask, and where to turn for help. Because of the unpredictable nature of drug abuse among adolescents, where there are few patterns and use can simply come and go because of fads and pressures, parents are often at a loss for guidelines in handling the problem. Unfortunately, there are also parents who are simply unwilling to look at or deal with the problem; many feel self-guilt, anger and embarrassment and refuse to cooperate. This unwillingness works at cross purposes with professionals who are trying to cope with the problem. There are other parents who simply want to turn the problem over to a counselor and expect him to deal with the issue without any cooperation on their part.

Each year 50,000 people die on U.S. highways and over half of these deaths are alcohol-related. Accidents involving alcohol also result in injuries to more than a half million people, more than $1 billion in property damage, insurance costs, medical costs, services, and several hundred thousand arrests. The majority of alcohol-related accidents occur at night and a larger proportion of men than women are involved. One of the biggest menaces on the highway is the problem drinker who has previous arrests for offences involving alcohol. Studies indicate that people with severe drinking problems are disproportionately involved in all kinds of crashes. Single vehicle accidents are alcohol-related 75% of the time. About 50% of all fatally injured drinking drivers are less than 30 years old. From 40-60% of all fatal crashes involving young people are alcohol-related. Not only are they inexperienced in both drinking and driving, they are more likely to combine alcohol with another drug. As a result of a rise in awareness about the risks to health, organizations have been formed to combat drug abuse. Helping those who are becoming addicted to alcohol has been of particular importance. Throughout the country, high school groups are being organized to help their classmates. Telephone numbers are available at all times for teenagers who have had too much to drink. They call a hotline, manned by their peers, and someone is sent to drive them home. As these groups are fairly new, there has been little evaluation of their effectiveness thus far, but the trend is encouraging.

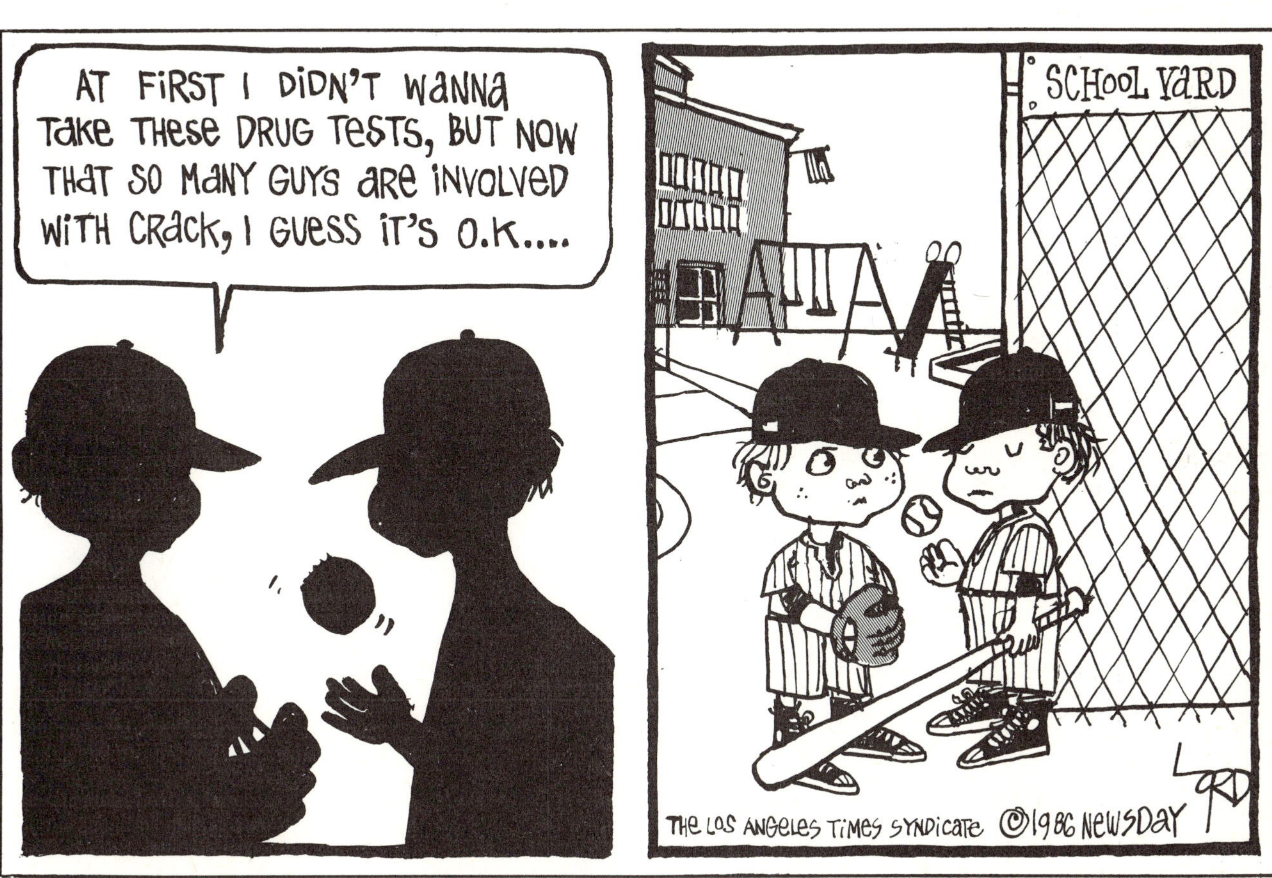

Education Plan Launched as Cocaine Use Sweeps Schools

The Reagan Administration November 20, 1984 announced a new plan to cut drug use among young people by 50% to 75% over five years. The program would stress drug education and would use professional and amateur athletes as spokespersons. "Professional and amateur athletes, coaches and schools are banding together to carry this message to our 60 million young people," said Federal Bureau of Investigation (FBI) Director William Webster at a Washington news conference announcing the program. The plan would involve a coalition of 40 drug organizations and would be coordinated by the federal government. According to the *New York Times*, drug professionals not involved in the Administration's program lauded the plan but thought that the 75% reduction sought might be overly optimistic. A spokesman for the Drug Enforcement Administration (DEA) said, "if we can't dent it by at least half, we will have failed."

In 1986 the Institute of Social Research at the University of Michigan released its annual survey which showed that the percentage of high school seniors who have ever tried cocaine had almost doubled since 1976, from 9% to 17.3. However the study showed that use of all other drugs—marijuana, stimulants, depressants, psychedelics and alcohol—has leveled off or declined in recent years, although researchers feared that the decline has ended. This would seem to contradict some of the findings from the institute's 1984 survey. But although the reality of school-age drug abuse in any given community cannot be inferred from national surveys, the vast majority of American high school students will pass through the turmoils of adolescence without succumbing to addiction. But it is also true that there is no other industrialized country in the world that has a comparable proportion of young people involved with illicit drugs. The national statistics on high school seniors have suggested that years of well-intentioned efforts have so far failed to eradicate drug use among the young. Cocaine's increasing availability, its glamour and its undeserved reputation as a low-risk high have combined to expand its allure to teenagers. It would seem that the strong mystique that cocaine offers is more powerful than society's ineffectual attempts to wean the young from drugs. Even many drug-abuse experts quietly concede that in-school drug-prevention programs have failed to reach their teenage audience, perhaps due to the widespread disagreement about the root causes of drug abuse and equally little consensus on the best tactics for prevention.

The Boston Globe
Boston, MA, December 1, 1984

A state study showing stunning rates of drug and alcohol use among Massachusetts students is cause for concern. However, assertions by students and teachers that drug and alcohol use are lessening may indicate that the problem is not out of control.

The study's statistics, which show that 60 percent of the state's high school students have used drugs and 90 percent have used alcohol, are no reason for panic. The statistics do not take into account that some students have used drugs or alcohol only once and that others may have quit.

The most important aspect of the study is that, for the first time, educators and state health officials have an idea of the extent of drug and alcohol problems among teen-agers. Governor Dukakis is moving quickly to launch a program aimed at preventing drug and alcohol use by the young.

The study was done by the state Department of Public Health, which surveyed more than 5000 students at 80 public and private high schools. It concluded that alcohol and drug abuse in Massachusetts exceeds national averages.

The findings are, as Dukakis says, "disturbing." However, they are not surprising, considering the extent of this abuse in society. A presidential commission was told last week that cocaine abuse has reached epidemic proportions, with one in every 10 Americans having tried the drug at least once.

Cocaine is marketed as the middle-class "drug of choice." It is not teen-agers but the "baby boom" generation that popularized drug use in the 1960s that is responsible for that unhappy trend.

Young people, whatever their reasons for using drugs – excitement, acceptance by their peers, experimenting – do not need encouragement from adults, whose own behavior seems to say that drug and alcohol use is acceptable.

The public-service campaign planned by the governor will be more effective if it stresses that it is no good to ask teen-agers to think about the harmfulness of drugs and alcohol, if adults are not willing to do the same.

DESERET NEWS
Salt Lake City, UT, February 23-24, 1984

Officials believe "steady progress" is being made toward reducing alcohol and drug abuse among Utah adolescents. That's encouraging, but the size of the problem is still alarming.

For example, an estimated 35 percent of all young people ages 12 to 18 have used alcohol or drugs to some extent in the past 30 days, state studies show. Among older teens, 16 to 18, that figure is 47 percent.

Such figures make it hard for parents to be complacent and feel it can't happen to their son or daughter.

Those frightening numbers are one of the reasons behind an all-day Alcohol and Drug Education Conference scheduled Saturday at the Salt Palace. Heavy emphasis will be on dealing with prevention and help for youth.

While the conference is sponsored by the Assistance League of Salt Lake, it will involve various state and local agencies and the Governor's Youth Committee on Alcohol and Drug Abuse.

Workshops at the conference include such subjects as parent-to-parent help, communication skills, how to teach values, developing positive peer support, how to help when there is trouble, dealing with stress, and effects of chemicals on the body, to name just a few.

The event is open to the public. Youth groups from more than 20 high schools in the Salt Lake area will be attending. The registration fee is $12 at the door.

For parents, young people, teachers, religious leaders, and others whose lives are involved with adolescents, it's an investment in learning that might help head off disaster for young people and their families.

The Hartford Courant

Hartford, CT, May 15, 1984

School administrators at Choate Rosemary Hall and Ethel Walker School missed an opportunity to perform a valuable public service by refusing to talk more openly about their recent expulsions of students discovered to have been using cocaine.

School officials at Choate said comment would be inappropriate because of related criminal proceedings. Officials at Ethel Walker have refused much public comment, although criminal proceedings there are apparently not at issue.

They can't be blamed for wishing to protect the privacy of their students, particularly if such students are minors or not under investigation. But that shouldn't prevent educators from publicly discussing the problem of substance abuse at their institutions.

The National Association of Independent Schools is considering drug information programs for member schools this summer, an example individual schools should follow.

It's a sorry fact that drug abuse today affects most schools, private and public. No matter what the circumstances, the more that school administrators, parents and students themselves air the problem, the more likely it is that prevention of abuse will be achieved and remedies to it will be found.

The number of young people whose lives are tainted or destroyed by drugs may even decrease as a result.

Herald News

Fall River, MA, December 4, 1984

The dimensions of the drug abuse scandal constantly escape our notice.

One reason is that in its initial phases drug abuse is easy to conceal.

By contrast, alcoholism is frequently obvious, even if its victims insist they are only occasional drinkers.

The alcoholic tends to betray his or her condition; the person on the way to becoming an addict may not, except to a skilled and careful observer.

This is no advantage. In fact, it makes detection and treatment of a person taking illegal drugs very difficult.

And this is true even when the person is a child.

Reportedly drug abuse in the high schools of this state is far more prevalent than supposed.

The results of a state study of the subject have been called "stunning" by education officials.

Not only is the use of these drugs extremely dangerous; it often leads those addicted to them into drug-related crimes.

The number of holdups and burglaries prompted by the craving for drugs is extremely large.

And on still another level, so is the number of crimes involved in transporting and distributing these substances.

There is a network of evil that has come into being as the drug habit has spread.

Onitially it involved adults, but now it has spread to adolescents and children.

It is imperative that the general public recognize its dimensions, even though doing so means becoming aware that it now touches the lives of youngsters from every social and economic level.

The school officials who call the report on drug abuse in Massachusetts high schools "stunning" have an obligation to make the full extent of that abuse known.

If they found the extent of the abuse grounds for dismay, so would many teachers and parents.

But if the abuse is as widespread as reported, then the facts about it should be known and faced directly.

Nothing is to be gained by dodging them or being very courageous about facing them somewhere else.

They should be confronted here.

That does not mean conducting a witch hunt, but it does mean that teachers should be made aware of telltale signs that could reveal a person who is using drugs.

And teachers should also be aware that there is a real possibility that some of their students may be using them.

The danger of drug abuse is too great to justify a sentimental approach.

Nor should parents resist knowledge of it if one of their children is taking drugs. The sooner they know, the better the chance will be that their son or daughter can be treated successfully.

Apart from its shock value, the most important benefit to be derived from the report of drug abuse in the high schools is to force schools and communities to take a more active role in fighting it.

If they continue to reduce its dimensions in their minds, the dimensions will grow still larger.

At this point, exaggerating the reality is less dangerous than underestimating it.

It is improbable that drug abuse can be as prevalent in the state's high schools as the report indicates and not be present to some degree in this area too.

The likelihood that there is some drug abuse in area high schools should be faced and acted on as soon as possible.

The future lives of a great many young people may well be at stake.

Rocky Mountain News

Denver, CO, March 1, 1984

USE of drugs in high schools appears to have declined substantially over the past five years, but far too many students still are numbing their minds with illegal substances.

The latest annual survey by the University of Michigan indicated that 5.5 percent of 1983 seniors nationwide smoked marijuana daily. That's the lowest since the survey began in 1975 and is nearly half the peak figure of 10.7 percent in 1978.

Another welcome finding was a lack of evidence to support the suspicion that teen-agers are substituting alcohol for illicit drugs. The 1983 survey showed a slight decline in daily use of alcohol to 5.5 percent.

While there is some comfort in the new statistics, it is still disturbing that large percentages of students are occasional users. Fifty-seven percent of the class of 1983 said they have smoked marijuana, 42 percent of them within the last year. Some 40 percent of seniors said they had tried an illicit drug other than marijuana, including 16 percent who had some experience with cocaine and 1.2 percent with heroin.

The survey director, psychologist Lloyd Johnston, said it would be a "serious mistake" to "lose track of how high the mountain is from which we're coming down. . . . It is still unacceptably high. . . . I know of no other developed country in the world where such a large proportion of youth become involved with drugs."

All told, 63 percent of the 1983 seniors surveyed said they had tried an illicit drug by the time they finished school.

That's proof enough of the continuing need for school personnel and parents to educate youngsters on the dangers of drugs and for legal authorities to crack down hard on persons who make the illegal substances available to young people.

Fort Worth Star-Telegram
Fort Worth, TX, March 6, 1985

This week is being observed as Drug and Alcohol Awareness Week throughout the United States. The project is being sponsored by the National PTA because studies have shown that most parents do not even know how to talk to their children about drugs.

Statistics show that some children begin experimenting with drugs in elementary school. The PTA says many children as young as 9 or 10 have knowledge of illegal drugs and alcohol, and by the time they are high school seniors, 63 percent will have tried an illicit drug.

More than 6,000 local PTA chapters across the nation are involved in promoting Drug and Alcohol Awareness Week in an effort to provide parents with suggested ways to help their children avoid drug use.

The proliferation of drug abuse on school campuses is made easy because younger children are easy victims to peer pressures.

The National PTA adopted the theme "Prevention Begins at Home" as a message to parents that they can influence their children's choices of whether to experiment with drugs or alcohol. It is suggested that parents begin talking to their children about drugs when they are as young as 5.

Many youngsters can be saved from becoming abusers if they are taught the dangers before they are exposed to drugs.

Drug and Alcohol Awareness Week is a worthy and worthwhile project and deserves wholehearted support. Officials and teachers of area public schools and parents with students attending these classes all would benefit by becoming involved in this project.

But best of all, these efforts might save some children from becoming victims of this dreaded evil.

The Seattle Times
Seattle, WA, August 12, 1985

THE Department of Education's recent attempt to clarify its ruling that schools must provide drug- and alcohol-addicted children with the same kinds of services offered to other handicapped youngsters only adds to the muddle.

According to Thomasina Rogers of the Department of Education's Office of Civil Rights, school districts are not obligated to offer special evaluations and programs for students unless their parents request it. That interpretation does not lessen the potentially devastating financial impact on school budgets.

If a parent were to request such an evaluation, for example, schools would be expected to have trained personnel available. Special programs cannot be created upon demand, but must be planned and in place when the need arises.

Rogers' explanation may relieve some of the worries of teachers who thought they were expected to recognize addiction in children. But the threat to school districts' resources remains.

Lake Washington school administrators had thought the Education Department's judgment against the district made schools responsible for identifying, evaluating and providing appropriate education for addicted children. Rogers' interpretation properly focuses on parents' roles, but apparently it is still up to the schools to provide programs beyond the drug-and alcohol-awareness programs now widely available.

It makes sense for parents, not harried teachers, to be responsible for monitoring the behavior of their children and acting if drug or alcohol abuse is suspected. It's a problem in which families should look not to the schools but to the medical profession when the occasion demands.

The Dallas Morning News
Dallas, TX, July 3, 1985

TIME was when the elementary school years were a period of innocence, when children could enjoy a breather before the turbulence of adolescent years.

Now surveys — by the *Weekly Reader* — show that at least a third of the country's fourth-graders are being pressured by their peers to try drugs.

As *Dallas Morning News* reporter Tom Howlett documented in a two-part series this week, the age at which youngsters are being introduced to drugs is alarmingly low:

At The New Place drug counseling program in Richardson, the average age of first use is 11. One-third of the young people surveyed by the Texas Drug and Alcohol Program in Oak Lawn reported experimenting with drugs when they were 10 or younger. Drug arrests of young people 14 and younger have jumped more than 40 percent in the last year in this state.

Just as shocking is the lack of adequate treatment and prevention programs for young people. The Texas Legislature, which authorized a full range of drug education and treatment programs in 1979, has not ever approved money to fund the programs. At present Texas ranks last in the nation in per-capita funding for drug and alcohol services.

Whether the cause is ignorance or fear or apathy, Texas in general and Dallas in particular have not faced up to the growing problem of substance abuse by young people.

There have been some tentative, encouraging developments locally, such as the organization in 1984 of Dallas Challenge, a non-profit agency for drug education-prevention-treatment. Then, too, grass-roots parents groups have been forming in local schools to sponsor drug-free parties for students. And in the government sector, Mayor Pro Tem Annette Strauss has put together a city drug task force to consider possible solutions.

The task force has the potential to shake the city out of its "denial" of the drug-abuse problem, if the group can zero in on an action plan that will excite the cooperation of the City Council, the county leaders, the medical community and the social services sector.

First, there's the need for a detoxification center and more inpatient and outpatient options for young people. School officials must be persuaded to expand their educational programs to younger grades. Private-public funding mechanisms must be created.

But just by its creation, the task force has started local leaders talking to each other about substance abuse. The next step is to get state leaders talking and caring so funds for needed programs can be approved. Requiring that drug treatment be added to group insurance and health programs would go a long way toward helping many families get needed assistance.

The problem is not that there are no answers to the problem of drug abuse by children and teen-agers. There are positive actions that can be taken. The problem is that too many adults don't realize there's a problem yet, while thousands of young people are chemically poisoning themselves.

The Dispatch
Columbus, OH, February 28, 1985

The National PTA has kept up with the times. It is about to launch a national campaign to help children deal with peer pressure to use drugs and alcohol.

The National Congress of Parents and Teachers is conducting a nationwide program, "Prevention Begins at Home," to increase parent awareness of the problem and to help them guide their children away from drug abuse.

The National PTA's Drug and Awareness Week, beginning March 3, will tell parents they can make a difference by talking with their children, as early as the age of five, about drugs.

All of us would like to think that our own children are not only drug-free, but free of pressures to use drugs. But the fact of the matter is that peer pressure in schools is so great it must be countered by parents at the earliest opportunity.

It is possible, through home education, to prevent significant numbers of youngsters from becoming abusers.

We join the National PTA in urging you to learn the facts about drugs and alcohol abuse and use that knowledge to influence your children away from potential tragedy.

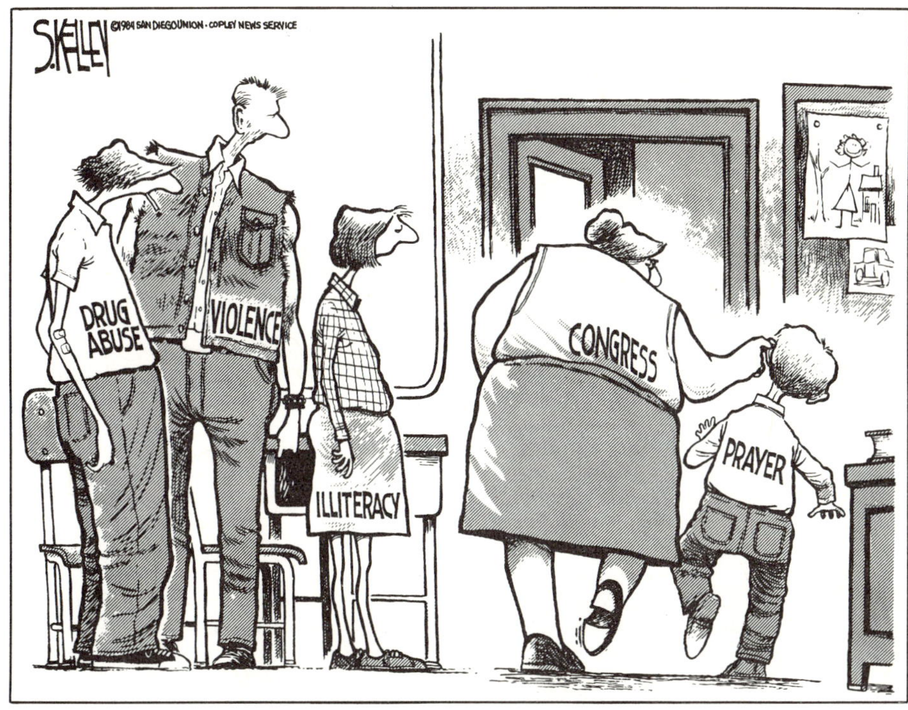

The Boston Globe
Boston, MA, August 8, 1986

Despite Nancy Reagan's interest in the drug issue, federal funding for drug programs has been sharply reduced during her husband's time in office. Drug-treatment programs in cities such as New York, where the use of "crack" is epidemic, lack sufficient resources to help all who need treatment.

President Reagan's belated offensive against illicit drugs gives Congress an opportunity to upgrade programs in drug education, counseling and treatment.

Traditional attempts to eradicate drug use by eliminating the supply and suppliers have failed. Law enforcement efforts cannot be ignored, but a consensus is building in Congress that the demand for drugs can be reduced through education.

The House Education and Labor Committee is examining a Massachusetts antidrug program, the Governor's Alliance Against Drugs.

The program has expanded from 18 communities to more than 200 in less than two years. It requires a memorandum of understanding between police chiefs and school superintendents, tough antidrug measures in school-discipline codes, expanded access to treatment for drug abusers, and drug and alcohol education from kindergarten through high school. The cost is about $5 a student.

Although the effectiveness of the program cannot yet be measured, Governor Dukakis makes a strong case for this approach. Studies show that 11½ is the average age for first smoking marijuana and 12½ for first drinking beer. "If you wait until high school, you've lost half of the kids," he told the committee.

Dukakis recommended a permanent commitment to fighting drug abuse. "Anyone who thinks a six-month PR campaign is going to solve this problem is kidding himself," he said. In searching for sensible solutions, Congress should look to Massachusetts for guidance.

The Chattanooga Times
Chattanooga, TN, August 25, 1986

Both houses of Congress and the Reagan adminstration are scrambling to come up with comprehensive legislation as part of a massive offensive against illegal drugs. House Speaker Thomas P. O'Neill Jr. has several committees working on the problem, and earlier this month President Reagan suddenly got involved with a televised speech calling for a "mobilization" to eradicate drug abuse.

Programs are fine, and mobilization will be necessary to make any kind of dent in drug usage in this country. But it's going to take a lot of money as well. Mr. Reagan acknowledged as much in a question-and-answer session with reporters after his speech. "We know that there's going to be a cost, and we're going to have to look at where we're going to find that money."

They're looking in a mighty funny place.

Mr. Reagan's eagerness to combat the drug abuse near-epidemic is unquestioned but it is putting the administration into a conflict between ideology and smart politics. Budget officials in the White House are having a difficult enough time dealing with the Reagan deficit without authorizing new spending for an anti-drug program. At the same time, the administration certainly doesn't want to lose any political points to the Democrats.

How convenient, then, for the Department of Education to agree to divert $100 million from other programs to the anti-drug effort. In a budget of $18 billion, a mere $100 million doesn't sound like much. But it's important to remember that while the department hasn't yet specified which programs will be cut to come up with the $100 million, the bulk of the budget is chiefly used to provide aid for college students, including the handicapped and the poor. How many students such as these will be denied college aid just because students elsewhere are snorting cocaine or smoking marijuana? Where is the fairness in that?

The administration seems to be saying that if Democrats insist on drafting new anti-drug programs that require extra money, then why not chop into existing education programs to get that money? But both programs are important. Educational scholarship and assistance programs should not be held up just to provide the money needed to combat a growing drug abuse problem.

IF CONGRESS decides to spend millions in federal funds on drug education, it should make sure that the nation's schoolchildren aren't the only pupils. Their parents — and grandparents — could also stand to learn a few things about substance abuse.

The Baby Boomers whose offspring now are approaching the age of experimentation, for example, ought to be told that marijuana is no longer the relatively tame weed they may have smoked in the early '70s. Drug researchers report that domestically grown pot has become up to five times more potent since then, and it's likely to produce effects far more powerful than a minor case of the munchies.

The National Academy of Sciences has found that today's strains of marijuana can cause such serious side effects as anxiety, delirium and confusion, plus short-term disruption of the learning process and possibly long-term health effects as well.

In short, smoking a joint is a much riskier and more intense experience now than it once was. Because of this, the differences between marijuana and cocaine may appear to be smaller than they really are.

Most people know it's dangerous to mix illegal drugs, not only because the outcome is tremendously unpredictable, but also because it's harder for paramedics and doctors to deal with overdoses. Many middle-aged adults, however, still need to be warned about the potentially deadly consequences of mixing many legal drugs, particularly barbiturates and alcohol — which most people don't realize is a depressant. Taken together, sleeping pills and booze can slow the body to the point where it quits functioning.

The elderly, too, could use a serious talking-to about prescription drugs. Counselors say many fixed-income seniors with minor ailments fall prey to the hazardous practice of trying to save on doctor bills by taking whatever medicine may be in the cabinet — even if it was originally prescribed for another person or a totally different problem.

The greatest benefit of drug education for all ages might well be a greater awareness by the average citizen that it's healthier to live with a little pain in our lives than to continually be seeking a quick fix — through alcohol, marijuana, pills or something even more dangerous.

Drug Use Down Among Teens

An annual survey conducted by the Institute of Social Research at the University of Michigan for the National Institute on Drug Abuse February 2, 1984 revealed that the number of high school seniors smoking marijuana on a daily basis had dropped to its lowest level since the survey began in 1975. Sixteen thousand seniors at 130 high schools took part in the survey. The number of daily users had dropped to 5.5% in 1983 from a high of 10.7% in 1978. Daily use was defined as smoking on at least 20 occasions during the month before the survey. Lloyd Johnston, a psychologist who directed the survey, stated that the study also showed a decline in the use of amphetemines, barbiturates, Quaaludes and LSD had also declined. Sixty-three percent of those surveyed said they had experimented with an illegal drug while they were in high school. Forty percent said they had tried an illegal drug other than marijuana. The survey also revealed that 16% of the seniors had some experience with cocaine, and that 1.2% of the seniors had tried heroin. The researchers noted that 80% of those who had participated in the survey disapproved of regular marijuana use, and that 61% disapproved of even the occasional use of marijuana. Cocaine use had apparently leveled off after an upsurge of popularity in the late 1970s, the survey found. The drinking level among high school seniors had declined slightly since 1978. There was no evidence, based on the results of the survey, that alcohol was replacing illicit drugs among teenagers.

The Dispatch

Columbus, OH, February 15, 1984

Steady decline in marijuana use by high school seniors was a bright spot in recent news.

In the annual survey done for the National Institute on Drug Abuse, among some 17,000 seniors in 180 representative U.S. high schools, figures on both daily and irregular marijuana use marked a continuing 5-year decline.

It was equally heartening that the seniors' daily and occasional use of alcohol showed a corresponding decline and that the students surveyed revealed increased awareness that drugs are harmful.

Use of other drugs — amphetamines, barbiturates, methaqualone and LSD — also declined, but PCP use increased slightly and use of heroin, cocaine and other opiates held at a low but steady rate little changed since 1979.

As Dr. William Pollin, institute director, commented, the figures show the "unparalleled increase" of the 1960s and 1970s has reversed to a "leveling and decline in drug use" in the 1980s.

The battle isn't won, nor will it be until teen-age experimentation with and use of drugs and liquor drop far lower. But the figures are encouraging, the trend is in the right direction and, best of all, the young people themselves are controlling the decline.

The Wichita Eagle-Beacon

Wichita, KS, February 20, 1984

Americans in general, and parents in particular, should be heartened by the latest report on drug use among high school seniors. A study commissioned by the National Institute on Drug Abuse reveals the percentage of seniors using drugs was down markedly, from 53 percent in 1979 to 47 percent last year. Marijuana use had declined even more, from 51 percent to 42 percent during those same four years.

Perhaps most encouraging of all was the finding that the number of those who smoke marijuana daily has been cut almost in half: from 10.7 percent of the senior population to 5.5 percent. Ironically, while researchers concluded alcohol abuse isn't really replacing marijuana use, precisely the same proportion of seniors, 5.5 percent, reported being daily drinkers.

Obviously, serious substance abuse problems persist — especially among those who are daily users — and organized treatment programs for individuals and their families, with educational efforts for larger groups, still are needed. But, due in no small measure to such efforts, the trend finally seems to be turning toward the positive. More and more, youth are becoming convinced that recreational drug use and alcohol abuse are harmful, and the inclination to indulge in that kind of behavior as a means of "acting out" the frustrations of adolescence seems to be abating.

Fortunately, that should work to reduce peer pressure to try drugs or alcohol, which is one of the primary motivating factors influencing young people. The problem may not be solved yet, but the prognosis appears better now than it has in years.

The State

Columbia, SC, February 10, 1984

AN ANNUAL survey of a representative group of American high school seniors turns up encouraging signs of a downward trend in the use of illicit drugs, including marijuana.

The survey, which is one of a series made each year since 1975, confirms there is still widespread use of drugs in that age group — 63 percent said they'd *tried* an illicit drug the previous year, and 47 percent said they *used* illicit drugs during the year.

The above figure on use of drugs is down 6 percent from the peak year of 1979, when 53 percent were regular users.

In 1978, 10.7 percent of the students said they used marijuana daily. The 1983 figure is almost half of that; 5.5 percent were daily marijuana smokers. The survey also revealed that 5.5 percent use alcohol daily, a slight decline from previous years.

The chief investigator for the National Institute on Drug Abuse project found the use of alcohol most alarming — 41 percent of those surveyed said they had taken five or more drinks in a row during the two weeks preceding the survey.

The data on alcohol use by high school seniors support the importance of raising the legal drinking age for beer and wine to 21. Teenage drinking drivers are responsible for 25 percent of the nation's traffic fatalities.

Indications that fewer high school seniors are involved with drugs today than before are welcome. There will be fewer tragedies in American homes. But the drug abuse problem is still a national disgrace.

OKLAHOMA CITY TIMES

Oklahoma City, OK, January 10, 1984

SURVEY evidence that today's teen-agers are too smart to fry their brains by smoking pot is welcome news for the nation. It's sad that the generation just ahead of them didn't learn the lesson soon enough.

The original "lost generation" made famous by novelists F. Scott Fitzgerald and Ernest Hemingway drowned its sorrows in booze in the decade after World War I. The new "lost generation" pickled itself on pot and other drugs during the 1970s as it sought to cope with a world turned upside down in the wake of the Vietnam war.

Many veterans acquired the drug habit while serving in Southeast Asia. Other young people of that era got into the drug scene because it was fashionable. Those who took up marijuana — which often was the first step toward hard-drug use — were led by false prophets, the do-your-own-thing crowd which insisted pot smoking couldn't hurt them and would "expand" their minds.

It has taken a number of years to demonstrate the fallacy of their argument. But now medical evidence is conclusive that using marijuana on a long-term basis does harm the body physically in a number of ways.

Unfortunately, many of today's adults — people who picked up the habit in their teen years — are inveterate users of marijuana. Some have advanced into cocaine and hard drugs and have made these so much a part of their lifestyle they apparently cannot see how they have been affected.

A case in point is the experience of an Alcoa aluminum plant in Vancouver, Wash. Personnel officials there report half of 750 job applicants were turned down because they failed drug tests. Evidence of marijuana use was the most prevalent, but about 1 percent of those rejected showed signs of being on hard drugs.

The unsuccessful applicants could not understand why they were not hired. And none promised to stop using drugs if hired. The personnel director offered the explanation that drugs are accepted so much in society they are treated "just as a lifestyle."

Tragically for themselves and for their country, many members of this drug culture may never be able to lead productive, useful lives. The cost will be borne not only by themselves and their families but by society at large through government treatment and rehabilitation programs.

Ironically, part of the tax burden will fall eventually on those now in their teens, who are said to be shunning the use of drugs. Surveys show the percentage of teen-agers who smoke marijuana has dropped dramatically from its peak in the late 1970s. The reports come from both private sources and government statistics.

The National Institute on Drug Abuse will release the results of its 1983 survey next month, and the downward trend is expected to continue.

The explanation seems to be that today's teen-agers are better informed about the health hazards of smoking marijuana and thus face less peer pressure. It's a shame it took medical science so long to come up with the proof.

St. Louis Globe-Democrat

St. Louis, MO, February 9, 1984

High school seniors may be much wiser than long-declining college entrance tests are showing.

One indication that the class of 1984 is brighter than the students who came before them can be seen in the fact that more and more of today's seniors are turning their backs on smoking marijuana or using other drugs.

Daily pot smoking by present-day seniors has dropped to 5.5 percent from 10.7 percent back in 1978. The annual study, conducted for the National Institute on Drug Abuse, surveyed 17,000 students.

The trend is encouraging since the use of marijuana among high schoolers has dropped for the fifth consecutive year. Last year's findings indicate the lowest level of usage since the surveys were started in 1975.

The study found that declining marijuana use is accompanied by a growing awareness by students that the drug is harmful. Medical experts in the federal government have been warning for years that if widespread marijuana use, especially among young people, is not curtailed society may find it will have to pay a big price in resultant health problems.

Disapproval of regular use of marijuana was expressed by 83 percent of the students questioned. That's an impressive gain; in 1978, only 68 percent expressed disapproval. Sixty-one percent of the students questioned disapproved of even occasional marijuana usage.

That hefty majority indicates today's seniors are on the right course and deserve more credit than some of the older folks have been giving them.

Portland Press Herald

Portland, ME, February 8, 1984

The problem isn't licked by any means but all the signs are encouraging. The use of drugs by high school students is dropping.

A report issued by the National Institute on Drug Abuse shows that the daily use of marijuana by students has been cut by about half since 1978—dropping from 10.7 percent then to 5.5 percent today.

That's the lowest level recorded for daily pot use since 1975, when the annual study was first conducted.

The study, developed by the University of Michigan's Institute for Social Research, also reports that the number of youngsters who have tried an illegal drug other than marijuana also continues to decline steadily.

Furthermore, the decrease in drug use and abuse by students has apparently not been accompanied by any appreciable rise in the use of alcohol as a substitute.

Changing social conditions and attitudes undoubtedly are playing a major role in the decline of drug use among students.

Parents and educators alike have shown a greater willingness to crack down on the problem, for one thing. Discipline has toughened and there has been a far greater effort to educate young people and their parents to the debilitating effects of drug abuse.

And students themselves, taking notice of the results of long years of abuse among their friends, have slowly been weaning themselves away from drugs or avoided their use from the outset.

Peer pressure, which played an important role in the popular spread of pot smoking and other drug use during the "permissive" years of the '60s and '70s, may now be working in the opposite direction to discourage abuse.

Federal Highway Funds Tied to Drinking Ages

Nineteen states currently have a minimum drinking age of 21 years, and more than a dozen states have raised their legal drinking age in the past decade. The momentum for the passage of these laws has come largely from such groups as Mothers Against Drunk Driving (MADD), who point to statistics on alcohol-related traffic accidents to focus national attention on the problem. MADD, is grass-roots group of drunk-driving victims and their relatives, was credited by many with providing the impetus that hurried the minimum-drinking-age proposal into law.

National studies have shown that teenagers are involved in proportionately far more car accidents than adults. Other studies have shown a correlation between reduced drinking ages—the general trend in the early 1970s—and greater numbers of car accidents involving young drivers. Regulation of the sale of alcohol had traditionally been the responsibility of individual states, and the Reagan Administration has sought to keep it that way. Recently, however, there has been a move to establish a national drinking age, in order to eliminate the widespread practice among teenagers of driving across state borders in order to buy alcohol and then driving after drinking. The House Energy and Commerce Committee February 7, 1984 approved a bill that would mandate a national drinking age of 21. A similar bill had been introduced in the Senate.

Herald News

Fall River, MA, February 16, 1984

Former Governor John Volpe, who is now the chairman of the National Commission against Drunken Driving, says New England has a long way to gobefore it can relax in the knowledge that the danger from drunken driving has been eliminated, or at least reduced to an absolute minimum.

Volpe, speaking at a two day seminar on the subject in Newport, urged much fuller education of youngsters to the dangers that arise when drivers have been drinking.

Although he is in favor of the stricter penalties for drunken driving in this state and others, he does not think the penalties alone will solve the problem.

He points out that there has been a decline in the number of alcohol-related accidents and fatalities since the new penalties went into effect, but that the decline has not been as steep as might have been expected.

Along with most New England governors, he recommends raising the drinking age to 21 throughout the region.

Certainly it is true that in a region made up of six relatively small states, unless the legal drinking age is the same everywhere, it is only too easy to evade it by crossing a state line.

When that happens, the whole point of establishing a legal drinking age is lost because the point is not puritanical restrictions, but increased public safety.

Furthermore, there is a statistical correlation between the legal drinking age and the number of alcohol-related fatalities in any given state. The higher the legal drinking age, the fewer there are.

In life and death matters like this, the statistical argument is virtually unanswerable.

Yet the most interesting point former Governor Volpe made was the need to educate young people, meaning school children under the age of 10, to the dangers of drunken driving.

It may indeed be true that this is the only way to reduce drunken driving appreciably, to make a firm enough imprint on young minds so that it will remain with them all through adolescence.

There is certainly no harm in introducing youngsters to the subject early on.

Drunken driving as a threat to everyone's safety is a reality they might as well be aware of as not.

The desire to protect youngsters from unpleasant realities is natural enough, but their ignorance may lead them, later on, to underestimate the danger from driving after drinking.

If they know from early childhood what that danger really is, they may avoid it.

Or, more probably, some of them will.

That is the best that can really be hoped, but in terms of drunken driving and the fatalities that stem from it, each person spared is worth the effort and expense that teaching youngsters to avoid it involves.

All of the current concern over drunken driving derives from the sense most Americans now have that something must be done to curtail the slaughter on our highways.

To be fair, there are fewer fatalities than there used to be. The national speed limit has helped, and now it is hoped that by making drunken driving a rarity, the fatalities will be reduced still more.

If that highly desirable goal can be attained by adding education in the perils of drunken driving to the school curriculum, then it should be done.

If the schools can help make drunken driving obsolete, then they should join in this extended campaign.

The San Diego Union

San Diego, CA, February 18, 1984

The Presidential Commission on Drunk Driving can take some credit for stirring interest in raising the legal drinking age to 21 in those states where it is now lower.

The drunk driving commission recommended the adoption of a uniform nationwide drinking age of 21, citing evidence that teenage fatalities have dropped off measurably in states which once permitted drinking at a younger age and then raised the minimum.

There are more reasons than traffic safety to fix 21 as the drinking age. What the commission has done is revive a recurring debate about maturity and the privilege of buying and consuming alcoholic beverages. State legislatures have been dealing with this issue ever since the repeal of Prohibition in 1933.

This leads us to take a dim view of the vote by the House Energy and Commerce Committee last week supporting a bill that would federalize the drinking age question. The bill seeks to establish 21 as the drinking age by federal decree. Congress would do so under its powers to regulate interstate commerce; in this case, alcoholic beverages.

Lurking in the wings is an alternative proposal that the federal government coerce states into adopting the 21-year-minimum drinking age by threatening to cut off their share of federal highway funds.

Can't the U.S. Congress leave any popular issue alone? Regulation of the sale of alcoholic beverages and regulation of motor vehicle traffic were both relegated to the states many years ago. State lawmakers are as capable as members of Congress of seeing a link between the drinking age and traffic fatalities, and their judgment on what to do about it is as reliable as a judgment made in Washington.

Regulating interstate commerce is a familiar dodge for federal intrusion into state affairs. So is the power of granting or withholding federal funds. Members of House and Senate should be required to stand by their desks at the beginning of each day's session and recite the 10th Amendment to the U.S. Constitution:

"The powers not delegated to the United States by the Constitution, nor prohibited by it to the States, are reserved to the States respectively, or to the people."

RAPID CITY JOURNAL —

Rapid City, SD, February 17, 1984

The dramatic decline in traffic deaths in the United States in 1983 is an indication that the campaign to crack down on drunken drivers is paying off.

Preliminary figures show there were 43,028 traffic deaths during the year, the smallest total in two decades. Moreover, the 1983 fatality rate of 2.6 deaths per 100 million vehicle miles was the lowest on record.

Much of the credit for the heartening news must go to citizen groups that have been pressing state legislatures and local courts to crack down on drunken drivers. According to the National Safety Council, 40 states strengthened their drunken-driving laws in 1983.

The organizations leading the campaign against drunken driving generally are of recent vintage. They include Citizens for Safe Drivers Against Drunk Drivers and Other Chronic Offenders (founded in 1977), Mothers Against Drunk Drivers (1980), Students Against Drunken Driving (1981) and Truckers Against Drunk Drivers (1982).

The aim of these groups is to get drunken drivers off the road and keep them off. To that end, they support such measures as laws requiring mandatory minimum punishment for people convicted of driving while intoxicated, programs to monitor drunken-driving cases when they come to trial, and efforts to prevent people whose license to drive has been revoked or suspended from obtaining a license in another state.

The American Automobile Association is advancing some pretty convincing facts in urging legislators to make 21 the minimum legal drinking age for all alcoholic beverages in the 31 states where it ranges from 18 to 20.

For instance, while drivers under 21 account for 10 percent of all licensed drivers, they represent more than 23 percent of all alcohol-related traffic fatalities. That's an indication that inexperience in driving and inexperience in coping with the effects of alcohol too often combine to bring about tragedy.

According to AAA, a study found a 28 percent reduction in alcohol-related accidents in eight of the nine states in which the drinking age had been raised.

To its credit, the American Automobile Association is presssing its case through individual state legislatures. That's a more palatable approach than the efforts being made to have the federal government mandate a minimum legal drinking age. Legislation introduced in both houses of Congress to establish a national minimum age of 21 is an unwarranted interference in an issue that should be decided by the states.

However if states don't take it upon themselves to raise the drinking age, they invite federal intervention.

Arkansas Gazette.

Little Rock, AR, February 15, 1984

Arkansas is among 19 states that set 21 as the legal drinking age, but the other 31 states have a hodgepodge of minimum-age drinking laws that range down to 18. Like most other state laws dealing with the sale of alcoholic beverages, consistency is sadly lacking.

A move is afoot in Congress, in any case, to make the minimum-age drinking laws uniform throughout the nation, and there is a certain appeal to the argument. In many cases it is a simple matter for someone under the age of 21 to drive across a state line into a state that allows the sale of alcoholic beverages to minors.

The danger is clear enough. A great many drinking teen-agers are put on the highways, commuting to border states, because of the lack of uniformity. In finding that there "is evidence of direct correlation between the minimum drinking age and alcohol-related crashes among the age groups" affected, the President's Commission on Drunken Driving has recommended that Congress set a legal drinking age of 21.

Arkansas is directly affected by the laws of its neighbors. Two of its six bordering states — Missouri and Oklahoma — set the legal drinking age at 21. But the legal age in Tennessee and Texas is 19, and in Louisiana it is 18. The age in Mississippi is 21, except for beer and table wine.

The immediate question is not whether the legal age be 21, or 18, 19 or 20. Whether 21 is appropriate is at least arguable. The question, instead, is whether all states should have the same legal drinking age and the answer clearly is "yes." The only way uniformity can be achieved, given the differing attitudes in the various states, is through Congress.

Everyone in the nation has a stake in reducing the incidence of driving while under the influence of alcohol. It is true that a uniform legal drinking age can address only one of many factors in drunken driving, but it should be a practical and effective way to eliminate at least some of the needless tragedy associated with the intoxicated driver.

The Boston Herald

Boston, MA, February 12, 1984

THE BEST thing about the new anti-booze bill just approved by a congressional committee is not that it would boost the minimum legal drinking age to 21, but that it would make it uniform throughout the nation.

As it is now, each state sets its own minimum — 21 in New Jersey and 18 other states; 20 in Massachusetts, Maine, New Hampshire, Connecticut and nearly two dozen more; 19 in a handful including New York, and 18 in Vermont.

The flaw is obvious, and dangerous. Young people in any jurisdiction with a minimum age of 20 or 21 need only drive over a nearby border — into Vermont for example — and buy just about anything they can get away with. When you consider that about 25,000 people die in alcohol-related highway accidents each year, and that drivers in their teens have a hand in some 6,000 of them, the enormity of that flaw becomes obvious. Making the legal age — whether 21 or 20 — the same for every state would do much to correct it.

If that is a federal intrusion in state affairs, the figures provide a persuasive argument for it being a warranted one. It would be unnecessary if Vermont and others in the lower half of the age scale raised theirs to where it should be. On another front of the war against drinking drivers, however, we believe Congress and the federal bureaucracy are being both unfair and unwise.

A law passed by the first and enforced by the second, which mandates that any motorist who fails a Breathalyzer test have his or her license lifted immediately, does violence to the "innocent until proven guilty" concept of justice — and penalizes Massachusetts and 38 other states which adhere to it.

We don't believe drinking drivers should be treated leniently, but we do believe they should be treated justly — and finding them guilty without or before a trial is on-the-spot "justice" such as might be meted out at a lynching.

To attempt to cow states which follow due process and their constitutions in prosecuting by threatening to withhold funds for fighting drunk driving from them until they bow to the federal dictates is wrong and short-sighted.

Wiser heads in Washington should — and we hope will — amend that law and policy before the Supreme Court does it for them.

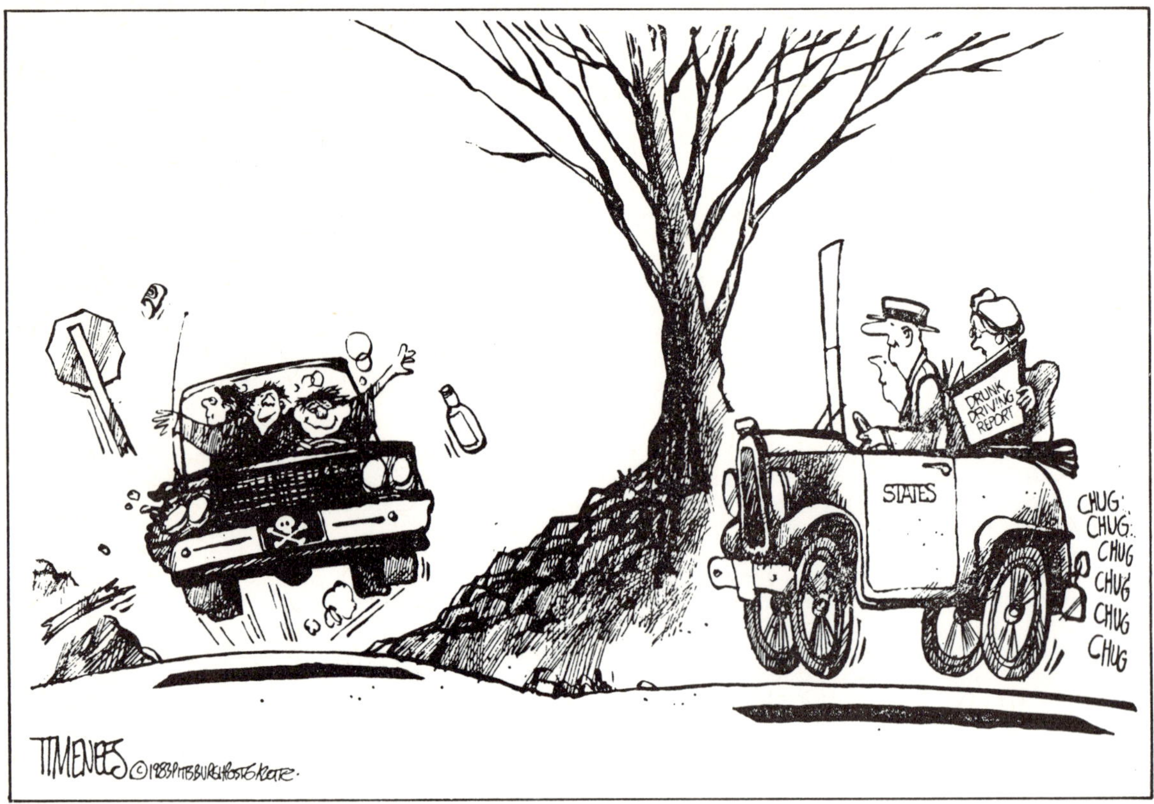

THE ARIZONA REPUBLIC

Phoenix, AZ, February 25, 1984

IMPATIENT with the checkerboard decisions of states in dealing with the legal drinking age, the House Energy and Commerce Committee has approved legislation prohibiting most bars and liquor stores from selling alcoholic beverages to anyone under 21.

The legislation is based on a far-fetched interpretation of the constitutional power of Congress to regulate interstate commerce.

Thirty-one states have drinking ages lower than 21 years. But some of them, including Arizona, are moving toward raising the age.

This is the approach the Reagan administration favors — states making the decision. So, even if the House committee's legislation sails through the House and the Senate — an exercise deemed not likely — the bill probably will be vetoed by the president.

But even if that occurs, a uniform federal drinking age undoubtedly will be proposed again, as proponents trot out impressive, emotional statistics of the slaughter on highways involving young people.

But a far more sensible approach in the meantime would be for states to be encouraged — through the carrot-and-stick approach if necessary — to enforce laws that already make drunken driving illegal and outlaw the use of alcohol by under-age young people.

New laws seem out of order until old ones are seriously enforced.

WORCESTER TELEGRAM

Worcester, MA, February 18, 1984

U.S. Transportation Secretary Elizabeth Dole has released preliminary figures on traffic deaths in the United States last year. Although 43,028 deaths on the highway is a horrendous toll, it is the lowest number in 20 years. Furthermore, the 1983 traffic fatality rate of 2.6 deaths per 100 million vehicle miles is the lowest on record.

The trend is encouraging. Much credit must go to those groups that have put such a blazing searchlight on the problem of driving and drinking. Citizens for Safe Drivers Against Drunk Drivers and Other Chronic Offenders, Mothers Against Drunk Drivers, Students Against Drunken Driving and Truckers Against Drunk Drivers have all heightened public awareness. Largely because of their efforts, 40 states tightened up their drunken-driving laws last year. Massachusetts was one.

Two years ago, President Reagan set up a special commission, headed by John A. Volpe, to study the drunken-driving issue. Its report, issued last December, urged Congress to deny federal highway funds to any state that fails to set the legal drinking age at 21.

"There is evidence of a direct correlation between the minimum drinking age and alcohol-related crashes among the age groups affected," the report stated. "The lack of uniformity among state laws is especially critical regarding the minimum legal drinking age because an incentive to drink and drive is established due to young persons commuting to border states where the drinking age is lower."

Two weeks ago, the House Energy and Commerce Committee approved a bill to establish a national minimum drinking age of 21. A similar measure is before a Senate committee.

So progress is being made. Yet, the battle for safer highways is far from won. Passing a national minimum drinking law will not be easy. Making people buckle their seat belts is even more difficult. Enforcing the 55-mph speed law varies according to regions and states.

But the figures to date show that something can be accomplished by determination. That determination must not weaken.

ALBUQUERQUE JOURNAL

Albuquerque, NM, February 23, 1984

Eventually time, stricter judges, tougher laws and even stronger law enforcement might cure what charitably can be called an outrageous hangover. The outrage comes with information that while more drunken drivers are being arrested, many of them manage to avoid completing court-ordered procedures.

For example, as many as 1,600 drunken driving warrants were outstanding in Albuquerque at the start of the month. That represented a 10-month backlog.

The problem became so severe that the Albuquerque Police Department assigned special teams to arrest drivers who failed to comply with court orders including arraignment, sentencing, failure to complete court ordered alcoholism-counseling and DWI classes. Those sweeps — which haven't been outstandingly successful, thanks to faulty information and other factors the police can't control — came after a one-week amnesty period where those with outstanding bench warrants could avoid arrest and jail by voluntarily making arrangements on outstanding bench warrants.

The APD sweep to find the DWI scofflaws emphasizes what seems to be an inherent weakness in the city's Metropolitan Court system. Warrants are not served in a timely manner. Recently, old parking citations were being dismissed in wholesale quantities, largely on the assertion that unpaid tickets purged from the current computer files were somehow "administratively dismissed."

The buildup of DWI warrants, however, is more serious. Drunken drivers are involved in a disproportionate number of fatal and injury traffic accidents. For example, last year in New Mexico, 324 traffic deaths were partly or wholly attributable to drunken driving. Another 5,700 persons were injured in accidents in which alcohol was a contributing factor.

Albuquerque recorded 13,885 accidents — as many as 7,900 of them alcohol-related — in 1983, including 31 fatalities, seven of which were attributed to alcohol.

In the United States, someone dies in a DWI accident every 20 minutes. That's approximately 500 a week and about 25,000 fatalities a year. More than 700,000 are injured each year in crashes where alcohol is involved.

Secretary of Transportation Eliabeth Dole describes drunk or drugged driving as "our most excused crime."

The toll taken by drunk drivers might be even higher than generally accepted. Pathologists say nine out of 10 fatal traffic accidents — double the accepted level — may be linked to alcohol.

New Mexico's concern with drunken driving is demonstrated by a bill passed by the Legislature this month and awaiting Gov. Toney Anaya's signature. It will permit arresting officers to seize the driver's license of any adult registering .10 percent blood alcohol or anyone refusing to take a blood alcohol test. Licenses of minors will be subject to seizure if a blood alcohol level of .05 percent is registered. That change in the law should deter many more motorists from driving after drinking.

Normally, fear of getting caught provides deterence to committing a criminal act such as drunken driving. Yet in Albuquerque, while police arrest and charge drunk drivers at a rate of more than 150 a month, the system of deterrence rather obviously is breaking down. An arrest and conviction is not as convincing if the consequences are not enforced.

Quite obviously, the system for deterrence needs improvement. There should not be a 10-month backlog of DWI case defendants who are not complying with various court orders. Driving safety would improve greatly if society could keep drivers who drink out from behind the wheel of their motor vehicles.

New Mexico's new law will help but follow up programs must not become lost in court and police paperwork.

The Seattle Times

Seattle, WA, February 21, 1984

TRANSPORTATION Secretary Elizabeth Dole had some happy news the other day. Dole announced that preliminary figures show there were 43,028 traffic deaths in the U.S. last year. That's happy news? Yes, when one considers it is the lowest total in two decades. Moreover, the 1983 traffic-fatality rate of 2.6 deaths per 100 million vehicle miles was the lowest on record.

The improvement is no mystery. It can be traced to the increased public awareness of the drunken-driving menace.

Further steps that can be taken are not without controversy. The problem is complex, to be sure. But statistics do point to one specific step that would further lower the terrible highway toll: the establishment of a national minimum drinking age of 21.

The House Energy and Commerce Committee has approved a bill to do that. A similar measure is pending in the Senate. Supporters of those measures are under no illusions that they would stop teen-age drinking. But they say a uniform legal drinking age would stop young people from crossing state borders to avail themselves of a lower drinking age and then climbing behind the wheel in an impaired condition.

Drivers under 21 represent about 10 percent of licensed drivers, but they were in the driver's seat in about one of five alcohol-related traffic deaths. Those figures tell a story.

Washington is one of 19 states with laws setting the minimum drinking age at 21. The whole U.S. should have that protection.

TULSA WORLD

Tulsa, OK, February 22, 1984

IF ANYONE doubts the link between teen-age drinking and highway deaths, he should consult a recent study by the National Bureau of Economic Research.

Economist Dennis C. McCornac studied teen-age highway mortality rates between 1970 and 1975, during which time 14 states lowered minimum drinking ages to 18. His conclusion: States which lowered their drinking ages experienced an increase in highway deaths among teenagers.

McCornac says if the minimum drinking age in all states had been 21 during the 5-year period, there would have been 700 fewer teenagers killed each year. Thousands more would not have been injured.

His findings are not surprising. The link between teen-age drinking and highway fatalities is well-established. In recent years many states, including Oklahoma, have raised minimum drinking ages to combat the problem. Already several states report a decline in teen-age highway deaths which they link directly to the higher drinking age.

The war on drunk drivers is a continuous battle. Oklahoma and other states have made substantial inroads in the problem by stiffening penalties for driving while intoxicated. But any penalty is in a sense an admission of failure — failure to prevent a drunk driver from getting on the road.

It's better to keep drunk drivers from getting on the road. Raising minimum drinking ages does that. McCornac's study shows 700 lives a year are saved as a result. That is a tremendous benefit from the minor cost of making teen-agers wait until they're 21 to drink.

Supreme Court Rules **S**tudent Searches Permitted

The United States Supreme Court January 15, 1985 ruled that it was legally permissable for public school officials or teachers to search students as long as there were "reasonable grounds" to think the search would yield evidence of a violation of the law or of school rules. In a 6-3 decision, written by Justice Byron R. White, the Court said school officials could search a student without a warrant and without the stronger "probable cause" to believe that evidence of a crime would be found, required generally for police searches. "It is evident," the majority opinion said, "that the school setting requires some easing of the restrictions to which searches by public authorities are ordinarily subject." The Court decided that students were covered by the Fourth Amendment protection against "unreasonable searches and seizures," but that the "substantial interest" of school officials in maintaining discipline must be balanced against the substantial interest of the student in privacy. Violent crime and drug use in the schools, the opinion said, had become "major social issues."

Justices William J. Brennan, John Paul Stevens and Thurgood Marshall dissented. All three agreed that the Fourth Amendment covered school searches, but objected to what they considered a weakening of the amendment's protection in this instance.

The decision, in *New Jersey v. T.L.O.*, arose from a 1980 incident at Piscataway High School in New Jersey, when a 14-year-old girl was accused of smoking in the lavoratory in violation of school rules. The student denied that she was smoking but a search of her purse produced cigarettes and also marijuana.

The Times-Picayune
The States-Item

New Orleans, LA, January 19, 1985

It is reassuring that the U.S. Supreme Court has just reinforced the value of discipline in the nation's public schools by giving discipline a higher priority than students' right to privacy.

The high court's decision came in a case involving Piscataway, N.J., school officials who searched a 14-year-old freshman's purse after she was caught smoking. They found cigarette papers and marijuana. The student later admitted to police that she sold marijuana cigarettes to classmates.

The U.S. Supreme Court's ruling reversed a ruling by the New Jersey Supreme Court, which had held that the New Jersey school officials lacked "reasonable grounds" for searching the student's purse.

With its ruling, the nation's highest court has not suspended within school environs students' Fourth Amendment protection against unreasonable searches. But it does not hold school administrators and teachers to the stricter "probable cause" standard applicable to police searches.

Writing for the majority, Justice Byron R. White observed, "It is evident that the school setting requires some easing of the restrictions to which searches by public authorities are ordinarily subject." The legality of the search of a student, he wrote, "should depend simply on the reasonableness, under all circumstances, of the search."

In supporting reasonable searches, the court acknowledged the almost universal problem — the "contemporary reality" —

of enforcing discipline in the nation's schools where drugs, weapons and violence have become part of the daily milieu.

While the stand is new for the Supreme Court, it basically reinforces a practice that had already become commonplace in many of the nation's public schools. The "reasonableness" standard had already been adopted by state and lower federal courts, including the New Jersey Supreme Court, that had considered the student search issue.

The broad acceptance of the Supreme Court's ruling among students, school officials, parents and others is at once encouraging and disturbing. It reflects widespread recognition of an urgent need to restore discipline in the nation's public schools. At the same time, it reflects a far-flung consensus on just how bad the "contemporary reality" has become.

That same reality, of course, is to be found in American society at large, where criminal violence is eroding such basic freedoms as freedom of movement without fear in one's own neighborhood. The court's response is to liberalize police powers, to turn from preoccupation with the freedom of the individual in an effort to restore the collective freedom of the community.

If the school decision helps to instill in the young a new appreciation of the value of discipline in their personal lives and in society, it will be well worth the small trade-off in students' slightly diminished right of privacy.

Richmond Times-Dispatch

Richmond, VA, January 21, 1985

Now that the U. S. Supreme Court has ruled that teachers and principals may search pupils they suspect of skulduggery without going through all the complicated legal process that restricts police operations, some national civil-liberties and children's-rights groups are complaining that the court has deprived students of constitutional protections. Soon liberal critics may add this case to those "proving" that this court is now only slightly to the left of Attila the Hun, and, given a few more Reagan appointees, will soon move to the right.

Such paranoia is unjustified. A reading of the text of the court's opinions in *New Jersey vs. T.L.O., a Juvenile*, should calm fears any rational person might have about overzealous school-masters conducting strip searches or demanding a student's pocketbook any time they want to rummage through it.

To begin with, the court unanimously rejected — that's right, *rejected* — New Jersey's argument that the Fourth Amendment ban on unreasonable searches and seizures applies only to police. School employees, too, are agents of the state, and accordingly are subject to restraint on their conduct. The court would have none of New Jersey's argument that teachers act *in loco parentis* — in place of the parents — and so could wield the absolute clout of Mom or Pop.

But while affirming that children do not shed constitutional rights at the schoolhouse door, a 6-3 majority of the court decided that because of the urgent need for discipline in the classroom and on school grounds, the rules for school searches should be somewhat less stringent than for those conducted by police. First (as even liberal dissenting justice William J. Brennan Jr. agreed), school officials need not obtain a warrant before searching a student under their authority. Second, in order to search, they do not have to have "probable cause" to believe that a crime has been committed. They need only have "reasonable grounds for suspecting" that a search would show that a student is violating either the law or the school's own rules.

"Such a search," Justice Byron R. White wrote for the majority, "will be permissible in its scope when the measures adopted are reasonably related to the objectives of the search and are not excessively intrusive in light of the age and sex of the student and the nature of the infraction."

That's a long way from authorizing searches unlimited, or from the fantasy of dissenter John Paul Stevens that the court had put shakedowns for heroin and gang activity in the same category with those for sunglasses and hair curlers. Certainly, interpretations of what is reasonable will differ and the high court will be asked to make more judgment calls. But the court was on the right track in balancing the privacy rights of pupils with the equally legitimate right — indeed, responsibility — of teachers and principals to maintain an orderly environment in which learning can occur.

As Justice White observed, drug use and violent crime in schools have become "major social problems." Arguably, that's at least partly the result of a string of judicial decisions that have eroded school officials' authority to crack down swiftly on wrongdoing. Call this decision one much-needed victory for authority, reasonably exercised.

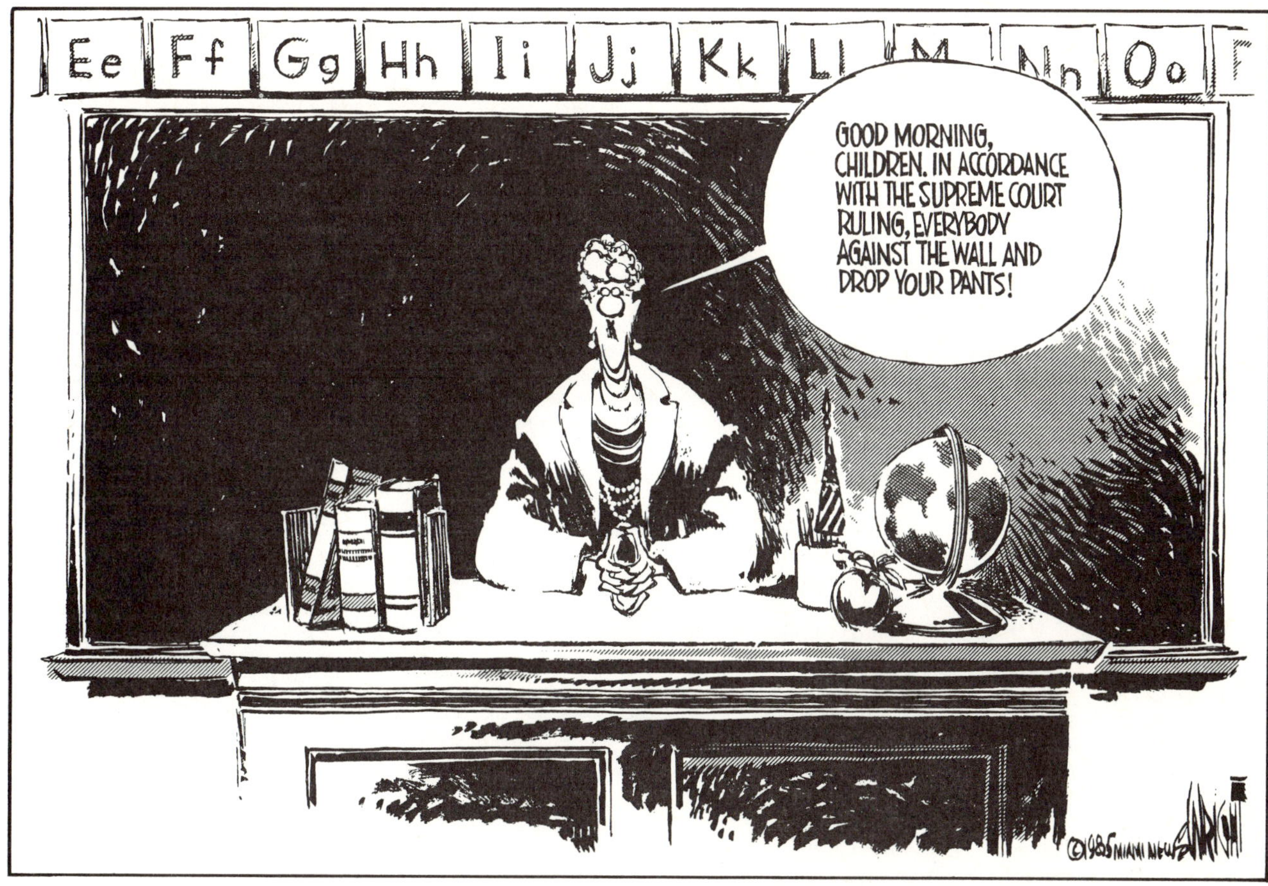

Rockford Register Star

Rockford, IL, January 19, 1985

With a ruling this week that raises more questions than it answers, the U.S. Supreme Court's blurring of the Fourth Amendment to the Constitution continues apace.

This time, the high court held in a split decision that public school officials may legally conduct searches of students without "probable cause" so long as there are "reasonable grounds." The case at issue involved a search of a student's purse for cigarettes, and the resultant discovery of marijuana therein.

That the differences between "probable cause" and "reasonable grounds" might be vague or confusing seems not to have occurred to the court's majority of six in this case. School authorities are left to guess the upshot of the ruling.

Does it mean school officials may legally search students at whim? Apparently not. The court warned against "excessively intrusive" searches.

Does it mean Fourth Amendment guarantees of privacy do not fully extend to students? Well, yes — or, at least, that would seem to be the court's drift. But to what extent, under what circumstances, at what age levels, in what kind of schools?

Does it mean evidence obtained in any school search is admissable in criminal action against the student? The court dodged that question in this case.

Then, too, questions remain as to whether students' privacy rights are the same for their desks and lockers as for their persons.

The best that can be said of this latest ruling is that it is consistent with other recent high court decisions on privacy, most notably the ruling that allows for "good faith" exceptions to the rule that bars evidence obtained by police in illegal searches.

School officials now face both procedural and academic quandaries with respect to the Fourth Amendment. How does it apply to their students as a practical matter? And what should they teach their students about the amendment's true meaning?

THE CHRONICLE-HERALD

Halifax, NS, January 18, 1985

THE SUPREME Court of the United States has ruled that public school teachers and administrators do not need court warrants nor the same justifications as police officers before searching a student suspected of being in possession of drugs.

It is an interesting decision which could have far reaching consequences. While it has been made in the American context, experience suggests that acceptance of the principle south of the border will herald its introduction in this country.

The idea of school administrations searching students is by no means new. It was not an uncommon practise a couple of generations ago. Those were the days when smoking among school students was frowned upon. Any youngster found with tobacco in his possession (there is no need to include the pronoun "her" in the observation because smoking among teen-age girls in those days was virtually unheard of) could expect to have the contraband confiscated and punishment administered.

A search today would be a very different matter. For one thing, it probably would not receive parental support and sympathy as once it did. For another, school administrations do not now have the authority to punish which once they possessed.

What happens, then, if a pupil is found to have drugs in his or her possession? Since a criminal offence has been committed, the matter is out of the hands of the school authorities. They have found out the guilty but dealing with the situation then becomes a matter for the police and the courts.

By giving teachers and administrators the right to search a pupil, the U.S. Supreme Court has considerably altered the nature of the student-teacher relationship. In the eyes of youth, school administrators and faculties are cast in the role of police informants.

That of itself may not be wrong but it does have the effect of widening the breach between those teaching and those who are taught. It will make no difference insofar as "good" students are concerned but it may make a world of difference among that group which most needs help and guidance.

The Supreme Court decision might have been more realistic and certainly would have been far more useful had it added to the right to search, the authority to administer punishment, corporal if deemed necessary. Much of the current unrest in the public school system had its origins in the relaxing of discipline which inevitably entered the picture when punishments were phased out.

The Record
Hackensack, NJ, January 18, 1985

The Supreme Court settled a most vexing question this week by deciding that teachers and administrators in public schools may search students without a warrant and without evidence of a crime. The ruling means that public-school pupils are only partly protected by the Fourth Amendment to the Constitution.

It was a New Jersey case, arising from a 1980 incident at Piscataway High School in Middlesex County. A teacher caught a 14-year-old girl smoking a cigarette, went through her purse, and found marijuana, drug paraphernalia, 40 one-dollar bills, and evidence of drug dealing. The girl was found guilty and put on a year's probation.

On appeal, however, the New Jersey Supreme Court reversed the conviction on the ground that the evidence was illegally obtained. A law-enforcement officer may not search an ordinary citizen unless he has good reason to suspect that he'll find evidence of a crime. In this case, the teacher had no such reason.

And so the question before the U.S. Supreme Court boiled down to this: Are teachers agents for the state or are they surrogates for parents? Since the Fourth Amendment applies only to law-enforcement searches, there's nothing unconstitutional about a search conducted by a private person — a parent, for instance. (This also means that the ruling does not apply to private schools.) The court could thus have ruled that teachers may search students without any constraint whatever. Fortunately, it didn't.

Had the court stopped there, this would have been a good decision. But it proceeded to open a giant loophole that seems guaranteed to make student searches more common. Where a law-enforcement officer needs "probable cause" of a crime to conduct a search, a teacher needs only "reasonable grounds" — a considerably weaker standard. As Justice Brennan noted in his spirited dissent, any erosion of the probable-cause guarantee "portends a dangerous weakening" of Fourth Amendment protections for everyone.

Moreover, the decision did not distinguish between serious and trivial matters. Drugs are one thing; but, as Justice Stevens pointed out in his dissent, teachers will now have license to conduct searches if they have "reasonable grounds" for believing that the dress code has been violated — to search kids for "sunglasses and hair curlers," as he put it.

Will this ruling make it harder for students to bring drugs and weapons into school? It seems unlikely. A principal in Paterson, where the schools have more than their share of crime problems, tells us that most students voluntarily submit to searches. If they don't, their parents are called in and they authorize a search so as not to get the law involved.

Let's not forget that students are citizens, too. They are protected by the right to free speech, the right of assembly, and all the other guarantees of the Bill of Rights. The Fourth Amendment is no less important. The high court's decision to weaken it for students is therefore both unnecessary and inappropriate.

The Burlington Free Press
Burlington, VT, January 17, 1985

In what must be considered a precedent-setting decision, the U.S. Supreme Court has ruled that school authorities may search students if there are "reasonable grounds" for suspicion that students have violated the law or school rules.

School officials thus do not have to use the same grounds as police to justify student searches, the court said. Under the Fourth Amendment, police must have probable cause before they can search individuals for evidence that a crime has been committed.

The court reversed a New Jersey Supreme Court decision which overturned a delinquency finding against a 14-year-old Piscataway High School girl who was searched by a school administrator in 1980 after she was caught smoking in a lavatory in violation of school rules. When she denied she was smoking, the school official asked to see her pocketbook and found a package of cigarettes, marijuana and written evidence that she had been selling the drug. She was turned over to the police and found to be a delinquent in Juvenile Court. The New Jersey high court reversed the judgment, saying the search lacked reasonable grounds.

But the Supreme Court said the pocketbook search "was in no sense unreasoable" and said probable cause was too restrictive a standard to apply in a school setting. Justice Byron White who wrote the opinion for the majority said that students' claim to privacy must be balanced against "the substantial interest of teachers and administrators in maintaining discipline in the classroom and on school grounds." "It is evident that the school setting requires some easing of restrictions to which searches by public authorities are ordinarily subject," he said.

However defensible the decision to allow school officials to conduct searches might appear to be, questions must be raised about the students' rights as compared to those of adults. It is one thing, for instance, for school authorities to search such items of school property as lockers for drugs or weapons when they suspect wrongdoing. It is quite another to search personal property of the students under similar circumstances. If incriminating evidence is found and turned over to police, such a procedure would seem to set a double standard for adults and minors.

In the final analysis, parents are ultimately responsible for the behavior of their children while on school grounds and they should exercise the necessary discipline in their homes to dissuade children from using or selling drugs. School officials at the same time should use available disciplinary measures to punish students who violate the rules. By making examples of the offenders, administrators might well persuade other students to comply with the rules.

If parents and school authorities took a stronger hand in the matter, it might not then be necessary for officials to search students.

Detroit Free Press
Detroit, MI, January 17, 1985

THE U.S. Supreme Court ruling to allow reasonable-grounds searches of students is reasonable indeed, given the current level of renegade behavior in too many schools. To sustain an atmosphere of learning, teachers and administrators need the power to examine purses and pockets when circumstances seem to justify it, as the court affirmed.

Does that mean the new search policy in Detroit schools is constitutional? 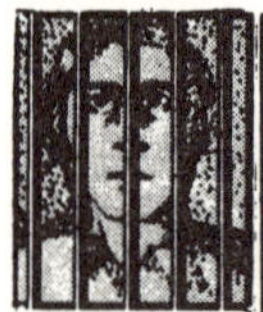
Superintendent Arthur Jefferson says the ruling supports his search procedures and Michigan's leading civil libertarian says it doesn't. The fact is, nobody knows for sure how far the decision allows schools to peer into desks and lockers or to conduct mass searches on the possibility that guns or drugs will be turned up. The precise answers await Supreme Court clarification.

But the high court majority plainly wanted to give school administrators some flexibility and to set a standard for student searches that is less rigid than what the Fourth and 14th Amendments require in criminal cases — reasonable grounds rather than probable cause.

Mr. Jefferson and school officials throughout Michigan have to pursue every reasonable effort against lawless student behavior. And Howard Simon and the American Civil Liberties Union have to keep in mind the rights and needs of an often-threatened majority of students to get an education, even as they pursue the legitimate matter of privacy rights.

The Supreme Court was careful to note that school officials are not surrogates for parents; they have no parental privilege to intrude into students' lives. The balance between privacy and security — in school and out of it — is not always easy to define. It sometimes shifts, depending on where society and the courts see the greater threat.

But a cautious reading of the decision shows the court still wrote large on the nation's blackboards: There's nothing wrong with reasonable discipline.

St. Petersburg Times

St. Petersburg, FL, January 17, 1985

The U.S. Supreme Court was right when it ruled Tuesday that public school students are protected by the Fourth Amendment, but it erred seriously when it cast aside the traditional standard for applying that protection.

Teachers and administrators surely need public and legal support in dealing with increasing violations of school discipline. But even that problem fails to justify such a broad exception to constitutional protections.

The Fourth Amendment is absolute: "The right of the people to be secure in their persons . . . against unreasonable searches . . . shall not be violated." That means a government official must have probable cause to believe a law has been violated in order to conduct a search.

In its 6-3 opinion, the court said that the probable cause rule did not apply to public school students as long as "there are reasonable grounds for suspecting that the search will turn up evidence that the student has violated or is violating either the law or the rules of the school."

WE AGREE with Justice William Brennan who in his dissent wrote that this "broad exception" is an "unclear, unprecedented and unnecessary" departure from traditional standards which "portends a dangerous weakening of the purpose of the Fourth Amendment to protect the privacy and security of our citizens."

What is reasonable to one school dean may not be reasonable to others. Today's exceptions to the probable cause rule for students become tomorrow's exception for every citizen.

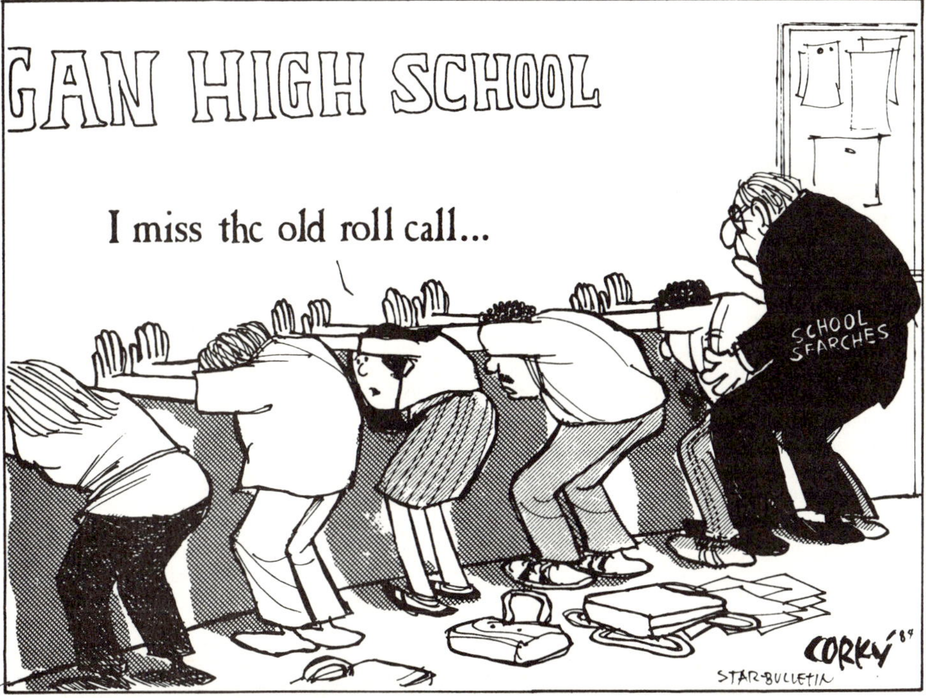

Minneapolis Star and Tribune

Minneapolis, MN, January 23, 1985

Public-school students have a constitutional right to privacy, says the U.S. Supreme Court, but only sometimes. The court ruled last week that privacy must give way when respecting that right could endanger student welfare. Though hedged with qualifying language, the decision opens the door a shade too far for school authorities and too nearly closes off individual rights.

Public-school teachers and principals must stop smokers, apprehend drug users, quell disruption and ward off violence. As agents of the state, they must also respect the constitutional right of students, as of other citizens, to be free from unreasonable search and seizure.

But what should suspicious school officials do when the only way to uncover serious wrongdoing is to conduct an immediate search? That was the question facing the court in the New Jersey case resolved last week. The 6-3 ruling offers a new tool to educators striving to maintain order. While they can't legally subject students to indiscriminate on-the-spot searches, the court said, they should be able to act quickly to find and confiscate dangerous drugs and weapons. The court ruled that school officials need not wait for a warrant before conducting searches; that, instead, they should be free to search students whenever they have "reasonable grounds" to suspect misconduct.

Justice Byron White's majority opinion rejected the notion that school officials should be free of constitutional restraint in conducting searches. School officials have an obligation, White wrote, to balance students' right to privacy against the need for school order. And the opinion noted that searches must not be "excessively intrusive."

Those warnings make clear the court's belief that the Fourth Amendment reaches inside the schoolhouse gates. But the opinion's vague language weakens it by granting school officials wide discretion to decide how much privacy students should enjoy. Students are thus left vulnerable to any search that a school administrator decides is reasonable.

Perhaps a sacrifice of student privacy is necessary to preserve order in public schools. But the court should have done more than open the door to all searches that school officials deem reasonable. It should have defined what constitutes a reasonable search. It should have assured that student privacy would be violated only when peace and safety are clearly jeopardized. Without such guidance from the court, school officials must strive to exercise their new power cautiously and sparingly.

The Honolulu Advertiser

Honolulu, HI, January 18, 1985

Hawaii school officials seem to be taking a common-sense approach to the U.S. Supreme Court ruling giving teachers more freedom in searching students. The court said public school officials and teachers may search students without a warrant or the stricter "probable cause" standard that applies to police.

Still, the court made clear that just as students are covered by the First Amendment (freedom of speech) and the 14th Amendment (due process), they are protected by the Fourth Amendment against arbitrary searches. It said that school officials must have "reasonable cause" to believe the law or a school rule has been violated in order to conduct a search.

THIS 6-TO-3 decision was a compromise between two views: one that students have all the rights and protections citizens enjoy in dealing with government authorities and the other that students surrender those rights when they go to school.

The ruling makes clear that students have rights, though somewhat modified. It balances the right of students to privacy against "the substantial interest of teachers and administrators in maintaining discipline in the classroom and on school grounds."

Of course, a safe, rule-abiding school atmosphere where learning is possible is also in the highest interest of the students as well.

The court's ruling has the potential for abuse or just petty, mean-spirited application. A lot depends on the intent and spirit with which searches are carried out, and civil libertarians should and will be vigilant to abuses.

HAWAII HAS its problems with violence and drug use on (and off) school grounds. They may not rank with those of some large, urban schools on the Mainland, but there is no question that weapons, drugs or anything else that disrupts academics have no place on campus.

While welcoming the ruling, Hawaii school superintendent Francis Hatanaka affirmed students' basic civil rights and cautioned teachers against misuse of their new authority. Some more detailed guidelines for teachers and students as to what constitutes "reasonable cause" would probably be appreciated by all.

Bennett Blasts **B** U.S. Colleges

Education Secretary William J. Bennett July 8, 1986 called upon America's college presidents to show "a little courage" and eliminate all drugs from their campuses starting in September. He made the remarks in Washington, D.C. before the Heritage Foundation, a right-wing research group.

Drugs laws on campus "could in fact be enforced," Bennett said. He asserted that no "parent or taxpayer" would object, but that "such a straightforward policy would require a kind of reinvigoration of our institutions, a recognition and resumption of their basic responsibilities." The secretary said he opposed student drug testing except as a last resort. But he also reiterated his suggestion that Congress give his office the power to withhold federal funds from colleges not adequately dealing with drugs on campus.

FORT WORTH STAR-TELEGRAM
Fort Worth, TX, July 14, 1986

Education Secretary William Bennett no doubt stirred up some dust in the academic community with his recent suggestion that colleges and universities get more involved in the fight against the use of illegal drugs.

But he does have a point, one that should be listened to. The campus is a place of tremendous influence, and some of that influence should be exerted in the direction of convincing young people not to use drugs.

Bennett would have the colleges and universities strictly enforce a campus ban on drugs. He said, "Such a policy could, in fact, be enforced. It should be enforced. And no parent or taxpayer would object if such a policy were announced and carried out."

The Cabinet member said colleges and universities have a responsibility to parents to take measures to protect their children from illegal drugs and drug pushers, just as they protect them against crime, fraud and exploitation.

He also said, "Parents do not expect colleges to be neutral as between decent morality and decadence."

As if that were not enough to put a burr under the saddle of those in the academic community, Bennett also remarked:

"Our colleges and universities often, and sometimes quite properly, call to task the rest of society for failing to live up to its stated ideals. They set themselves the role of moral gadfly, moral conscience. But what of them?"

Colleges and universities will want to carefully examine Bennett's suggestion to determine if there is more they can and should do to reduce drug abuse.

But the need for stepped-up, corrective action certainly is not limited to the college and university campus.

Indeed, every segment of the nation's society must be called into action to find more effective ways to wage war against the use of illegal drugs. That heightened effort must be waged in the homes and in the public schools. It must be waged on the job and in the churches.

The reason is that what is being lost to illegal drugs — lives, minds, property, the well-being of individuals and families and so much more — is robbing us all.

Better ways must be found to teach that and to learn better what to do about it. That message must be spread on the college and university campus, as the education secretary said, but it also must be spread wherever it must be heard. And, given the epidemic proportions to which illegal drug use has spread and in view of its toll, that means everywhere.

THE ARIZONA REPUBLIC
Phoenix, AZ, July 27, 1986

EDUCATION Secretary William Bennett, never one to mince words, has proposed a simple, straightforward course for our nation's colleges and universities. The alternate route is a course of disaster.

Citing the alarming statistics indicating increasing drug use among our nation's future leaders, Bennett, speaking before the conservative Heritage Foundation, asked college presidents to send a simple message to returning students this fall:

"Welcome back for your studies in September; but no drugs on campus. None. Period. This policy will be enforced — by deans and administrators and advisers and faculty — strictly, but fairly."

As everyone knows, that letter probably will not be written. After all, many of our nation's hallowed institutions of higher learning have higher priorities than restricting and policing the "individual liberties" of students — making the Final Four and bowling on New Year's Day.

Drug use and abuse on campus is nothing new. Even before Dr. Timothy Leary and *Reefer Madness*, another drug, alcohol, besotted some of the nation's finest minds to the point where fish-swallowing became a sliding scale of college achievement.

But Bennett is correct. America needs to delcare war on drugs, and the battle needs to be launched and carried out in America's institutions — the churches, the schools, the family.

Whether students are star athletes or top scholars, a lesson in upholding the basic values of our society might be of more benefit than any other course offered.

Liberal *intelligentsia* protestations aside, there is a moral and ethical link between education and society that weaves the entire fabric of our nation's culture — now, and for the future.

Make no mistake, America's drug problem is not confined in ivy-covered walls or inner-city ghettos; the issue is neither conservative nor liberal — both first lady Nancy Reagan and the Rev. Jesse Jackson repeat the same message: "Say 'no' to drugs!"

But if, as Bennett says, we watch as though helpless as "our social and cultural institutions drift away from their moorings," we then abdicate our responsibilities — intellectually and morally — to future generations.

A mind is, indeed, a terrible thing to waste. And the ash heap of history is just a short trip down the path of intellectual banckruptcy.

St. Louis Review
St. Louis, MO, July 11, 1986

In the weeks before the Liberty weekend two talented athletes, Len Bias and Don Rogers, both died of cocaine overdoses. While their tragic deaths surprised many people, deaths of famous people such as these two seem to have little deterrent effect on others caught up in the same addiction. Cocaine is apparently the thing to do right now among the rich and famous and also the kid on the corner.

A study recently concluded by the University of Michigan reported that 30 percent of college graduates try cocaine before they graduate. Despite the highly publicized deaths of entertainment and sport stars using this drug, only one-third of those surveyed said that they saw much risk in using it. In light of this we might suspect people's intelligence, but we all tend to think that tragedies happen to other people and not to us.

It is a sad commentary on American life just when we are celebrating liberty as a national treasure. For many liberty means what the philosophers used to call "license" or the freedom to do whatever I please. As a result we are ending up with many immature adults unable to focus their talents in any useful direction.

Pope John Paul II touched on this topic of drug use last week during his visit to Colombia, where much of our cocaine originates. The Pope on this occasion referred to the slavery of drug addiction and called drug dealers "traffickers in freedom." He is pointing out just what taking drugs does to us. It takes away our freedom — our freedom to be human.

Secretary of Education William Bennett this week called on college and university administrators in this country to declare their campuses drug-free zones and to take steps to keep drugs off campus. That idea has a lot of merit. We have a great aversion nowadays to telling other people what to do. Too often therefore we stand by, as it were, while innocent lives are being ruined "letting everyone find out for themselves." We forget that friends don't let friends ruin their lives.

TULSA WORLD
Tulsa, OK, July 24, 1986

THE PROPOSAL by U.S. Secretary of Education William J. Bennett to cut off federal funds to schools that do not enforce an absolute ban on illegal drugs was greeted with appropriate criticism by state university leaders.

The very idea of being able to punish an entire institution for the foolish acts of a few is unacceptable.

Bennett asked Congress to provide him with the power to withhold federal aid from schools that "do not protect their students from drugs," and invited university presidents to enforce an absolute ban on illegal drugs on their campuses.

Surely Bennett doesn't actually believe that responsible university leaders are unaware of drug problems on campuses. And, how would such a power be enforced? Who would be the judge of what an absolute ban would be?

Any kind of illegal activity, including drugs, has been discouraged at universities. Enforcement, however, is just as difficult on a large campus as in the streets of any city. And, there are legal limits to enforcement.

As University of Oklahoma President Frank Horton said: "We can't go into a student's dorm room and search for drugs."

Drugs are a problem. Not just in universities, but everywhere.

Strict measures must be taken to curb drug use. The threat of cutting off much-needed federal funds, however, is not the answer.

The Washington Post
Washington, DC, July 12, 1986

SECRETARY of Education William J. Bennett had some suggestions for college administrators the other day about dealing with drugs on campus. They have an obligation, he told the educators, to care for the moral and physical well-being of their students and to protect them from certain influences, including drugs, criminals, fraud and exploitation. Mr. Bennett says he has been criticized for expressing these views and told that he sounded like "a small-town PTA president." We don't think that's necessarily a pejorative, since PTA presidents tend to be the kind of people who care about children and public institutions. But why is this admonition to the colleges derided as "simplistic"?

It would be wonderful, the secretary told his audience, if every college president would write the following letter to his students this summer: "Welcome back for your studies in September; but no drugs on campus. None. Period. This policy will be enforced—by deans and administrators and advisers and faculty—strictly but fairly." That sounds fine to us. We agree with him that most parents, and students who are not involved with drugs, would welcome such a clear policy announcement and would support its enforcement. Does this necessarily mean calling in the local police to handle every problem? Of course not. But a commitment to combat drug use on campus will go a long way toward creating a climate where this behavior is viewed as risky, foolish and, eventually, unacceptable to a large majority of the students.

Colleges can't solve the drug problem alone, for students of that age are free to make decisions about their own lives. But just as university health services encourage fitness and deplore smoking and alcohol abuse, they have an opportunity and an obligation to campaign vigorously against drugs. And as administrators would act quickly in cases of theft, violence or racial discrimination, they should not hesitate to move against offenses involving drugs for the simple reason that these acts are both illegal and wrong.

University leaders have some authority and much responsibility in our society. It is not unreasonable to ask them to take a strong stand against drugs on campus.

THE BLADE
Toledo, OH, July 14, 1986

IN THE wake of the cocaine-related deaths of sports stars Len Bias and Don Rogers, some governmental officials are calling for sweeping programs to discourage drug abuse. Some of their plans are questionable, though well-intended.

Secretary of Education William Bennett is urging colleges and universities to enforce a strict ban on drug use. Mr. Bennett would like Congress to give him the power to withhold federal funds from schools that do not protect their students from drugs.

But there is no reason to believe that the drug-abuse problem on campuses is necessarily worse than elsewhere. Many persons, young and old and regardless of whether they attend a university, go to high school, or live in an urban ghetto, are using illegal drugs. To be consistent, Mr. Bennett would have to propose a Draconian enforcement campaign aimed at all levels of society.

Colleges and universities have taken at least modest steps to discourage drug abuse. However, it is difficult to enforce university policies and city or state laws in areas where thousands of students study and live in close confines. Short of daily urinalyses of all students, there is no way to completely prevent drug abuse.

Trying to withhold federal money would create problems of its own. Complex rules and an enforcement bureaucracy would have to be created. Consider, for example, the difficulty in trying to define the point at which federal support could be cut off.

Drug abuse is a fitting target for attack, considering the tragic consequences that often flow from it. But inevitably the Federal Government would be a clumsy, coercive partner in this war, duplicating efforts already under way by college and local law-enforcement authorities.

The Burlington Free Press
Burlington, VT, July 16, 1986

As heads of institutions that closely resemble small cities or towns, college presidents must accept the responsibility for governing those communities in such a way as to protect the welfare of their students.

Evidence of increasing drug usage on campuses should alert college heads and other administrators to the need for bringing the situation under control.

By setting strict rules against use of drugs by students, the schools can assure parents that their children will be protected from the serious consequences that could result from drug abuse.

The time has long since passed when college presidents can ignore such problems on campuses.

Following the drug deaths of two young athletes, Education Secretary William J. Bennett declared that every college president in the nation should begin and strictly enforce a ban on drugs on the campus.

"Such a policy could, in fact, be enforced," he said. "It should be enforced. And no parent or taxpayer would object if such a policy were announced and carried out."

Colleges and universities have a responsibility to parents "to protect their children from illegal drugs and drug pushers," he said. "Parents do not expect colleges to be neutral as between decent morality and decadence."

College presidents certainly cannot look the other way — as they did in the 1960s — when there is a danger of broader drug usage on campuses.

They must take drastic steps to prevent the sale and use of drugs on the grounds of their schools and must set harsh penalties for those students who disobey the rules.

The deaths of Len Bias, University of Maryland basketball star, and Don Rogers, Cleveland Browns football player, from the effects of cocaine should be a warning to college presidents of the tragedies that can occur on campuses if they do not act to end drug usage by their students.

California Girl Turns in Parents

Deanna Young, a 13-year-old Tustin, Calif. girl who had fought with her parents over their use of drugs, walked into the police station in the Orange County community early August 14, 1986 and gave officers a trash bag containing pills, marijuana and cocaine she said she had found at home. The estimated street value of the drugs was $2,800. The girl's parents, Bobby Dale Young, 49, a bartender, and Judith Ann Young, a U.S. bankruptcy court clerk, were charged later that day with one count each of cocaine possession. They faced a possible sentence of three years in prison. Their daughter was taken to an Orange County shelter for abused children. "Every action Deanna took," said Bob Theemling, director of a county foster-care facility, "was to make things better at home and to have good things happen to her parents." Theemling called Deanna's actions "a genuine act of love."

The teenager reportedly made her decision after attending an antidrug lecture at the Peace Lutheran Church near her home. After turning the evidence over, she told the police that she had already attempted less drastic methods to persuade her parents to give up drugs such as confronting her mother with what she thought were telltale marijuana seeds and pleading with her father to stop. A juvenile court judge in Orange County, Calif. September 8, 1986 accepted a recommendation from the Orange County Department of Social Services that Deanna be allowed to move back home with her parents. A social worker who interviewed them had concluded they would not harm their daughter in reprisal for her actions.

Most studies of children of drug dependent individuals deal with alcoholics but it is possible to generally predict the future drug abuse patterns of a child by studying the drug abuse pattern of his of her parents. One of the most negetive effects of having a drug dependent parent is that it predisposes a child to drug abuse. Daughters of alcoholics, for instance, become alcoholics 20-50% of the time and alcoholic mothers seem to exert more influence in this way than alcoholic fathers. Studies have also shown that even if a daughter of an alcoholic parent escapes becoming an alcoholic, she is likely to marry one. The exact connection between child abuse and drug use is not known but studies have shown repetitive cycles from generation to generation. If an adult has been abused as a child, he or she will be more apt to continue the abuse pattern.

The Pittsburgh PRESS

Pittsburgh, PA, August 18, 1986

If President Reagan is looking for a symbol, a shining ray-of-hope, a love-thy-parents kind of symbol, for his war on drugs, he has one in 13-year-old Deanna Young of Tustin, Calif.

Deanna is like many other junior high school students, with many of the same fears and worries that normally confront teen-agers. But she had a burden that she couldn't dismiss.

She suspected that her parents were using drugs.

She pleaded with them to quit and, after finding marijuana in her home, she flushed it down the toilet. Then she found cocaine vials in her parents' bureau drawers.

She really didn't know what else to do but she made up her mind after attending a church lecture by a police officer on the effects of drugs.

From her home she collected about an ounce of cocaine, some marijuana and pills and drug packaging equipment. With her evidence, she went, apprehensively but purposefully, to the police station and turned her parents in.

Her parents were charged with possession of cocaine. Deanna is being cared for in a shelter for abused and abandoned children.

"It's really the reverse of what we hear of parents fighting and fighting to keep their kids off drugs," said Tustin Police Capt. Fred Wakefield.

It is that, certainly. But it's more. It's concern. It's love. It's doing the right thing.

We hope Deanna's parents, when their situation is resolved, realize that, whatever they have done wrong, they have done one thing extremely well.

They have raised a good kid.

The Washington Times

Washington, DC, August 29, 1986

Judging by the media response, you'd think Deanna Young, age 13, had blown the whistle on the Rosenbergs. But it was her parents she fingered, turning them into the police, along with a trash bag filled with marijuana, a quantity of unidentifed pills, and about $2,800 worth of cocaine.

Deanna has been lionized for her "courage." Nancy Reagan went so far as to say that she "must have loved her parents a great deal." Deanna's attorney says she and her folks have talked and that "they are very supportive of her." Dickering has begun for the film and TV rights. And never mind that, as Michael Kinsley pointed out in *New Republic*, we are witnessing a real-life remake of Orwell's *1984*.

Under Stalin it was a source of pride to snitch on one's parents for "anti-party" activities. The same was true during the Third Reich. Even New York Mayor Fiorello La Guardia urged youngsters listening to him read the Sunday-morning comics on radio to report their parents' drinking and gambling habits.

This celebration of Deanna is another indication of the public confusion over drugs, and of the moral dilemma occasioned by habitual and widespread disregard of the law. Why else would the anti-drug bill cranked out of the House, with its tough penalties for pushers, and all the publicity surrounding the Army's participation in the Bolivian anti-drug campaign, make little or no fuss about drug users themselves?

And the problem is more widespread than supposed. The spotlight continues to fall on teen-agers, but they appear to account for only 5 percent of crack users. The rest are in their 20s (54 percent) and 30s (36 percent). More than a quarter of all crack users make $25,000 a year or more. They're yuppies.

So what to do? Nothing would make a yuppie's gums recede faster than the possibility of BMW-size fines and a taste of life in the Big House. Hitting the producers and distributors of drugs is fine, but we should crack down on the crack-pots as well, though fingering one's mother may be carrying law enforcement a bit far.

The Sunday Record

Hackensack, NJ, August 24, 1986

The erratic behavior and the pungent smoke in the hall were Deanna Young's first clues that her mother and father were using drugs. She pleaded with them to stop. They didn't. She found marijuana hidden around the house and flushed it down the toilet. They bought more. Then she found the vials of cocaine stuffed under the living-room couch. That's when she decided she'd had enough.

One night earlier this month, Deanna walked into the police station in Tustin, Calif. — a suburb 30 miles southeast of Los Angeles — carrying a trash bag. Inside the bag were more things that Deanna had found hidden around the house: some unidentified pills, a handgun, $1,500 in large bills, and almost an ounce of cocaine. Police arrested Deanna's mother when she came to the station to fetch her daughter and picked up Deanna's father a few hours later.

The story of the 13-year-old girl who stood up against drugs in her home cheered the nation. "She must have loved her parents a great deal," said an admiring Nancy Reagan. Nine Hollywood producers called the Orangewood Children's Home, where Deanna was sent after her parents' arrest, to bid on the rights to her story. "Deanna has become a national symbol," the home's director said.

Deanna Young is indeed a symbol — a symbol of the misery and frustration endured by the millions of American children whose parents abuse alcohol or drugs. Yet Hollywood will need a lot of creative license to make her a hero. Heroes are meant to be celebrated, and there is nothing to celebrate when a child turns her parents over to the police — not in a culture that treasures family life as highly as ours does. This story of a child's desperation and her elders' failures has many victims, but no heroes.

Naturally, the gravest failure was that of Deanna's mother and father, who apparently did not understand either their responsibility as parents or the strength of their example. But Deanna may also have been failed by the social-service agencies that are supposed to come to the rescue of families in trouble. She should have had some place to turn for comfort, support, and advice — some place besides her local vice squad. Children like Deanna shouldn't have to squeal on their parents in order to get help.

Turning from California to New Jersey, however, that's essentially what state rules require. County mental-health centers have counselors trained to assist children growing up in families with drug or alcohol problems. They understand the misplaced guilt and feelings of powerlessness that afflict these children, and can work with them to develop strategies for dealing with addicted parents. But they can do so only if the parent agrees or if the child initiates a formal investigation by the Division of Youth and Family Services (DYFS).

State officials say the regulations are necessary to protect the rights of competent parents to decide what types of professional care are appropriate for their children. Unless DYFS finds that a parent's behavior constitutes illegal abuse or neglect, the officials maintain, the state has no business stepping in.

That position seems insensitive on two counts. First, it asks children to assume a heavy burden: It says they cannot obtain professional guidance without the risk of putting their parents behind bars. That is too much to ask; few children have Deanna Young's nerve. Second, it does nothing to help the children of parents whose drug and alcohol problems are not yet so severe that DYFS can prove unlawful abuse or neglect.

State law already allows children to seek counseling for their own drug-abuse problems without permission from their parents. Allowing them to obtain advice about their parents' drug problems, free of concerns about sparking an official inquiry, is a reasonable next step that can only make families stronger.

The State

Columbia, SC, August 19, 1986

IT TOOK real courage for that 13-year-old Tustin, Calif., girl to turn her drug-using parents into the local police, and First Lady Nancy Reagan's praise should be reassuring to her. She will need strong support for what is coming.

Deanna Young had pleaded with her mother and father to stop using drugs, police said, and after attending a drug abuse lecture at her church "she felt she had to do something. She didn't want that kind of family life." She collected all the drugs she could find in the house while her parents were out, and went to the police.

She brought in a plastic bag containing several gram vials of cocaine valued at $2,800, a small amount of marijuana, unidentified pills, cocaine cutting equipment, $1,500 in $100 and $50 bills, and a .25 caliber pistol. Her parents were charged with possession of cocaine and released on their own recognizance until a Sept. 23 appearance in court.

Deanna was placed temporarily in a children's center until a juvenile court decides what's to be done with her. Authorities said she was "in a state of anguish" but relieved that it was over.

It isn't over, of course. What happens next is up to her parents. If convicted, they will be eligible for a drug rehabilitation program in lieu of a jail sentence. But a critical question for the family is whether they can handle a new relationship with their daughter. They all will have to deal with the pressures of national publicity.

That's quite a switch, isn't it? Usually it is the parents who are worried about drug-abusing sons or daughters. As Mrs. Reagan said, "She must have loved her parents a great deal, and I hope they realize how much she loves them."

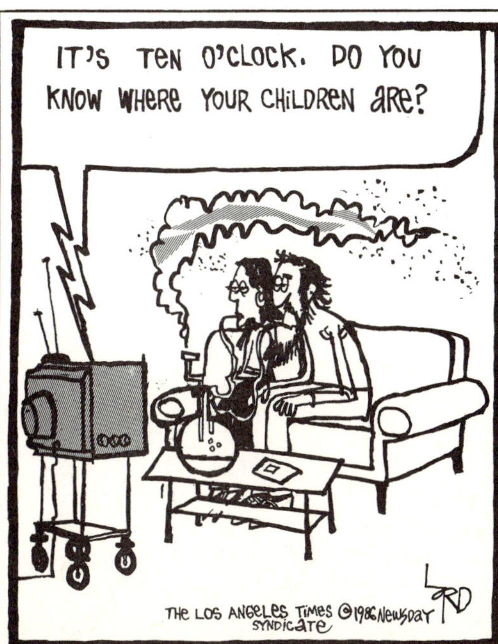

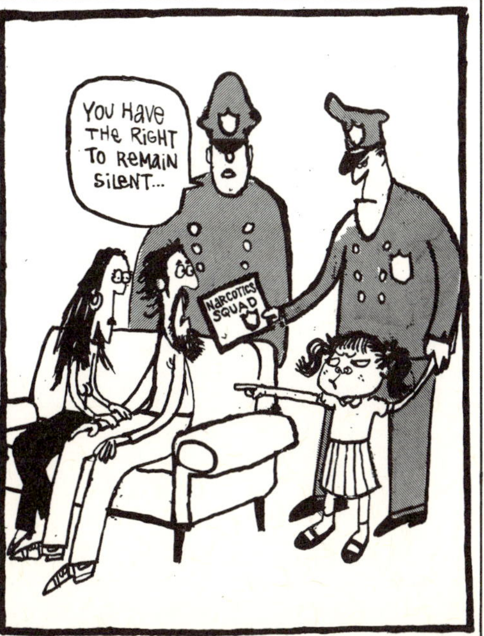

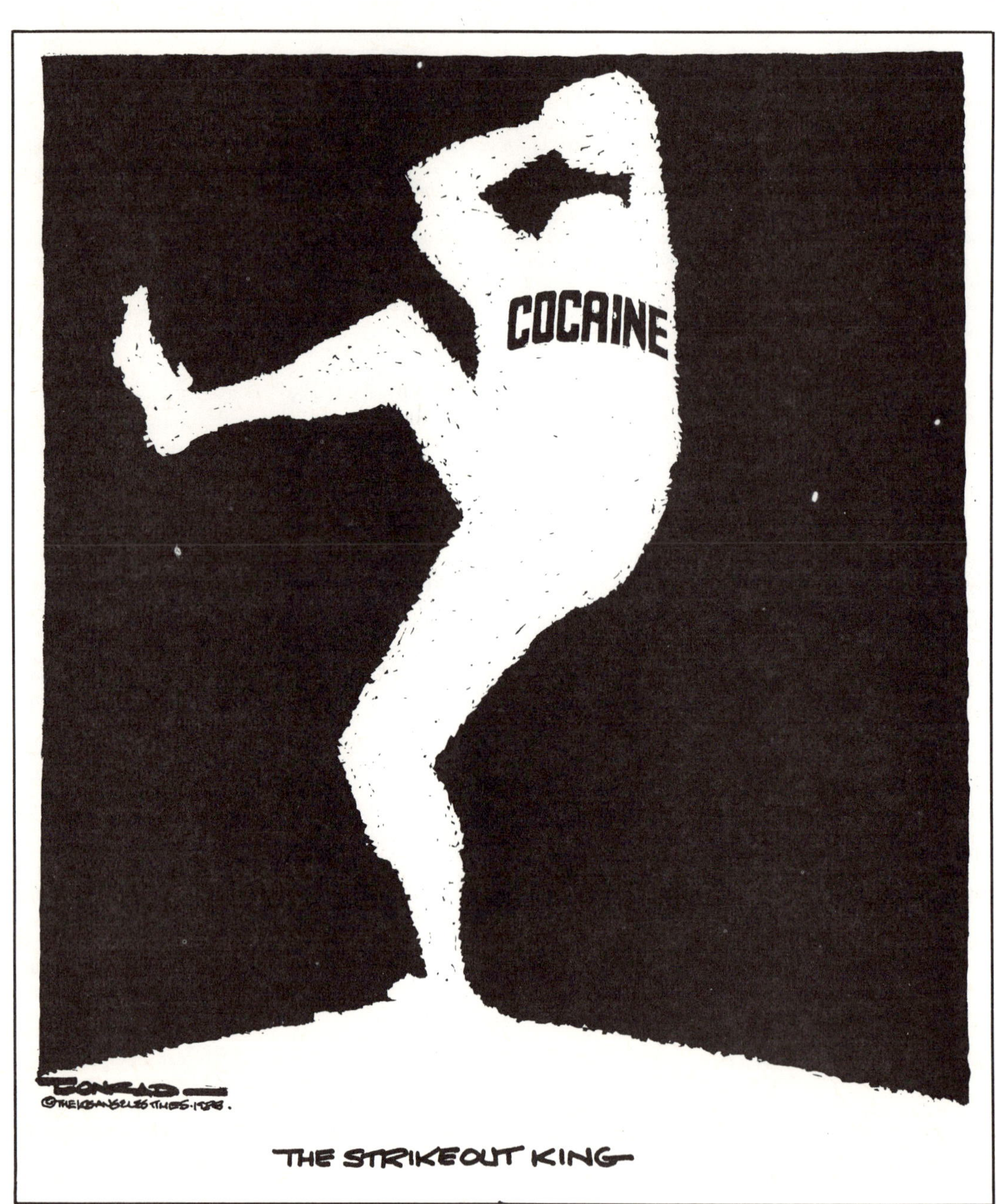

THE STRIKEOUT KING

Part V: Sports and Drugs

The use of drugs by competing athletes dates back a hundred years or more when the popular drugs to use for increased performance were alcohol and caffeine. Today the use of drugs by athletes is far more widespread and while any number of drugs are used, the most popular are amphetamines, steroids and cocaine. Drug use is not limited to professional athletes; it has also been found on both the college and high school levels.

The reasons for drug use vary. In some sports they are taken to diminish pain or fatigue and increase strength and endurance; in other sports they are taken to provide greater concentration, intensify aggressiveness and the desire to achieve, or to reduce tension and anxiety. Steroids are taken by athletes in order to gain weight and increase body mass.

There has been a recent campaign among athletic organizations, particularly the National Football League (NFL), Major League Baseball and the National Basketball Association and the International Olympic Committee, to eliminate the use drugs. Olympic contestants are aware that they will be tested for evidence of drugs during the games; in professional football the testing is sporadic and the players are never sure when they will be tested. The use of drugs by football players was prohibited in 1972. Up to that time it had been common practice for team doctors and trainers to hand out amphetamines.

In a June 1982 Sports Illustrated article, former Miami Dolphin, New Orleans Saint and San Diego Charger Don Reese described in graphic detail the course of his growing dependence on cocaine during his career in the NFL. Stating that cocaine "controls and corrupts" professional football players, Reese told the painful story of how he acquired an expensive habit and how it involved daily "freebasing" with other players and memory blackouts during games. Cocaine is readily available to NFL players, he said, not only from dealers who sometimes attend practices but also from respected veteran players. Typical reactions to Reese's confession included accusations that he must be mentally unbalanced to have fallen prey to such a habit and that, accordingly, his allegations must be dismissed. Nevertheless, insiders' reports reveal that as many as 60% of pro football players may regularly snort and freebase cocaine. Coaches and players consistently deny the existence of any drug problem yet continue to oppose urine tests to detect the presence of drugs. The result, as Reese points out, is that "what you see on the tube Sunday afternoon is a lie. When players are messed up, the game is messed up. The outcome of the game is dishonest when playing ability is impaired."

Enormous profits are generated by sports events in the United States. While sports fans encourage and demand victory and condone aggressiveness from athletes, it is not difficult to understand why competitors use drugs to to achieve what the public wants. Nor is it hard to see why owners, trainers and officials in the various sports want to please the public. Until competitors and management are educated to the dangers of drug use, it will probably continue to grow worse.

Pan American Games Marred by Disqualifications for Drug Use

The IX Pan American Games were held August 14-28, 1983 in Caracas, Venezuela. The event, held every four years, featured 4,000 athletes from 35 countries in North and South America. As in the 1979 games, the United States, Cuba, and Canada took the top three positions in medals. But the athletes' achievements were overshadowed by a scandal involving the apparent use of anabolic steroids by several athletes. Anabolic steroids are chemical compounds that contain either natural or synthetic testosterone, the male hormone. The drugs was used medically to promote the growth of muscle fiber. Steroid use is banned from most national and international sports events.

The Pan American Games crackdown was aided by sophisticated computer-enhanced urinalysis equipment never before used at so high a level of athletic competition. Using this equipment, the officials were able to identify substances taken by the athletes several months before the games. The crackdown resulted in the disqualification of 11 athletes from nine countries; the disqualified athletes were also subject to disciplinary action by the International Weightlifitng Federation, including suspensions that could keep them out of the 1984 Summer Olympic Games. In addition, 13 members of the U.S. track and field team left Caracas Aug. 23 before competing and returned home. The members, all men, denied that they had taken steroids but some admitted using antihistamines and caffeine, which had also been banned at the Pan American Games. The U.S. Olympic Committee, embarrassed by the hurried departure of the athletes, issued a statement Aug. 23 saying that the actions "should not be taken as an implication of guilt, or interpreted in any such manner."

FORT WORTH STAR-TELEGRAM

Fort Worth, TX, August 27, 1983

Sports in America didn't really need another black eye, but it suffered a king-sized shiner this week when more than a dozen American athletes fled the Pan American Games in Caracas, Venezuela, rather than face new, and effective, tests for drug usage.

Their departure came after several athletes — including at least one American — were forced to forfeit medals they had won in the prestigious international competition, an important forerunner to the 1984 Olympic Games. The forfeiture was ordered after tests for illegal drug use were positive.

Unlike their professional counterparts, whose use of cocaine has created a major scandal in American sports, athletes in the Pan American Games have been whistled down for using anabolic steroids, which increase the growth of body tissue and possibly make an athlete stronger.

But doctors warn that steroids can be dangerous, too. Their use has been linked to kidney and liver failure and sexual impotence. Several deaths have been blamed on the drugs.

Participants in international sports have been suspected for some time of taking steroids, but testing procedures designed to weed out offenders have been haphazard in both application and results. But a new process is being used in the Pan American Games. Officials say it is accurate enough to pinpoint the use of steroids by an athlete anywhere from six months to a year prior to testing.

The sudden exodus of a number of athletes before they had even competed is a tribute — albeit a sad one — to the efficacy of the test. By leaving, the Americans squandered a great deal of money, much of which had been donated by ordinary citizens anxious to help their country do well in next year's Olympic Games.

What effect their actions will have on the American Olympic team remains to be seen. But something good may yet come from all this.

Although the sordid episode indicates that drug abuse among athletes is more widespread than many previously suspected, those who believe in the importance of international athletic competition can take heart in the fact that something is finally being done to control an outrageous, and potentially dangerous, situation.

For years, athletes have relied on steroids to give them a real, or imagined, boost in performance. If the new testing procedure is as effective as officials claim, international athletic competitions will once again be won by the best athletes. And that's the way it should be.

The Washington Post

Washington, DC, August 25, 1983

ACCOMPLISHED ATHLETES from several nations, including the United States, have been stripped of medals won at the Pan American Games in Caracas, Venezuela. They flunked the new, improved tests designed to catch "dirty" competitors —common parlance for those who have used any of several prohibited drugs, most notably the male hormone testosterone and related steroids thought to facilitate more intensive training and muscle development. Several more competitors left rather than risk expulsion. Olympics officials plan to use testing equipment at least as sensitive and to be just as strict in enforcing the drug prohibitions in 1984.

But why all the fuss? If competition and winning are so important to the athletes and to national prestige, what's wrong with juicing up the players a little bit so that they give the most their bodies and minds can produce? After all, everyone does it, say some U.S. athletes defensively. The East Germans are notorious in this regard, having been fast off the starting block in both good and bad uses of high-tech sports training. The romantic ideal of the unspoiled human machine seems a bit out of place in today's amateur athletics industry. It's hardly an unambiguously glamorous enterprise. Does it make sense for competition to have become so intense, and so profitable, that prepubescent kids are up before dawn, swimming, running and skating for miles, year after year, foresaking childish ways in search of . . . something? And if that's okay and natural, why not a couple of pills to help get the most out of weight training? Sure, the drugs have dangerous side effects, but the sports themselves pose risks.

It must have something to do with spirit, which cattle are presumed to lack, but athletes are supposed to exemplify. Steroid injections and chemically laced food are the staples of Iowa feed lots, and there's nothing spiritual about producing prize-winning physical specimens that way. The protests against East German practices and the adoption of drug prohibitions were partly a counter to unfairness, but more a counter to sheer ugliness. A medal is a testament to the best of body, mind and spirit. Test-tube technology spoils the romantic glory, which is what we need from world class athletics. The expulsions at the Pan American Games are good training for the Olympics.

TULSA WORLD

Tulsa, OK, August 25, 1983

THE PAN-AMERICAN games have turned the spotlight on amateur sports' dirtiest little secret — athletes' abuse of anabolic steroids. A dozen members of the U.S. track team left the games Tuesday without even competing after they learned they faced strict new drug tests.

Eight medal winners were stipped of their awards after tests showed they had been using steroids.

Improper use of steroids has been going on for some time. The drug is a synthetic derivative of a male hormone. It is used by athletes who wish to build muscle quickly or increase recovery time.

Not only does use of steroids destroy the purpose of athletic competition; it is dangerous. Long-term use of steroids can contribute to heart disease and blood pressure and prostate problems.

The use of such drugs defeats the whole purpose of athletic competition. The idea is to test the athletic capabilities of man. There is no sense of human accomplishment in watching someone win a competition because of chemicals which transformed his body and increased its capabilities. We might as well be watching competing robots.

Amateur athletics was meant to test the limits of human ability, not the frontiers of science.

The Chattanooga Times

Chattanooga, TN, August 31, 1983

Twelve track and field athletes from the United States left the Pan American Games in Caracas, Venezuela, last week just after officials there had launched the biggest crackdown on drugs in the history of international athletic competition. Whether those American athletes left to avoid having to submit to tests to detect the use of illegal substances, only they know. Considering the circumstances of their departure, however, it is reasonable to suggest that they were worried about exposure. The episode is an embarrassment for the United States' amateur athletic organization; one of our athletes, a weight-lifter, was among those whose medals were rescinded after tests showed they had used competition-enhancing drugs. The embarrassment is compounded when you consider that for years, the United States has lodged numerous protests against the use of anabolic stereoids and other drugs by athletes from the Soviet Union and Eastern Europe.

The irony is that it is debatable whether such drugs actually improve the athletes' stamina and performance. And even if they do, the benefit is probably counterproductive; medical tests have shown that using stereoids over time can produce undesirable and severe side effects. Worse, their use mocks the purpose of amateur athletics, which is to ensure that individual athletic skills are pitted honestly against others.

The drugs' disputed effectiveness and the effects of their use aside, no athlete can ignore the fact that the drugs are strictly prohibited by the board that governs international track and field competition. Athletes found to have used the drugs are suspended from competition for life.

Some good has emerged from the Pan American Games investigation into drug use. The United States Olympic Committee has directed that drug tests be performed in all events where American athletes have qualified to represent this country. Since sophisticated testing can uncover the use of more than 100 banned drugs, and since the message of the Pan American actions won't be lost on Olympic officials, the outlook, we hope, is for a relatively drug-free competition in Los Angeles in 1984.

In years past the U.S. has blamed the lack of an effective drug testing program on the costs involved. That fails to persuade, considering that other countries have managed to finance such a program. The need to protect our athletes' health, not to mention avoiding another embarrassment like the one in Caracas, should be sufficient reason to put such a program into effect, no matter what the cost.

Portland Press Herald

Portland, ME, August 27, 1983

A dozen or so U.S. track and field athletes must have set world-record times in conjunction with the Pan American Games in Venezuela this week. There'll be no medals, however; the speed attained in flight to avoid drug detection isn't recognized as an international event.

The use of steroid drugs by athletes has been banned internationally for years, first, because steroids give users an unfair training advantage over non-drug users and, second, because of their potentially dangerous side effects.

Years ago it used to be fashionable to claim that athletes from European Communist-bloc countries were the principal drug offenders. But the spectacle of American athletes hightailing it back to the U.S. indicates how pervasive the illegal use of drugs has become.

Until now, apparently, athletes felt free to use steroids in training up to a few weeks before actual competition, secure in the knowledge that the drugs wouldn't be detected.

All that changed in Venezuela. The Pan American Sports Organization began using state-of-the-art testing equipment said to be capable of detecting evidence of steroid use as long as a year ago. The exodus began after a number of weightlifters were disqualified when urine tests revealed evidence of drug use.

The athletes had good reason to run for cover. Discovery of drug use carries an 18-month suspension—long enough to bar a user from participation in the 1984 Olympic Games.

All in all, the flight from Venezuela by American athletes hardly presented an attractive picture, either to the world in general or to those who place a high value on fair play in international amateur athletic competition.

Lincoln Journal

Lincoln, NE, August 31, 1983

The IX Pan American Games at Caracas, Venezuela, will be historically marked as the place where a firmer line was drawn against athletes using illegal drugs, mainly synthetic derivatives of the male hormone testosterone.

Awarded Pan American Games medals were revoked when very sophisticated post-competition medical testing disclosed traces of proscribed drug use. Some of it was chronologically ancient, too. Like months before.

The Caracas crackdown landed harder on athletes from Latin-American nations than it did on U.S. entries. Perhaps one reason for that was the sudden departure of a dozen Yanks prior to their scheduled competition. Having been found out in Caracas as a drug user could lead to disqualification from future participation.

In any event, the U.S. Olympic Committee now says it plans to give unannounced, random drug screening tests to men and women trying for places on the 1984 team.

Medical testing "equal or better" than that in use at the Pan-American Games also has been promised for employment at the Olympics in Los Angeles next year.

Athletes ingest the steroids with the belief the hormones will increase muscle size and therefore give them a competitive edge. Weight lifters and throwers, trackmen, wrestlers and cyclists are said to be particularly keen on the illegal drugs. East German athletes were among the first to put chemistry to use for the greater glory of the Marxist puppet state,

Doctors have sound reason to suspect the drugs can result in heart disease, reduced tolerance to cancer, liver tumors, sterility and impotence. That has not seemed to frighten the international sports community, to this point. Maybe what happened at Caracas finally will — but only if the international federations and governing bodies hang just as tough in their testing practices.

The shame of having Olympic honors jerked because of the certain discovery of past drug consumption should be constant and alarming prospect for all nations with teams at Los Angeles. Leave the steroids, properly, to postoperative patients and geriatic cases.

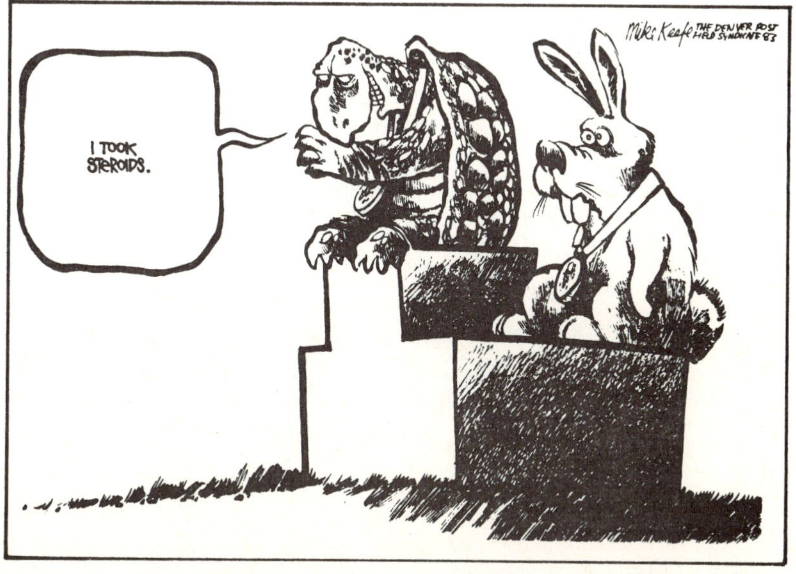

RAPID CITY JOURNAL—
Rapid City, SD, August 31, 1983

In a competitive world, it's not surprising that athletes spare no efforts to excel. Nor is it a surprise that those efforts sometimes include the use of anabolic steroids, the banned muscle-building chemicals that enhance their performance.

Most steroid users got away with it until officials at the Pan American Games in Caracas, Venezuela, launched a long-overdue crackdown.

Armed with a state-of-the-art drug laboratory, technicians from West Germany were able to detect steroids taken within the past six months to a year. The less sophisticated method normally used in evaluating urine samples in international competitions detected only the drugs taken up to three months prior to the competition.

In two days, steroids were detected in 11 weightlifters, eight of whom had to return medals they had won. Athletes who only hours earlier basked in glory were shamed and embarrassed.

Thirteen American athletes left the games shortly before competing. Despite their silence and denials, skeptics assumed they departed because they knew they would flunk the drug tests.

Some competitors grumbled that the new testing methods were overly strict. However, unless what appears to be a veritable epidemic of steroid use is halted and the ban against that use is strictly enforced, competitive pressures will lead hundreds of others to take steroids, feeling they won't stand a chance without them.

Athletic heroes who are role models for the young are expected to set high standards. They should care enough about their own health to avoid potentially dangerous substances.

The same sophisticated tests used in Caracas will be used at the Olympic Games in Los Angeles next year. They should be. The International Olympic Committee has spent far too much time fussing over the issue of a competitor's amateur status and not nearly enough making sure the competition itself is fair.

The gold which symbolizes excellence should go to natural talent and not a chemically-strengthened robot.

The Dispatch
Columbus, OH, August 25, 1983

The word "drugs" in the news from Caracas was shocking — particularly since the foregoing reports had been so pleasant.

It had been a good feeling, in the late-summer doldrums, to escape from grim events like wars and hurricanes and assassination, to watch the superb young athletes perform — and to see the tally of U.S. medals mount steadily as the Pan American Games continued.

We had a short reprieve. The report of the first athletes found to have used banned steroid drugs was bad — but they weren't our athletes. Then the first group of U.S. contestants flew home from Venezuela without competing, and the cloud of scandal came with them.

It is the first time since the Western Hemisphere games began in 1951 that participants have been suspended and medalists stripped of their honors for using drugs — and that is deeply regrettable.

The positive result is that the practice was exposed, that Pan American Games officials acted promptly and decisively, and that Olympics' officials have pledged, with a year's fair warning, that drug detection methods will be at least as efficient, and penalties as prompt, for the Olympic Games in Los Angeles next summer.

The "why" of the scandal is not so clear-cut. Why would talented athletes, who spend years training and conditioning their bodies, risk their health and their future for a temporary "boost" of questionable value?

Anabolic steroids, synthetic derivatives of the male hormone testosterone, have been used increasingly by sports participants over the last three decades. Athletes who use them think they "bulk up" muscles with more protein, but some medical experts say no evidence supports this and that any beneficial effect is probably psychological.

More easily documented, and leading to the ban of the drugs in international sports competition, are side effects that can include altered liver function, sterility and impotence.

Good can come from the unsavory blight cast on the Pan American Games.

First off, it might prompt a fresh look by athletes and those who coach and train them not only at anabolic steroids but at any and all artificial means being used to affect an athlete's performance. That seems advisable.

Certainly, it will strengthen the resolve and stated purpose of those in charge that the Olympics will tolerate no drug use and that next summer's games will be a showcase — as they should be — for the natural talents of the world's best.

If the athletes in turn cán be a lesson and example to thousands of other young people around the world, against the awful influence of drugs, then the Caracas experience, startling and shaming as it is, will have been worth it.

THE ANN ARBOR NEWS
Ann Arbor, MI, August 25, 1983

Little white lies.

That — and not the talent of world athletes — is what has put the spotlight on the IX Pan American Games, being held in Caracas, Venezuela. This week, a drug scandal involving steroids (growth hormones) has overshadowed the games and raised questions about the integrity of 13 U.S. athletes who abruptly returned home after seven medal winners (including U.S. weightlifter Jeff Michels) failed to pass two drug analysis tests and were ordered to return their awards.

It was the first time in the 32-year history of the Pan American Games that athletes were stripped of their medals for drug use.

There is no question that the athletes knew the rules: no drugs. But in the past, it had been acceptable practice among some athletes to use steroids up to three months before the games then discontinue the drug so that it would not show up in tests taken at competitive events (ergo, the little white lies).

Steroids, it is alleged, improve muscle strength. Several doctors disagree, however, saying that tests have failed to prove the drug is useful for anything more than psychological stimulation, and one claimed that two cups of coffee provide more sting. The potential side effects of steroids are of great concern: temporary or long-term sterility, impotence, premature heart disease, liver malfunction and tumors.

Winning, however, appears to be of greater importance to some athletes. Using steroids, one athlete flippantly declared on Tuesday, is no worse than girls using makeup.

Now, the drug charade is over. A German firm has come up with a test that can determine what drugs an athlete has used over the past year, perhaps even longer. Athletes, coaches and managers were even warned about the sophisticated test being used in the Caracas event prior to the opening of the games. Next time, the warning will be clear: The same test is planned for the 1984 Olympics.

It's difficult to determine how widespread is the use of steroids. It is definitely unfair to presume that because a handful of athletes have been caught that all of the 5,000 competitors in the Pan American games are drug users.

But the scandal has had its positive effects:

"We have known for some time (drug use) was a problem...," admits William E. Simon, president of the United States Olympics Committee. "I frankly welcome this. The justice has been swift and severe and the international governing bodies will decide the sanctions."

The U.S.O.C., he promised, will "take whatever steps possible to see it does not occur in the Los Angeles Games."

James King, an American intermediate hurdler at the Caracas games, said: "I think this is going to scare a lot of people into changing their training habits between now and the Olympics. You may not see any more world records for a while. A lot of the time in the Olympics might be bad, but they'll be honest."

The IX Pan American Games, said King, "may be the first clean track and field meet ever."

We hope it isn't the last

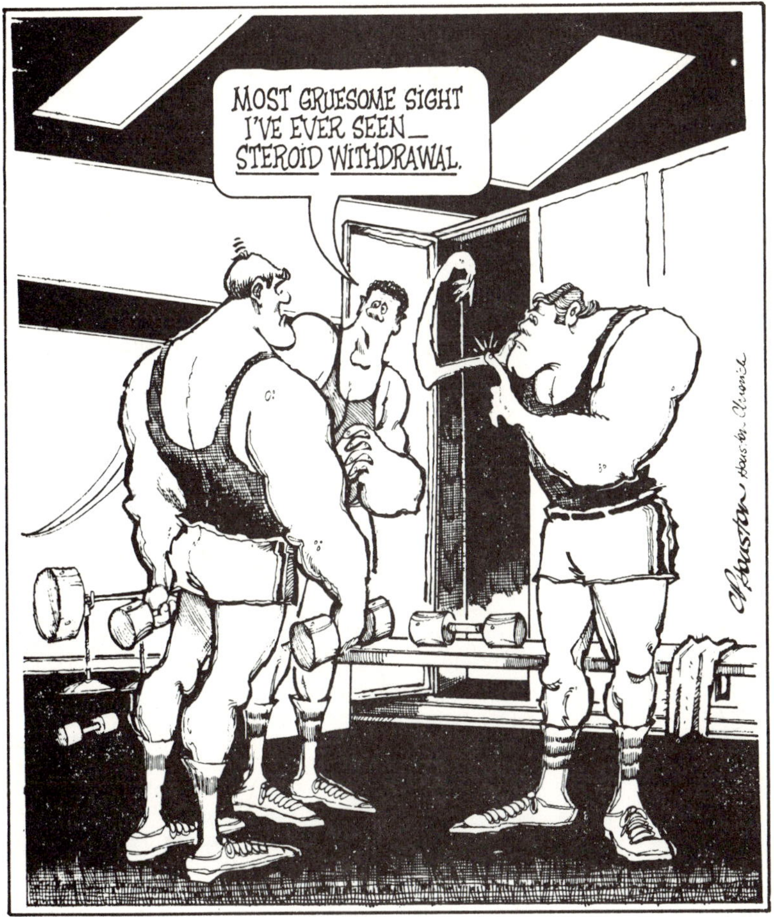

The Hartford Courant

Hartford, CT, August 25, 1983

There's something pathetic about the effect of a gold medal on that symbol of physical and mental purity, the amateur athlete.

The lure of the gold can do strange things to a competitor — and to those who run amateur sports. It can make men and women compromise their principles and defile their bodies in hopes of winning.

In pursuit of the prize, athletes will take dangerous and illegal or banned drugs which can improve their performances at the next meet, but which can shorten their lives and ruin their reputations. In pursuit of the prize, coaches and other officials will actually encourage illicit drug use or tolerate it.

Nearly 100 substances are on the banned list for amateur athletes. Many can be purchased over the counter. Some, like anabolic steroids, can be very dangerous. Over the short term, such drugs can build muscles, improve endurance and allow athletes to train at a faster pace. They can also dramatically lower life expectancy.

But, despite official sanctions against the use of drugs and medical evidence which warns of harmful long-term effects, many athletes continue to turn themselves into so many Six Million Dollar men and women — part human, part synthetic substitute. They become spurious superhumans unfairly playing a human game.

The practice is defended by some Americans on the basis that everybody, especially Soviet bloc countries, does it. The world of international amateur athletics finds itself using the same kind of logic that impels the crazy arms race and threatens humanity.

Now, as the scandal at the Pan American Games in Caracas illustrates, there is a seemingly reliable means to test for the use of banned chemicals, even those used well before a competition begins. Thus far, 11 athletes have been reprimanded or stripped of medals for failing the drug test, and a number of competitors, including 13 Americans, have withdrawn from the games.

Those who love the ideal of amateur competition and who have concern for the athletes as human beings ought to insist on rigorous testing (perhaps the concept of mutual verification would also be appropriate here) for chemical abuse by athletes before they are allowed to compete in international events. Those who refuse or flunk would be banned from competition for life.

Americans who support amateur athletics should let competitors and coaches know they reject the use of harmful chemical stimulants as a means to win. Consideration might be given to more rigid controls governing the manufacture and sale in this country of the most harmful drugs.

If anyone can't understand the controversy over human athletes using steroids, consider the strict prohibition against chemically doctored mounts at the race track.

They disqualify horses, don't they?

The Boston Herald

Boston, MA, August 30, 1983

THE MOST noteworthy news at the just-concluded Pan American Games was not the overwhelming number of medals won by U.S. athletes but the determination to ban anabolic steroids from events such as these.

That action makes it certain that the same sophisticated tests which detected use of the muscle-building chemicals by some competitors at Caracas will also be used next summer at the Olympic Games in Los Angeles.

The crackdown at Caracas cost eight weightlifters, including an American, medals they'd previously been awarded, and apparently prompted more than a dozen members of the U.S. team to leave the games before tests could be run on them.

But the use of steroids, despite knowledge of their serious side-effects, has become increasingly prevalent among athletes to whom winning is all that matters — whatever the cost.

The officials at the Pan American Games, and those planning the 1984 Summer Olympics, have served notice on competing nations that resorting to steroids — or any other chemical enhancer or stimulant, is too high a price to pay for success. They deserve the world's applause.

THE INDIANAPOLIS STAR

Indianapolis, IN, August 27, 1983

The departure of 13 U.S. amateur athletes and the de-medaling of another at the Pan American Games is sad business, but it could help clear up a mess that has been a long time in the brewing.

Our athletes were not the only ones in the spotlight of the international drug scandal. Three Latin American weightlifters were stripped of their gold medals and three were reprimanded for using anabolic steroids, an illegal muscle-building drug. Steroids were also detected in the system of Chile's leading cyclist.

The U.S. Olympic Committee insisted the Americans' exit was not to be interpreted as evidence that drug rules had been violated. But the decision came after word went out that drug testing at the Pan Am Games was being done with sophisticated new detection equipment.

William Simon, USOC president, called drug abuse "an evil that must be stamped out" and added that what happened was "ample warning to the athletes that the (drug use) game is over."

He's probably right and if he is, well and good. Drug use defeats the whole idea of fair competition. When a drug does produce the "winning edge," the victory belongs properly to the drug, not the athlete. Losers if they have not been on an equal amount of drugs are justified in feeling cheated.

There have long been grounds for suspicion about the purity of communist athletes. Greed for Olympic gold does not seem to be exclusively a capitalist sin. Beefy Red women athletes whose virility would put John Riggins or Bubba Smith to shame surely did not get that way on borscht.

It made sense to add the male hormone, testosterone, to the Olympic list of banned drugs, which was done this year. Caffeine, which concentrated has a stimulatory jolt of magnitude, also was added to the list of nearly 100 forbidden drugs.

Unfortunately, cheating to win is not universally condemned in a society where plenty of jaded characters think anything goes if it brings Olympic medals or megabucks — which tend to go together. Removing stimulatory and "edge-giving" drugs is necessary to return sports to pure competition under fair rules.

The sophisticated new testing equipment and drug bans, as the unfortunate but hope-giving episode at Caracas seems to be proving, can do a necessary cleaning job and make the future of international games shine as it should.

Point Shaving Scandal Brings End to Tulane Basketball Team

A grand jury in New Orleans April 4, 1985 indicted eight people, including three members of the Tulane University basketball team, on charges connected to point shaving in two games during the 1984-85 season. In response to the indictments, the president of Tulane announced that the university was ending its basketball program. The eight people were indicted under Louisiana's sports bribery laws. The three indicted Tulane players, and two players who were granted immunity, were charged with conspiring to hold down their team's score in order to benefit gamblers betting that Tulane's opponents would beat the point spread against Tulane. Among the indicted players was John (Hot Rod) Williams, the team star and top pro prospect. Three other students were indicted, including one who was also charged with distributing cocaine to Tulane players. Another of the indicted men was a convicted sports bookmaker. According to Tulane president Eamon Kelly, the school's head basketball coach had admitted making illegal cash payments to some of his players. He and two assisstant coaches resigned from the university. Kelly said he had reason to believe that the coaches were involved in the alleged point shaving.

Gary Kranz, the alleged mastermind of the basketball point-shaving scandal at Tulane University, was sentenced December 16, 1985 to three months in jail, fined $45,000 and ordered to perform 1,500 hours of community service. Kranz had pleaded guilty and cooperated with authorities in return for having charges that he supplied cocaine to Tulane players dropped. Williams was acquitted of five counts of sports bribery connected to charges of pointshaving during the 1984-85 season. The verdict was reached by a jury in New Orleans after a six-day trial. A previous trying of the case had ended in a mistrial. Williams was then free to play with the Cleveland Cavaliers of the National Basketball Association.

The Dispatch

Columbus, OH, April 13, 1985

When the adjuster came to look at the wreckage of the Tulane University basketball program, he determined it was total. The program was consigned to the scrap heap.

The adjuster, in this case Tulane President Eamon M. Kelly, really had no other choice. The program was rotten to the core. Rehabilitation, however well-intentioned and conscientiously pursued, could not have lifted the cloud of doubt and cynicism.

With players shaving points for profit at the behest of big-time gamblers and coaches making illegal payoffs of their own, the program clearly was living on borrowed time.

Critics of the tendency of colleges and universities to put accomplishments in the highly visible arenas of sports competition ahead of the more significant but less noticed achievements in academic excellence will applaud Kelly's decision.

When Kelly said the academic community would not tolerate the violations and actions uncovered in the Tulane basketball program, he was serving notice on the forces that, if unchecked, would likely attempt to corrupt all major collegiate athletic programs. By affecting the outcome of games, shaving a point or two here and there, gamblers cash in big. The enticements they offer college athletes, some struggling to meet expenses, are enormous.

Tulane University put its integrity first and its corrupters out of the business of buying its basketball players. If you have to bulldoze the building to get rid of the rats, so be it.

It was too late for Tulane. Basketball had to go. For the alumni, who relive the college experiences by cheering on and often supporting the teams of their alma mater, it will be a bitter pill. But most will see the necessity. They don't want to be greeted with a smirk when they identify themselves as Tulane graduates.

The university president would like the basketball ban to be permanent. That may not be necessary. But Tulane should and no doubt will allow whatever time is needed to completely distance itself from the basketball scandal.

In fouling out of basketball, Tulane University has made a tough decision, one that will cost money and prestige. At the same time, the university has said integrity will come first, whatever the cost.

The Times-Picayune
The States-Item

New Orleans, LA, April 5, 1985

Local reaction to Tulane University's announcement that it will no longer participate in men's intercollegiate basketball must surely be one of compounded sadness.

Sadness, first, at the allegations of sports briberyand point-shaving among Tulane students and violations of National Collegiate Athletics Association rules by Tulane players and coaches that has become a nationwide news story. Sadness, further, that the scandal should have reached such proportions that the university judged that its response must be to abolish a basketball program with a long history of excellence and public support.

The Orleans Parish Grand Jury has returned indictments in connection with the point-shaving allegations.

Now Tulane President Eamon Kelly, citing newly discovered NCAA rule violations, said he will accept the resignations of head basketball coach Ned Fowler and assistant coaches Mike Richardson and Max Pfeifer and recommend that Tulane immediately drop its men's basketball program.

Although Mr. Kelly said he has no reason to believe Coach Fowler or his staff were involved in the alleged point shaving, he announced that among NCAA violations uncovered by the university's own investigation "are some cash payments by head coach Ned Flower to players on the basketball team."

"I will not allow anything to impede our progress or compromise the mission of the university," Mr. Kelly said, noting that Tulane is first and foremost a distinguished university committed to high standards of teaching and research. "The only way I know to demonstrate unambiguously this academic community's intolerance of the violations and actions we have uncovered is to discontinue the program in which they originated."

Thus the problem as far as Tulane's potential vulnerability goes, is simply abolished. But the problems in collegiate sports nationwide — of clandestine payments to student players, of the insistent pressures of big-time gambling on sports, of student players who are, for all practical purposes, not students at all — remain to be solved.

One must hope — one must insist — that they will be solved and that collegiate sports can attain the high standards of honesty and good sportsmanship they were designed to exemplify. One may hope, too, that a new Tulane basketball team can, in some not too distant future, take to the courts again.

The Philadelphia Inquirer

Philadelphia, PA, April 7, 1985

For collegiate basketball, last week held flowers and ashes. As Villanova's proud Wildcats were receiving presidential accolades in the Rose Garden, bad news surfaced in New Orleans.

Tulane University president Eamon M. Kelly has moved to terminate the school's basketball program, the target of an ugly point-shaving scandal. It was an unwelcome subplot of corruption in what has been one of the sport's finest hours.

Said Mr. Kelly: "I think its critical that we do reaffirm the university's primary mission as an academic institution in terms of teaching, in terms off learning and in terms of research and indicate our unwillingness to permit this kind of activity in our intercollegiate programs."

To do less would rob college sport of the honest joy and healthy competition it is hard-pressed to preserve.

Tulane's tragedy serves notice again that coaches, university presidents and professional team owners must redouble their efforts to have players constantly on guard against crooks who would bribe them with money or drugs to throw a game or shave points. And they can't do too much to make their players aware of the consequences now closing in on three Tulane players who have been indicted on charges of violating Louisiana's sports bribery law.

ST. LOUIS POST-DISPATCH

St. Louis, MO, April 8, 1985

Intercollegiate basketball is on the way out at Tulane University. Its president, Eamon M. Kelly, decided to ask Tulane's board of administrators to drop the program permanently following indictments against eight people (including three members of the basketball team) that charged them with point-shaving and disclosures that Tulane's basketball coach had been making under-the-table cash payments to some of his players on a regular basis.

To college presidents around the country — to say nothing of the faculty, alumni and students for whom college without sports verges on the unthinkable — Mr. Kelly's decision bespeaks an unwelcome heresy. Team sports have become so closely linked with school image, pride, and even attractiveness to future students that any move affecting intercollegiate athletics at a given institution will inevitably have quick and tangible repercussions in nearly all other areas of school life. The extreme step of eliminating a program that had been a source of much institutional pride may well result in curtailed alumni support, which runs the risk of harming many more — and more important — programs than those involving varsity competition.

Mr. Kelly is aware of this risk, and it is to his great credit that he has stood up to it. "I think it's critical that we do reaffirm the university's primary mission as an academic institution . . . and to indicate our unwillingness to permit this kind of activity in our intercollegiate programs," he said in announcing his decision. That primary function — to teach — is one that too often seems to take a back seat to others. For having had the courage to set things aright at Tulane, Mr. Kelly has set an example that his colleagues elsewhere, should they find themselves in similar straits, would do well to follow.

Roanoke Times & World-News

Roanoke, VA, April 9, 1985

TULANE University President Eamon Kelly has announced plans to drop the school's basketball program. The announcement comes after the indictment of three players for accepting gamblers' bribes to shave points, and the firing of Coach Ned Fowler and two assistants for making under-the-table cash payments to several players.

For the university, it is a question of maintaining institutional integrity.

The only private school in the Metro Conference, of which Virginia Tech is also a member, Tulane is not Jock U. or Podunk State. It is one of only six institutions in the South (and the only one in the Metro) that belong to the academically prestigious Association of American Universities. Tulane's admissions policy is selective. Several of its undergraduate and graduate programs are considered among the best in the region, and among the better in the nation. Giving up intercollegiate basketball is a small price to pay for restoring as quickly as possible the university's overall reputation.

But there are questions, too, for the collegiate sports establishment in general. Here are three:

● How can public confidence be maintained in the honesty of intercollegiate athletic contests — particularly in football and basketball, which seem to draw the most gambling interest?

The task of policing the colleges is tremendously difficult, if not impossible. The National Collegiate Athletic Association (and its smaller cousin, the National Association of Intercollegiate Athletics) is composed of hundreds of schools, public and private, big and small, intellectually vibrant and intellectually asleep. In professional sports, the job is easier: Of the major professional organizations, only the National Football League has as many as 28 teams, and members of the professional leagues are similar in the size and goals of their operations.

Moreover, intercollegiate athletics must contend with the tendency for the odor of scandal to spread, justified or not. New Orleans authorities presumably have some evidence, else there would be no indictments, but the fact remains that point-shaving is devilishly hard to detect. For honorable athletes and their coaches, the problem is this: Because such wrongdoing is hard to spot when it *does* exist, there's a temptation for the public to suspect wrongdoing when it *doesn't* exist. Every missed shot, every turnover, every defensive lapse — each an inevitable part of every game — becomes cause for speculation.

● Is the integrity of intercollegiate athletics helped or hindered by its role as a farm system for the pro leagues?

When salaries for professional athletes skyrocketed, the theory arose that college players would become less susceptible than in the past to the blandishments of gamblers. Why would a collegian risk the potential for millions in future earnings by accepting a few hundred bucks in bribe money?

Sadly, but not surprisingly, the Tulane case has undermined that assumption. Some blame it on illegal drugs, noting that they can be an inducement even when money isn't. But that seems to beg at least part of the question: Why would an outstanding athlete risk a pro career by using illegal drugs any more than by accepting cash bribes?

A better explanation may lie in the fact that college athletes are very young men who are put under intense public pressures that most people don't experience until much later in life, if at all. The fact that some 18-, 19-, or 20-year-olds respond in immature ways to sudden fame and the potential for sudden fortune really shouldn't come as a surprise. Moreover, it is often the best athletes — fawned over as schoolboys, assiduously wooed by college recruiters sometimes two or three times their age — who are least prepared for what they'll face.

● Does the structure of big-time college athletics today foster rather than discourage disrespect for the law and for traditions of honor?

The question is not easy to ask, because it implies doubts about certain venerable and convenient beliefs — that participation in sports "builds character," or that amateur athletics is "purer" than professional athletics. But one can accept such beliefs, at least in part, and still recognize hypocrisy for what it is.

There may be an old-timer or two, coaching mainly for the fun of it and holding fast to the idea that athletics is but a peripheral adjunct to academic life, still around. The species even may be flourishing at those schools which deliberately keep athletics low-key, and in those sports usually labeled "minor." But in the revenue-generating sports at NCAA Division I schools, the species is close to extinction. In such programs today, the standard-model coach enjoys a big-bucks contract, administers a big-bucks budget, and knows full well that his team's record is the main criterion for determining how long he'll keep his job. Coaches are paid to win games, not build character.

As for the "student-athletes" on "scholarships," it is hardly accurate to say that they, unlike the pros, do not play for pay. They play for pay, all right; it's just that the wages are paltry. In doling out cash to his players, Tulane's basketball coach violated an NCAA rule and gained an unfair advantage over his competitors. But he didn't turn "amateur" players into "professionals." That was done entirely within the rules, as it is elsewhere, when his athletes agreed to play at Tulane in return for the costs of tuition, fees, and room and board.

Tulane's coaches have not been implicated in the point-shaving scandal. But who the worse sinners are — youngsters who accept gamblers' bribes, or their adult mentors who show them how to break rules to gain advantage — is an arguable issue. Clearly, both actions are wrong, and the considerations above, while they might help explain those actions, do not excuse them.

The real test of honor comes not when temptation is light but when it is intense. Even in a system that values winning above all else, many coaches pass the test: They abide by the rules, and some of the brighter ones actually take an interest in the academic lives of their players and of their university communities. Even in a system with hypocrisy at its heart, many players pass the test: They respect the game, their teammates and themselves too much to consider doing business with gamblers.

At Tulane, evidently, the test proved too stiff. President Kelly is right: Kill the basketball program there. Put it out of its misery.

The State

Columbia, SC, April 12, 1985

THE POINT-SHAVING scandal at Tulane University not only shocked the Green Wave campus, it has cast another shadow over college basketball everywhere.

And in South Carolina, still reeling from athletic trauma at Clemson University, the shock waves reverberated since the University of South Carolina is a member of the Metro Conference with Tulane. The conference will have to be restructured if Tulane carries out the president's decision to drop men's basketball.

In fact, Tulane's mess inevitably cheapens the league. Any new conference faces tough going in its young years, and a scandal invites cynics to brand it as an outlaw league.

The Tulane disgrace has a twist. The players are accused, not of throwing games, but of rigging the point spread to help gamblers. And the offense transcends the Metro. It throws unwarranted suspicion on any program where teams have performed erratically or not lived up to expectations, as did the most recent point-shaving outrage in 1981 at Boston College.

The Tulane scandal was marred by other sordid elements — cocaine, which was used to lure the offenders into the conspiracy, a mysterious shoebox that contained thousands of dollars, and possibly other dark forces that Tulane's president has hinted at. The money supposedly was a reward for John (Hot Rod) Williams for deciding to play at Tulane.

The case shatters many illusions. Tulane is an institution highly respected for its academics; at his high school in Lousiana, Williams was named most popular boy, most likely to succeed and most talented; resigned coach Ned Fowler, who has not been implicated in the point-shaving scheme, but has admitted making cash payments to several players, was called "a man of impeccable reputation" by *Sports Illustrated.*

It is understandable and, probably wise, that President Eaman Kelly decided to drop men's basketball. He felt it was critical that the 150-year-old private institution reassert decisively that "our primary values are academic, and that academic integrity is essential to university life." Thus, he forthrightly opted to drop a sport that the school has competed in since 1912. His decision has angered many Green Wave students and athletic boosters.

Although Tulane's scandal dwarfs the one which surfaced at Clemson and is vastly different, both reflected similar syndromes that have commericalized college athletics and made winning everything. President Kelly cited the problems of media pressure, drugs, and gambling. And they add up to societal problems.

Columnist Nicholas Von Hoffman, in a moment of outrage, observed: "Despite the blah-blah about how important our colleges and universities are supposed to be in the struggle to catch up with the Japanese and defend us against the Russians, board members, alumni and sports morons around the country continue to believe their schools' primary mission is to have the young, ignorant oafs on their team beat the unlettered empty heads from 300 miles away on the interstate."

Perhaps Robert Mayard Hutchins, who took Chicago University out of big-time sports, went too far when he claimed a university can have either a great football team or a great university, but not both. But at least, the Tulane and Clemson affairs point to the desperate need for universities to re-examine their missions.

THE PLAIN DEALER

Cleveland, OH, April 6, 1985

The president of Tulane University took a drastic but courageous course in moving to drop intercollegiate basketball from the school's sports program. The action has been criticized as being too extreme. No other action, however, could better have demonstrated the notion that a university sport plagued with scandal is expendable.

Dropping basketball—Tulane's administrative board still must approve President Eamon M. Kelly's recommendation—will hurt players not involved in either point-shaving or illegal payments, and will be a blow to avid followers of the team. It will hurt the university financially. But with players alleged to be involved in one scandal and coaches in another, the program was rotten.

Reform rather than disbandment was one possibility. That would have answered the doubts of cynics, who contend that Kelly acted to forestall action against the school by the National Collegiate Athletic Association and/or the Metro Conference. But there is every indication that the school president was appalled, shaken and saddened by revelations about the basketball squad's possible involvement with drugs, bookmakers and under-the-counter payments.

The move should be taken for what Kelly said it was, "the only way I know to demonstrate unambiguously this academic community's intolerance of the violations and actions we have uncovered . . ."

All big-time sports schools are vulnerable to the double menace of drugs and gambling, as well as the temptation to extend illegal payments to some athletes. What allegedly happened at Tulane might be going on elsewhere. Coming as they did when the nation was applauding Villanova's marvelous victory over Georgetown, the events at Tulane cast a shadow over collegiate basketball, which otherwise was enjoying one of its finest hours.

Tulane basketball might be back, although Kelly wants a permanent ban. For various reasons, other universities have dropped one or more intercollegiate sports and have prospered, and Tulane will as well. Unfortunately, illegal gambling and its ally, the drug racket, are out there—muscular and cash-laden— ready to prey on any school aiming for the top in sports.

THE KANSAS CITY STAR

Kansas City, MO, April 8, 1985

The pitiful state of affairs surrounding Tulane University's basketball program points to a larger problem: It's getting extremely difficult to agree on the precise role athletics should play at this nation's colleges and universities.

To proponents, sports programs are wonderful things. They provide scholarships to needy and worthy young people, and teams the students can rally around. To opponents, sports programs merely take advantage of many gifted but dumb athletes. They also get too much attention and money to the detriment of worthier, scholastic-related efforts.

At Tulane, the opponents are winning. What started as an embarrassing point-shaving episode has turned into a depressing scandal. In the last few days several Tulane players and students have been indicted for shaving points during basketball games in return for money and drugs; the school's basketball coach has resigned amid charges he gave cash to players on a routine basis; and the school's president wants to drop the basketball program.

Those are drastic actions. But they were drastic problems. Yet it's amazing how these numbing developments seem almost accepted by some Tulane students. "This goes on everywhere. We were just dumb enough to get caught," one student said.

Does it go on everywhere? Certainly the temptations to be greedy are there. Betting on football and basketball contests have become accepted as part of the intercollegiate sporting scene. So lots of gambling money is riding on the outcome of games played by young men 18 to 22 years old. Is it really surprising the gamblers try to control the actions of these often-naive athletes with bribes and inducements of drugs? Unfortunately, no.

Certainly not all schools suffer from such shoddy practices. But the incident at the New Orleans school, once best known for its academics, will get the attention of athletic directors everywhere. College sports should not be the breeding ground for tainted games and ill-gotten money.

They won't be if punishment in the Tulane case is swift and severe. They won't be if persons concerned about college athletics, including money-giving alumni, make it clear they want decent and clean programs.

The Wichita
Eagle-Beacon

Wichita, KS, April 8, 1985

WHAT went wrong with Tulane University's basketball program? The drugs, payoffs and point-shaving that have come to light are depressing symptoms of a larger sickness within collegiate athletics today: An attitude that winning — at any cost — is more important than how you win, or lose. An attitude that universities are built around athletics instead of academics. Tulane University President Eamon Kelly took the courageous and proper action last week by announcing the end of TU's basketball program.

The Tulane scandal should prompt other universities to put their priorities in order. Granted, a strong, honest athletic program can be a big boost to a university, bringing it attention, support and prestige that often translate into academic excellence. But when a university's sports obsession leads to unethical or criminal behavior, this tarnishes the entire university. Wichita State University, once involved in unethical recruiting of basketball players, well knows how long it takes to repair the damage caused by such incidents.

Colleges must ask themselves: Is a compromised athletic program worth the cost of an institution's academic reputation? One college president who answered "no" is the Rev. John J. LoSchiavo, president of the University of San Francisco, who disbanded the school's nationally-ranked basketball program in 1982 following scandals involving payoffs to athletes. Wrote President LoSchiavo at the time: "Turning our heads and pretending that violation of rules is permissible under any circumstances jeopardizes our institutional integrity. If universities dismiss their principles in one area, how can their other purposes be respected?"

Universities must apply strict ethical standards to sports programs, and enforce them vigorously. Otherwise higher education will be the big loser.

ALBUQUERQUE JOURNAL

Albuquerque, NM, April 12, 1985

That's overly strong medicine Tulane University President Eamon Kelly has prescribed for the university basketball program. He proposes to euthanize the patient for a disease that could be cured.

Kelly says the basketball progam at Tulane will be dropped because of the point-shaving scandal at the university and because the head basketball coach admitted making cash payment to basketball players.

It is a severe, but honest, response to a situation some school presidents might be inclined to conceal, or, failing that, to play down with the excuse that everybody does it.

"The only way I know to demonstrate unambiguously this academic community's intolerance of the violations and actions we have uncovered is to discontinue the program in which they originated," Kelly said.

Fine. Tulane will go without basketball, but the earth will continue to rotate around the sun. But what is Kelly's purpose?

If it is to punish the wrongdoers, dropping the basketball program is too drastic. The harm has been done, and there is no program left to benefit from the punishment or the example.

The University of New Mexico apparently runs a winning basketball program by the book in the aftermath of our own Lobogate transcript forging scandal.

If Kelly's action was meant solely as a philosophical statement, which is what he apparently intends, one questions if the severity would be consistent throughout the university. Will Kelly excise any and all non-academic programs where illegal activity is detected?

Such questioning is by no means intended to take the violations at Tulane lightly. Indeed, sanctions and firings often seem to have no effect, particularly in college football.

But the underlying questions remain unanswered: Do college athletics serve a useful function? And if so, how can intercollegiate competition be cleaned up without being eliminated altogether?

Those are the basic questions Tulane has avoided.

The Idaho STATESMAN

Boise, ID, April 11, 1985

The integrity of college sports is at stake and only tough action by the NCAA will prevent further erosion of an already sullied amateur image.

Rocked by the recent point-shaving scandal at New Orlean's Tulane University, the NCAA has scheduled a special convention in New Orleans June 21-22 to discuss stricter sanctions than those now in effect. These could include longer probations and forcing schools to drop sports programs.

The Tulane scandal is only one in a long series of major and minor problems at dozens of universities. Tulane President Eamon Kelly plans to abolish that school's basketball program.

That's sad for the school, its players and boosters. But President Kelly is right to come down hard and fast on a program wracked with scandal. Often, as when the University of San Francisco dropped its basketball program a few years ago, it's the university president, not the NCAA, whose punishment is the toughest.

Also disconcerting are the results of an NCAA survey which shows college presidents are worried about the integrity of college sports and that a quarter doubt they have the authority to ensure their sports programs are run honestly. A special NCAA presidents' commission plans to sponsor resolutions at the June meeting to bring athletic budgets under college presidents' control and to overhaul the rules for policing athletic violations.

Idaho schools have been relatively scandal-free, although Idaho State University's athletic program currently is under NCAA investigation. Big Sky Commissioner Ron Stephenson said the problems of money and amateur athletics are "getting frightening."

The problem stems from the bizarre nature of college athletics. Individual athletes are supposed to be amateurs, but are paid with "full-ride" scholarships, and sometimes receive cars, stereos and summer jobs from over-zealous boosters. Meanwhile, the universities make thousands from lucrative television contracts while alumni scream for better players and more championships.

Unless the NCAA elects to shed pretenses and allow colleges to buy and sell players as in the pros, it had better begin policing its own with a vengeance or watch amateur athletics become a hapless joke.

Cocaine Trial Rocks Major League Baseball

After a 14-day trial, a federal district court jury in Pittsburgh September 20, 1985 convicted former caterer Curtis Strong on 11 of 16 original counts of selling cocaine to major league baseball players in Pittsburgh between 1980 and 1983. The jury had seen and heard seven current and former major league players, including current stars Dave Parker of the Cincinnati Reds and Keith Hernandez, a New York Met, testify that they had purchased the drug from Strong. The other players who testified were: Lonnie Smith, an outfielder for the Kansas City Royals; Enos Cabell, a utility player with the Los Angeles Dodgers; Dale Berra, a New York Yankee infielder; Jeff Leonard, a San Francisco Giants outfielder; and John Milner, formerly with the Mets. The players testified under immunity from prosecution. Their detailed accounts of narcotics transactions, often implicating players on their own and other teams, provided a startling picture of widespread cocaine and amphetamine use among Major League members. Each count upon which Strong was convicted carried a maximum penalty of 15 years' imprisonment and a $25,000 fine. He was one of seven men who were indicted for selling cocaine to baseball players, and the first to come to trial.

After the jury had announced its verdict, the presiding judge in the case, Gustave Diamond, held Strong's lawyer, Adam Renfroe, Jr., in contempt of court for "reprehensible behavior." Throughout the trial, Renfroe's strategy had been to portray the testifying players as "junkies" who should not be believed because they were testifying to protect themselves. Diamond had ordered the jury not to consider the government policy of immunity in reaching its verdict.

THE ARIZONA REPUBLIC
Phoenix, AZ, September 15, 1985

THERE is no joy in Mudville. Baseball has struck out.

Not since the 1919 Chicago Black Sox betting scandal has America's national pastime been rocked so uniformly and decisively. An omen to the game's current sickly state was evident in 1983 when four Kansas City players were sentenced to jail on cocaine charges.

Today, unfolding in a federal courtroom in Pittsburgh, is the ugly revelation of widespread drug use among high-priced professional ballplayers, an unseemly situation so pervasive that baseball commissioner Peter Ueberroth regards it as the No. 1 problem facing the sport.

One after another, major league players are pointing the finger at Curtis Strong, a former Philadelphia Phillies caterer charged with 16 counts of cocaine distribution, as a man they did business with.

Strong is just one of seven men who've been indicted on 165 drug counts. The players have been granted immunity from prosecution in return for their incriminating testimony that not only details the purchases involving Strong, but the sordid world of major league baseball in the 1980s and the wretched abuse of the minds and bodies of athletes earning an average salary of $350,000 per year.

In short, baseball itself has been indicted and is on trial.

A three-month investigation by *The New York Times* turned up, among other findings, that "scores of players" have been implicated as cocaine users, purchasers and sellers in criminal investigations, yet the players usually aren't prosecuted nor are their identities revealed. Almost all 26 teams have been affected, *The Times* said, dispelling the notion that drug use has been confined to just those that come out of the closet and seek treatment.

The Justice Department is repeating its highly questionable investigatory tactic of granting blanket immunity in return for ballplayer testimony, just as it did in its investigation of the illegal check overdrafting scheme by middle managers of the E.F. Hutton & Co. brokerage firm which resulted in no charges being filed against those culpable.

Those baseball players now furnishing details of their cocaine habits are just as guilty as those that they say sold them the drug. It is bewildering to law-abiding citizens why a litany of athletes must receive immunity. Certainly, it doesn't take more than a few to build a credible case with corroboration against cocaine sellers and distributors.

Ueberroth, fearful of cocaine's image-sullying impact on baseball — including the inevitable mingling of ballplayers with criminals and gamblers — took a page from his successful stewardship of the 1984 Summer Olympiad and proposed in May a random drug urinalysis program. It covers all baseball personnel except those seemingly the most addicted — the players. Their union, the Major League Baseball Players Association, rejected the plan, saying their own voluntary program is working and mandatory drug testing is an invasion of privacy.

The Pittsburgh trial shows that the voluntary drug rehabilitation program is an abject failure. Players have abused not only their God-given minds and bodies, but an implied trust bestowed upon them by American youngsters.

Ueberroth should start handing down severe suspensions. The player's union should accept Ueberroth's drug program. Both are prerequisite initial steps if America's national pastime is to rid itself of insidious drug abuse and recoup its unique spot in the eyes of the public.

ARGUS-LEADER
Sioux Falls, SD, September 13, 1985

Lonnie Smith. Keith Hernandez. Dale Berra. Joaquin Andujar. Enos Cabell. Dave Parker. Gary Mathews. Lee Lacy. Bill Madlock. Willie Stargell.

The names of major-league baseball players are popping like popcorn from the witness stand of a drug trial in Pittsburgh.

Editorial

It's the first of several court cases expected to involve professional ballplayers. Names already are being dropped like balls lost in the lights.

By the time the drug-peddling trials are finished, there probably will be enough players implicated by fact, hearsay and outright speculation to start a new league.

"Baseball is on trial," defense lawyer Adam O. Renfroe Jr. pronounced to the jury.

Wrong.

No player is on trial. Some should be, perhaps. But the only person on trial now is Curtis Strong, 38, a former caterer for the Philadelphia Phillies.

Strong is accused of selling cocaine to players. Players have been given immunity from prosecution in exchange for testimony, and they're singing like cardinals.

For example, Berra, a New York Yankees infielder, testified that former team captains Madlock and Stargell provided him amphetamines while all three played for the Pittsburgh Pirates.

And Kansas City's Smith said that Pete Rose was once among the players supposedly taking amphetamines — a charge that Rose, baseball's career hit leader, says is false.

The stories could go on and on, and no doubt will — with players, not the pushers — at center stage.

Illegal drug use certainly cannot be condoned. It should be discouraged in all professions and in all layers of life. Baseball reflects society, but professional athletes are heroes and role models for youth. So there is nothing wrong with holding ballplayers to an abnormally high standard of conduct to keep the game clean.

But let's not get carried away.

If the Strong trial is an indication of what's to come, baseball is on the verge of a witch hunt reminiscent of Sen. Joseph McCarthy's search for communists in the 1950s.

Baseball players who violate drug laws should be punished. But let's not fall in love with the hunt.

Let's not forget the presumption of innocence until proven guilty. Let's not allow ambitious government prosecutors and glory-seeking defense lawyers to run amuck in their actions and words.

Baseball is not on trial, at least not yet.

The Honolulu Advertiser

Honolulu, HI, September 26, 1985

Everyone seems to agree that major league baseball has a problem with drugs and that something should be done.

How many players, who have an average salary of $360,000, use illegal drugs is uncertain. Estimates range from just a handful to "there is a lot more to the problem than the public knows."

BUT WHAT to do? Commissioner Peter Ueberroth's answer — that players voluntarily submit to three tests a year — is troubling.

It assumes a player is guilty until proven innocent. It places an unfair onus on those who, for perfectly legitimate reasons, choose not to take the test. It bypasses the Major League Players Association, the union, which has a Joint Drug Agreement with owners that should serve as a foundation for any anti-drug effort.

The initial response indicates that the majority of ball players will not accept Ueberroth's Friday deadline to agree to voluntary testing. They want the union involved.

However, Ueberroth is right when he warns that unless pro ball does *something* itself, Congress or others will take over the responsibility. Lawmakers who seriously consider devising a censorship system for rock music would not stop at intruding into the national pastime.

Baseball does not need to have its drug problems aired in congressional hearings. The just-completed Curtis Strong trial in Pittsburgh and the upcoming Robert McCue case there are doing enough to drag baseball's reputation through the mud. (Strong was convicted of supplying cocaine to players; McCue is charged with supplying drugs.)

WHAT THE public needs to see is an indication that professional baseball is cleaning up its image.

There are problems with the commissioner's approach but not with his concern. The Major League Players Association needs to make a counter-proposal that will take its concerns into account but still ensure that baseball is shaking its drug habit.

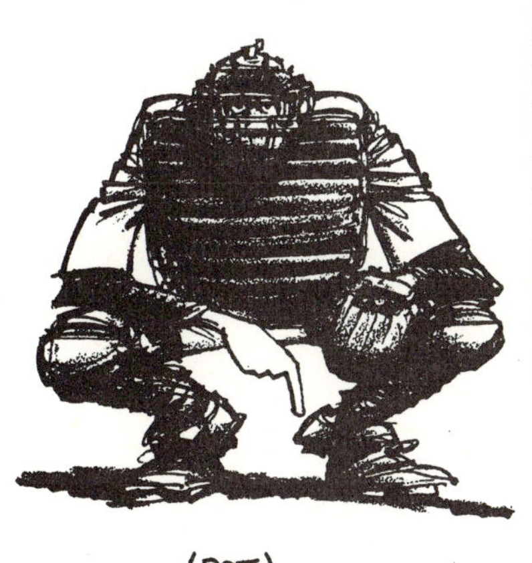

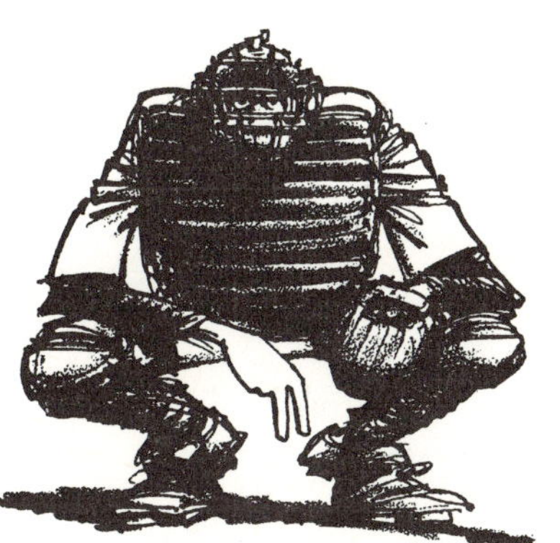

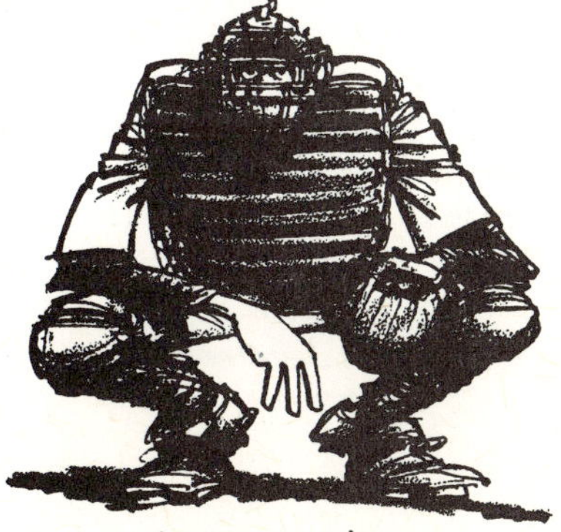

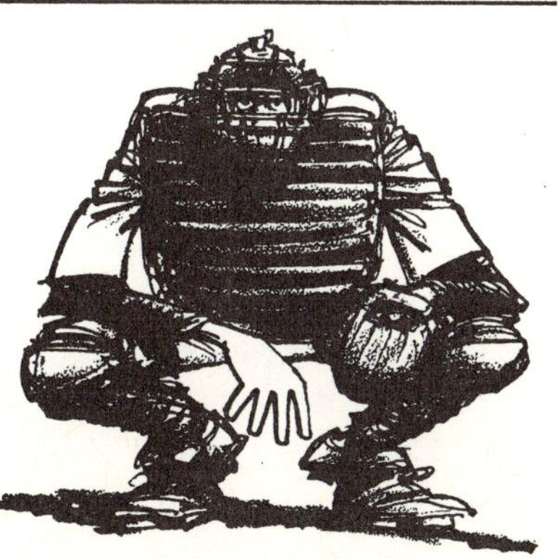

Richmond Times-Dispatch

Richmond, VA,
September 17, 1985

The cocaine-trafficking trial in Pittsburgh is, or should be, baseball's worst scandal since the Black Sox of 1919. Granted immunity from prosecution, seven big-name players have been singing like birds, not only admitting their own cocaine use but implicating dozens of other prominent players in illicit drug use. But a baseball-loving public seems hardly scandalized.

A short time after testifying that he had regularly snorted coke from 1980 to 1982 as a member of the St. Louis Cardinals, Mets' first baseman Keith Hernandez received a standing ovation from fans at New York's Shea Stadium. He also drove in the winning run in one of the Mets' showdown games last week against the Cards, with whom they are locked in a tight pennant race. We wonder what the message was to TV-watching children, who saw Mr. Hernandez go from hero to goat to hero again literally overnight. We fear it was: Drugs can't hurt you. Nobody's touched Keith and, heck, he even used cocaine in 1982, the year the Cardinals won the World Series. And never mind what he testified as to the deleterious effects on his body — the sweats, shakes, nosebleeds, etc.

Pete Rose of the Cincinnati Reds provided the wholesome, Horatio Alger, role model for youth when he toppled Ty Cobb's all-time hit record last week — an achievement built on the natural high of hustle and determination. But consider that the next batter up after Mr. Rose's Ty-breaker was league runs-batted-in leader Dave Parker, who testified in Pittsburgh that when he was a member of the Pirates he had not only taken drugs but arranged drug deals between a pusher and members of three major-league teams. Without a grant of immunity, Mr. Parker could have landed years of hard jail time for such an admission. Yet, there he was back in the lineup on baseball's starriest night, as though the blizzard had never occurred.

Declaring that his intent is to "fight drugs, not players," baseball commissioner Peter Ueberroth has proposed to implement random drug tests for all major-leaguers. The U. S. Olympic Committee used a similar procedure effectively this summer at the National Sports Festival to check athletes for steroid or cocaine use. The major-league players' union has resisted Mr. Ueberroth's plan, deeming it an invasion of privacy. Continuing revelations out of the Pittsburgh courtroom may bring new converts to testing, however. Tommy Herr, player representative for the Cardinals, is one who believes that ballplayers, the majority of whom don't do drugs, are becoming "tired of protecting drug users" and thus may become receptive to random testing.

Testing would at least offer some assurance that a championship had not been decided because a player was too stoned to steal a base — or because another player had obtained a chemical edge. But maybe instead of more tests, baseball needs less tolerance — less tolerance, that is, of players who take their million-dollar salaries and stick them up their noses. If Mr. Ueberroth began handing baseball's junkies stiff suspensions, or even lifetime expulsions, from the game, the attitudes of players as well as the message sent to youth might change drastically.

THE BISMARCK TRIBUNE

Bismarck, ND, September 22, 1985

If there were any lingering doubts whether drug abuse is a pervasive and possibly growing problem in U.S. society, they have been dispelled by the news events of the last few weeks.

In one instance we have had a continual parade of professional baseball players taking the witness stand in Pittsburgh to recall — with immunity from prosecution — how they and fellow athletes bought and used drugs. The names of some of the players implicated in baseball's cocaine scandal reach all the way to the Hall of Fame. It has been a sorry and sometimes sorrowful spectacle.

At another trial, on the West Coast, witnesses have recounted how the late comedian John Belushi spent his last days with a few friends, getting shots of mixed drugs to reach new "highs."

Oh, how could the mighty sink so low?

These two courtroom cases have illustrated, as never before, that drug abuse — once associated with poverty, crime and young people — has become accepted behavior for a lot of upper and middle class Americans.

Maybe the recent stories of lost fortunes, careers and even lives will finally shake some sense into people; at least those who should know better.

Then, if America's successful people will go out of their way to set examples and try to educate others, maybe some headway can be made in coming to grips with the nation's drug problem.

Once we all recognize that there is a problem, and that it is serious, the solution becomes simple: Quit using drugs.

EVENING EXPRESS

Portland, ME, September 26, 1985

The boss of the Major League Baseball Players Association is way off base in rejecting as "silly" the plea of Commissioner Peter Ueberroth that all players submit voluntarily to drug tests. Drug abuse by professional athletes is injuring not only the players but sports themselves.

Seven active or former baseball players recently testified in a Pittsburgh court to having purchased cocaine from a man later convicted of drug trafficking. The testimony revealed that some of the players used drugs directly before and even during games.

One player testified to doing a drug deal in the clubhouse between innings. Another told of sliding headfirst into a base out of fear that he might damage a packet of cocaine in his hip pocket.

Yet Donald Fehr, acting executive director of the players association, asked for his reaction to Ueberroth's drug-testing proposal, says: "Am I in favor of it? No. I think it's silly, I think it's counterproductive and I think it's likely to provoke confrontation."

As matters stand now, everybody involved in professional baseball—the owners, the coaches, the scouts and umpires—are subject to drug testing, except for the players themselves.

Ueberroth's recommendation is a sensible one. Major league players are required to pass physical examinations to prove they are fit enough to earn salaries which average more than $350,000 a year. Testing for drugs is only a logical extension of the physical; why should owners be expected to pay big salaries for damaged goods?

Only those players who take drugs have anything to fear from Ueberroth's proposal. In rejecting the idea, Fehr only succeeds in creating the impression that drug use by players is far more extensive than anyone imagines.

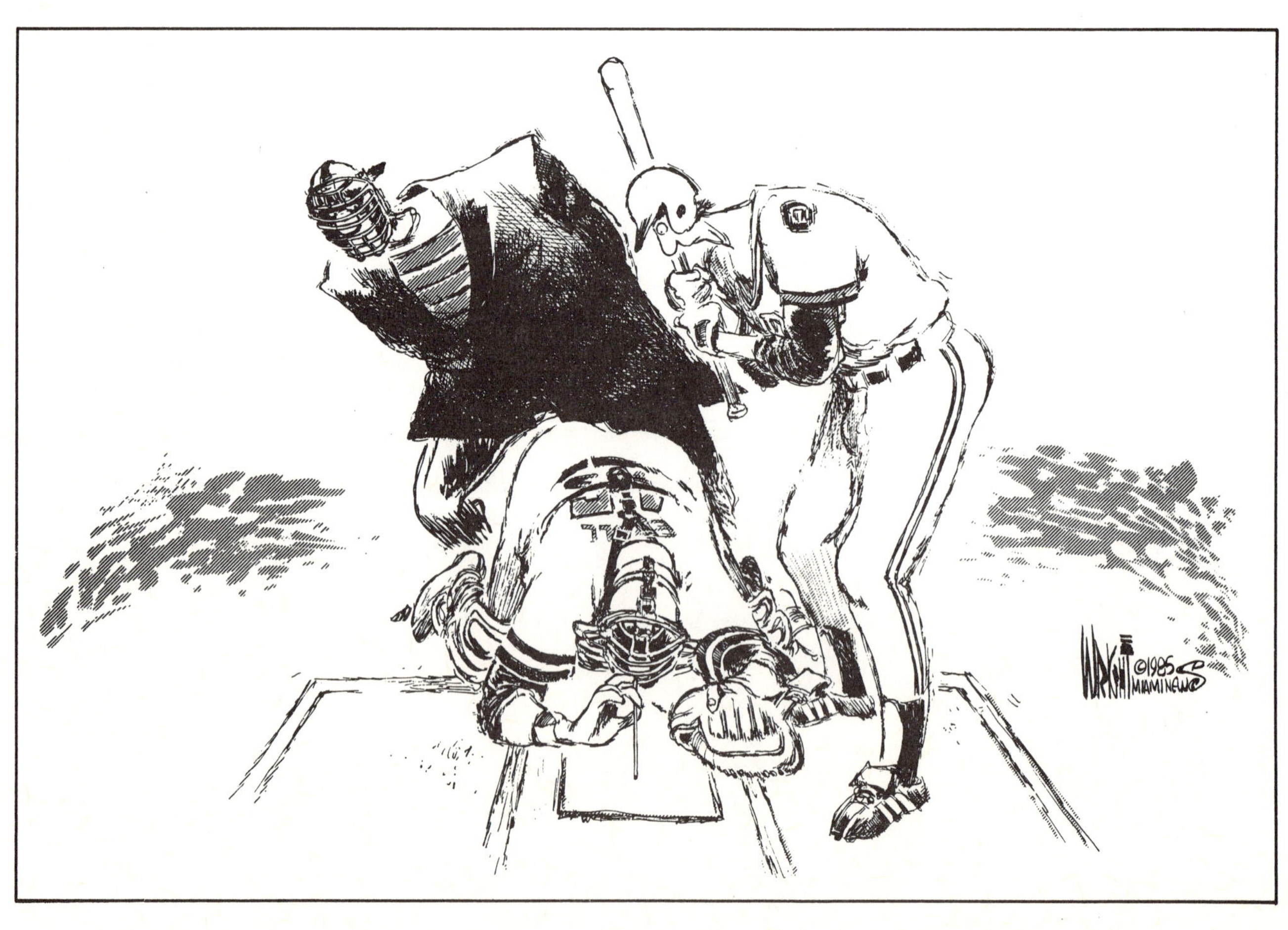

AKRON BEACON JOURNAL

Akron, OH, September 29, 1985

IN LATE September, spring's promise of a new baseball season is harvested in the closing days of the pennant races. Autumn is a good time for the sport — even for the losers who are already thinking about next year. But Major League baseball has been preoccupied with things besides pennant races this year, leaving some of its most ardent fans despairing about the state of their heroes' art.

The problem is drugs. Last week, a jury in Pittsburgh convicted Curtis Strong, a caterer who hung close by the Pittsburgh Pirates' locker room, of 11 counts of selling cocaine to players over a three-year period. One Pirate reportedly left the dugout during games to snort cocaine in the dressing room. A Montreal Expo outfielder actually stashed it in the hip pocket of his uniform and took it onto the field with him.

All this, of course, has properly raised questions about the extent to which drugs have stained the ballplayers and thus, the game itself. Reacting quickly to shore up baseball's sagging image, Commissioner Peter Ueberroth has called for voluntary drug testing of the players — an appeal that is gaining some support by the athletes themselves. "Baseball," Mr. Ueberroth said, "is in trouble."

Throughout its history, all professional sports have experienced one problem or another with some of its participants, whether it was alcoholism, public rowdyism, questionable personal conduct or drugs. But the same could be said about other professions, and it would be wrong to damn athletes as the world's only sinners.

Still, we have come to expect more from our high-salaried Goliaths, perhaps because they represent the highest physical skills that can be produced by the human body. And millions upon millions of fans, young and old, pay to see what often seem to be superhuman performances. We routinely refer to winners as world champions and All-Americans.

In other words, we take our athletes seriously even though the games were never intended to be anything more than games.

Those are the conditions facing baseball today. We, like millions of others, love baseball. But like Mr. Ueberroth, we think that for the health and glory of the sport, it's time for baseball to clean up its act.

Pittsburgh Post-Gazette

Pittsburgh, PA, September 28, 1985

Shame and scandal have come to settle firmly on the reputation of professional baseball. In the Pittsburgh drug trials, two sets of convictions have now been returned for the crime of selling cocaine — judgments that still leave the game of baseball in the dock.

For many people, the guilt of the accused has not seemed so far removed from that of their accusers — baseball players who have admitted their own drug use and who testify against dealers only under a grant of immunity. It comes to this: The two defendants who have been found guilty will pay their debt to society; what will the game of baseball do?

Baseball players can count themselves extraordinarily fortunate. For their ability to bat and pitch balls, skills that count for little in the wider world, they reap fame and riches. For the most part, those who pay their way, the fans, are not so lucky — they have to work in jobs that are anything but games, and for a fraction of the reward.

At a fundamental level, the players owe something to the fans, and it is implicit in every ticket that is sold. What the fans have a right to expect is just this: that the players use their natural gifts to the best of their ability.

The testimony in federal court indicates that this simple bargain has been broken too often. In taking amphetamines and cocaine, certain players have put their natural ability in jeopardy. They want to cheat nature, but they end up cheating themselves and, ultimately, their fans. What heroes are these?

Perhaps it is only a few who are guilty of drug-taking, but suspicion, like a fine powder blown in the air, has settled on all. Now, only a combined response will blow it away. This week, Baseball Commissioner Peter Ueberroth suggested what should be a first step. Mr. Ueberroth appealed to each player to agree to voluntary drug testing three times a year. The program, which would be similar to the mandatory one that already exists for players in the minor leagues and for non-player Major League personnel, would not be punitive. It would be a confidential way of suggesting treatment for those who need it.

If anything, Mr. Ueberroth's anti-drug suggestion was the softest of pitches. After all, the only penalty for those who did not take part in the testing would be moral suasion. Yet because the Major League Players' Association was not approached directly, this benign suggestion raised immediate resentment at the union-management level.

Of course, the subject should be worked out in direct negotiations at the top level. But the fact is that baseball players have as much a stake in cleaning up the game as the baseball commissioner. In this regard, it was heartening that members of the Pittsburgh Pirates, the club at the center of the current drug controversy, supported the idea of testing provided that the union agrees.

In many Olympic sports, testing for other sorts of drugs is conducted routinely, and nobody seriously argues anymore that the athletes' civil liberties are being violated. If baseball is being singled out, then it is only because a few players drew attention to themselves by their own behavior. Now the whole game has something to prove: that it is *not* guilty. Voluntary drug testing is needed urgently — and mandatory testing as soon as possible.

The Star-Ledger

Newark, NJ, September 30, 1985

The highly damaging—and disturbing—testimony of a recent drug trial has prompted the commissioner of baseball to urge major league players to submit to voluntary drug testing. That seemed to be a reasonable enough request by Commissioner Peter Ueberroth, but it was brushed off by the head of the Players Association as "silly, counterproductive and likely to provoke a confrontation."

The negative reaction by the players' group may be precisely the reason why big-league baseball now finds itself, as the commissioner aptly noted, with a "cloud hanging over its head." And, it follows, too, that baseball's drug problem undoubtedly will worsen if its representatives persist in pursuing a protective, defensive course.

The testimony at the trial, in which seven players admitted buying cocaine from the drug dealer and implicated other players, had unsettling implications of widespread drug abuse in baseball. It also confirmed earlier reports of the prevalence of drug use among players.

The defendant in the drug trial has been convicted for possession and sale of cocaine, and now faces a jail term. His customers, who happen to be highly paid baseball players, are off the hook because they were granted immunity for testifying. Presumably, their punishment is that their addiction has been given public exposure. But indulgent fans are quick to forgive and forget.

Worse still, little has been done about the problem itself. There have been isolated incidents where players admitted their addiction and voluntarily entered drug rehabilitation programs. But there has been a self-serving resistance by the players' union against remedial measures to curb drug use among its members. Team owners have been put on notice by the union that it is opposed to drug testing on constitutional grounds that it would invade players' rights to privacy.

In fact, George Steinbrenner, a principal owner of the Yankees, was sharply chastized by union leaders after he disclosed that one of his players had voluntarily submitted to testing. The player later testified at the trial that he had had a drug habit for several years, which critically impaired his skills.

What has emerged from the Pittsburgh court proceeding is that baseball—not the alleged small-time drug dealer—was on trial. Ball players like to picture themselves as role models for youngsters. Instead, they now have grossly miscast themselves as self-destructive "druggies." It is not a pretty picture.

It should be fully apparent that the Players Association cannot continue to blithely tolerate a serious drug problem, hoping that it will go away by itself and ultimately be overlooked by its fans.

This is a problem that must be responsibly addressed by all its principals—the players, their union, the owners, and, above all, the baseball commissioner, who can take a tougher stance by penalizing the players named as drug users in order to deter their colleagues.

NCAA Votes Drug, Academic Tests

The National Collegiate Athletic Association (NCAA) January 13 and 14, 1986 voted to institute academic eligibility requirements for student athletes and to implement drug testing at championship events. The actions came at the NCAA's convention in New Orleans.

The convention voted overwhelmingly to implement random drug testing at 18 major college football bowl games and selected championship events in football and other sports. The tests would check for illegal recreational drugs as well as for anabolic steroids and amphetamines. Athletes testing positively would be barred from the championship or bowl games and suspended from competition for 90 days. A second positive testing would result in a sterner penalty. Costs of the tests would be covered by the NCAA, the schools involved and gate receipts from the bowls and championship games.

The eligibility standards, contained in Proposition 48, were adopted by the convention Jan. 13. The rules would, by the fall of 1988, require entering freshmen athletes in Division I schools to have achieved a combined score of 700 on the Scholastic Aptitude Tests or a 15 score on the American College Test. In addition, entering freshmen would have to have compiled a grade point average of 2.0 or better in a core curriculum during high school. Students not meeting these requirements would be ineligible for participation in sports as freshmen.

Chicago Tribune

Chicago, IL, January 24, 1986

The National Collegiate Athletic Association's Division I, the major sports schools, has taken some steps to rid athletic programs of drugs, gambling and academic fraud. Although none of the measures approved will be able to clean up the athletic programs alone, they are important because at least the NCAA finally has admitted it has some problems.

Lacking police powers, there is little the NCCA schools can do by themselves to control gambling. However, the association, because it controls the eligibility of athletes, has considerably more power over drug abuse, which has become epidemic in American sports, and the academic performance of athletes.

Give the NCAA the following grades:

- A for drug control.
- C for academics.
- Incomplete for gambling.

The gambling issue was punted to Congress. An NCAA resolution urges tougher federal laws against gambling on college sports.

The antidrug program, which includes testing of athletes before championship events and a list of proscribed substances, is by far the toughest stance the association took. If enforced, it should greatly reduce the drug problem.

The academic program is a somewhat smaller step toward solving another big problem. The NCAA, despite the objections of some predominantly black institutions, has decided to require more stringent academic requirements of freshmen athletes. Starting in 1988, freshmen must have certain minimum scores on standard college entrance tests as well as 2.0 grade averages in high school to be eligible to play in college.

The minimun test scores will not certify anyone as a genius, but by requiring them the NCAA has at least started to address the problem of the academic performance of athletes. The program also should put pressure on secondary schools across the nation to upgrade their academic performance.

Although the nation's major colleges, with a few exceptions, have continued to delude themselves that their athletic programs were populated only by student athletes, a succession of scandals across the country in recent years clearly indicated that many of the schools had become little more than ivy-covered farm teams for professional sports franchises. Too many college athletes were leaving school illiterate, without degrees or without having taken courses much more demanding than Volleyball 101.

Now that the NCAA has acknowledged that this is wrong, it ought to consider reinstating its ban against freshmen playing in any sport and take a serious look at the practice of redshirting that enables an athlete, usually at the behest of his coach, to prolong a four-year college career by an extra year. Redshirting may have had a few legitimate reasons when it was instituted, but as a practical matter it has evolved into a system that allows a coach to overcome his recruiting mistakes. If he gets too many tight ends on the roster, he can redshirt a few for a year until graduation pares the surplus.

There is no reason that a disadvantaged athlete, if he needs an extra year to complete his work for a degree, can't spend the fifth year studying.

No one expects all college athletes to earn Phi Beta Kappa keys, but they at least should be held to the same academic standards as the rest of the student population. Colleges should have the reasonable expectation that the athletes their coaches recruit are capable of college-level work. Anything less is a cruel hoax on both the institution and the athlete.

The Birmingham News

Birmingham, AL, January 22, 1986

The National Collegiate Athletic Association has taken an overdue step to eliminate the drug menace from college sports.

Beginning next fall, athletes competing in the association's 78 championship events and the 18 major-college postseason football games will be subject to drug tests.

Not every competitor will be tested but enough of them will be to make the program effective. For example, 36 players from each team will be tested before football bowl games. The five players who play the most minutes and two others chosen at random will be tested from each team after the second round at basketball tournaments. All medal winners and some others selected at random will be tested in track and field competitions.

Perhaps more important, the NCAA's plan will encourage more individual colleges and universities to conduct their own anti-drug programs. No college will want to be embarrassed at championship events or bowl games by having one or more players kicked off its team.

Drug abuse among college athletes has been a problem for years, particularly the use of so-called performance enhancers, such as anabolic steroids and amphetamines. Often these substances are taken to increase chances of getting contracts with professional teams.

Campus scandals involving the use, even the selling, of "street" drugs — marijuana, cocaine, heroin — also have increased in recent years.

The anti-drug rules adopted at the NCAA's annual convention covers 81 substances, ranging from steroids to hard drugs.

The NCAA's action should have a beneficial effect beyond college athletics. It could discourage drug use among high school athletes who want to participate in college sports. And weeding out abusers at the college level should reduce the number of drug users getting on professional teams.

NCAA delegates deserve commendation for recognizing that stern measures are needed to combat a problem that has been ruining the lives of many athletes and tarnishing the image of educational institutions.

The Christian Science Monitor

Boston, MA, January 31, 1986

AFTER the humiliation of their Super Bowl defeat, the New England Patriots have embarked on an even stronger test of courage — eradication of drug use among the football team's players by the new season. This could make a greater contribution to sports than winning the coveted Lombardi Trophy.

The Patriot players, after Sunday's game in New Orleans, voted to accept a drug testing program. They became the first professional football team to do so. The Patriots were not blaming drugs for their defeat. They were under some pressure to respond to reports of drug use among as many as a dozen of the team's 58 players: A news story was delayed by agreement — itself a subject of controversy — until after Sunday's game.

There are problems with the Patriots' solution. It is already under challenge. The agreement holds only as long as the current coach, Raymond Berry, and the current management, the Sullivan family, retain their positions, and the Sullivans are expected to put the team up for sale in the next few weeks. The agreement lacks leaguewide sanction. The league's players association strongly objects: Such programs can, if handled injudiciously, tarnish their careers and wipe out their livelihood.

Getting leaguewide cooperation is essential. Dallas Cowboys president Tex Schramm calls for leaguewide, mandatory, unannounced testing of players. This can best be described as the management's opening bargaining position. The professional baseball and basketball leagues have adopted drug programs that include testing and treatment, with salary cuts and suspensions as sanctions, depending in part on whether players are convicted of drug use or come forward voluntarily. Suspected cases can trigger panel review and a recommendation of testing. Testing, however, is not mandatory — a situation that baseball commissioner Peter Ueberroth would remedy.

Civil liberties issues are also raised by testing. Unless one agrees to testing on a truly voluntary basis or as terms of a contract, it is a violation of privacy. Search of one's home or auto for drugs cannot be random; the same holds true for one's person. The Constitution protects against governmental intrusions of this sort — efforts by a New Jersey school district to require drug and alcohol testing of students have been stalled in the courts. Nonpublic entities like pro sports teams can make testing subject to collective bargaining, even though individuals may object as a matter of principle.

In competitions like the Olympic Games, testing is a condition the athlete accepts upon entering. The National Collegiate Athletic Association earlier this month authorized drug testing for athletes entering its championship events and the 18 major college postseason football bowl games. The NCAA will test for 86 drugs, with suspensions as penalties.

Required testing of athletes should have its limits. It should be directed at eradicating the problem, helping the athlete, and ensuring a drug-free athletic climate. Tragically, the market among young athletes seems to be building for mood-altering, "competition enhancing," and size-building drugs — an array far broader than the few drugs singled out by pro sports.

Patriot coach Berry told the Boston Globe: "I knew all along, . . . when I began to realize this issue would be part of my job, that what we're talking about is not going to be easy. The mind-set is such that it's like playing a real tough football team. It's a real tough battle, but it'll be worth the battle somehow or other. Maybe eventually a program will come out of this that will be a tremendous help to a tremendous number of people."

Professional athletes have a responsibility to themselves, their families, and the impressionable youths following them in the game to agree to stop drug use in its tracks.

Fort Worth Star-Telegram

Fort Worth, TX, January 20, 1986

Drug abuse among sports figures is probably no more prevalent than it is in society as a whole, but the prominence of sports figures makes it more noticeable and, because youngsters have a tendency to view athletes as heroes, more reprehensible.

Professional sports have been grappling with the problem of drug abuse for some time now, with only limited success. Major league baseball was rocked by revelations from a sensational drug trial in Pittsburgh last summer, and stories about basketball or football players being hooked on drugs appear with disturbing regularity in the nation's newspapers.

Only the most naive fan would believe that the problem doesn't also exist among collegiate athletes. That's why the announcement that the National Collegiate Athletic Association has authorized the testing of college athletes for drugs comes as welcome news.

The NCAA, by an overwhelming vote of its members during its recent convention in New Orleans, approved legislation that will allow the association to examine at random athletes entered in championship events and major-college football bowl games.

Athletes testing positive for any of 79 prohibited drugs will be barred from the event and suspended from further competition for at least 90 days. More severe penalties are called for if athletes test positive a second time. In addition, athletic staff members and employees of the school will face disciplinary action if they fail to report knowledge of a student-athlete using banned drugs.

The new regulation undoubtedly will spur regular testing by member institutions to avoid the embarrassment of having players declared ineligible for important championship competition because of drug abuse. Currently, only 98 of 790 NCAA schools conduct regular drug testing.

The new policy appears to be a realistic, reasonable and effective approach to a growing problem. The NCAA and its college members are to be commended for taking a more active role in combating drug abuse than are the nation's professional sports organizations.

The Dispatch

Columbus, OH, January 23, 1986

The National Collegiate Athletic Association took two much-needed steps last week when it approved its most sweeping set of academic rules for new college athletes and ordered drug testing of athletes at football games and at all NCAA championship contests.

The college presidents who sponsored the new academic rules say they are designed to keep colleges from recruiting athletes who have almost no chance of earning a degree. The rule's supporters tried to take into account objections by the heads of some predominantly black colleges by temporarily lowering the standards slightly in hopes that more than half of all black athletes will not be excluded from playing.

As Ira Heyman, chancellor of the University of California at Berkeley, noted, requiring a minimum score on SAT or ACT tests gives colleges "some objective, outside measure" of the student's ability.

Heyman also noted that the rule's two-year phase-in period "will permit us to gather further data on its impact." If a large percentage of athletes is still being eliminated, he said, the NCAA could revise the rule again in 1987.

But the message to student athletes should be clear: The main purpose of America's institutions of higher learning is learning, and if they want to play collegiate athletics they will have to demonstrate at least some ability in the classroom.

The NCAA's anti-drug plan, which received near-unanimous approval, also doesn't mince words. It bans a long list of street drugs and performance-enhancing substances, including anabolic steroids and caffeine.

Any athlete who tests positive will face an immediate 90-day suspension of eligibility, and coaches and school employees can be penalized for knowing about drug usage and not reporting it.

That's the way it should be.

THE LOUISVILLE TIMES
*Louisville, KY,
January 15, 1986*

To the disappointment of many academically minded presidents of colleges that go in for big-time sports, the NCAA has backed down slightly on its new resolve to be concerned for the minds as well as the physical skills of those who get "scholarships" in return for their services to college athletic programs.

Still, the resolution, as passed Monday by the NCAA's Division One members, is an important step toward draining the swamp of disrepute into which college athletics has sunk over several decades. It delays until the fall of 1988 a rule that incoming freshmen, to be eligible for varsity sports, must achieve a 2.0 grade-point ("C") average in high school, on a curriculum that includes specific core studies.

He or she also must score a combined minimum of 700 (of the possible 1,600) on the Scholastic Aptitude Test, or 15 (of the possible 37) on the other widely used entrance examination, the American College Test. Those are minimal scores — about as low as a student can measure if he's to have any reasonable hope of doing bona fide college work.

That's the root of the matter — competition between *students* is what college athletics is supposed to be all about. These days, at many institutions, that's a complete fiction. Tales of universities that seldom graduate *any* of their athletes who participate in big-time sports abound. Stories of those who do graduate — but remain functionally illiterate — are scarcely less common. The rule at such schools is to use athletes for their box office value, and, except for the rare few who find profitable careers in professional sports, cast them aside as ill-prepared for life as they were on arrival.

Black athletes are the chief victims. That's why it's shocking to find predominantly black schools opposing the rule. The rule doesn't say black athletes who may be academically below par can't play. It simply means they'll play o repair their academic deficiencies efore entering the time-consuming ield of varsity athletics. More responsible schools sometimes do that now, by requiring remedial work for athletes before they enter.

In fact, the NCAA's commitment to reform would have been much more impressive if it had returned to the rule that prevailed before commercialism got out of hand. *No* freshman should be eligible for varsity sport, with its requirements for traveling and other activities that prevent a student from getting a proper start in college.

Still, the new rule is bound to inspire many young athletes to realize that their lives can't be tied completely to playing with a ball. Those who opposed this rule should turn their energies toward remedying the ills that made it necessary.

The Miami Herald
Miami, FL, January 17, 1986

THE **NATIONAL** Collegiate Athletic Association (NCAA) was formed 80 years ago to rescue college sports from that era's abuses — including football brutality so notorious that President Theodore Roosevelt intervened personally to save the sport.

For awhile the NCAA fulfilled its mission well. It generally upheld the ideals of amateurism and the primacy of education. As a result, collegiate athletics grew and prospered.

With prosperity came problems, however. And in recent years the lure of television money made winning more vital than ever to budgets strained by demands to support women's teams and a full array of men's sports. Meanwhile, the NCAA — originally an organization run by college presidents and nominally still that way — became dominated by coaches and athletic directors.

As a result, the NCAA has ceased to be a source of solutions for the serious problems of college athletics — among them drug abuse, gambling, recruiting violations, academic cheating, and cover-ups of assorted other offenses.

In fact, the NCAA's timidity has become a part of the problem. This was demonstrated anew at the NCAA's

NCAA Misses Opportunity

annual meeting this week in New Orleans. The Associated Press describes its climax: "The convention was to end [Wednesday] but adjourned with business concluded Tuesday."

Business concluded? Hardly. The NCAA may have completed its agenda, but a lot of unfinished business remains. Granted, delegates did stiffen admission standards and approve testing athletes for drugs. They also approved a resolution against sports betting.

Yet the NCAA continues to duck two issues basic to restoring the sullied reputation of college sports: putting teeth in the enforcement of NCAA rules, and curbing the excesses of "boosters." Such boosters spawn much of the current mischief in college athletics.

Its inaction in these areas signals subtly that the NCAA still cowers before the major-college coaches who bring collegiate athletics so much money — and so much grief. Until it comes to grips with the issues of enforcement and boosters, the NCAA's credibility in dealing with other issues will suffer.

THE SACRAMENTO BEE
Sacramento, CA, January 20, 1986

The pooh-bahs of the National Collegiate Athletic Association have approved tougher academic eligibility standards for varsity athletes, though not without a little point-shaving here and there.

The rule was first approved by the NCAA in 1983, then challenged by a group of black college presidents who argued that the criteria, particularly the minimum total score of 700 on the verbal and math portions of the Scholastic Aptitude Test (out of a possible 1,600) that the rule required for freshman eligibility, was too tough and discriminated against blacks. The vote the other day reaffirmed that standard, but postponed its full application for another two years. In the meantime, college freshmen with scores lower than 700 will be eligible if they had more than a 2.0 grade point average in high school: the higher the high school GPA, the lower the SAT score has to be. The 700 rule goes into effect in 1988.

That's a small step toward progress in a system which routinely recruits athletes, then drops them like worn-out equipment when their eligibility expires — often without either a degree or even the beginning of a real education. But it's hardly a triumph for academic distinction; roughly 85 percent of all students who take the SAT score over 700; a student who answers no question right gets 400. Combine that with the fact that other academic eligibility rules are frequently violated, sometimes in the most cynical and blatant form, and the NCAA is a long way from fielding the "student athletes" that the blurbs on the Saturday afternoon college football games like to proclaim.

One doesn't have to go far to find illustrations. Just the other day a lawsuit went to trial in which a group of teachers at the University of Georgia testified that administrators at the university had changed the grades of football players in remedial classes over the teachers' protests to protect their athletic eligibility. The suit was brought by a former teacher who said she was fired because she protested. The attorney for the university agreed that athletes get favored treatment, then added (incredibly) that "we may not make a university student out of him, but if we can teach him to read and write, maybe he can work at the post office rather than as a garbageman when he gets through with his athletic career."

As he was speaking, the NCAA had before it a proposal, eventually put over until next year, to lengthen those athletic careers by extending athletic eligibility, now four years, to five. The proponents of this travesty offer the preposterous argument that it will enable more athletes to finish their studies by (it is said) lengthening their scholarships and keeping them in school longer, which is like the old argument that since most often it's the last car on the train that's involved in railroad accidents, the accident rate can be reduced by eliminating the last car. By the same logic, one could argue that eligibility ought to continue indefinitely, until the old boy can't run or throw a football anymore — or until he gets a better offer from the Chicago Bears — at which time he can go home and work for the post office like the Georgia lawyer said. Assuming, of course, that they've taught him to read and write, which is not always the case.

THE INDIANAPOLIS NEWS
Indianapolis, IN, January 16, 1986

The National Collegiate Athletic Association says it's a move designed to put "student" back into the term "student-athlete" in America's major universities.

Many black educators, however, are calling NCAA's move a step toward athletic apartheid and are threatening legal action.

The "it" provoking the controversy is the NCAA's Proposition 48, an academic rule adopted this week. Proposition 48 will set new academic standards for incoming freshmen athletes before they can compete in college.

The standards include scores on the standardized ACT and SAT college placement tests high school junior and seniors take and grade point averages in a core curriculum of math, science and English. As the rule stands, the standards are set on a sliding scale so that a high grade point average can offset low standardized test scores. Thus far, these standards apply only to large Division I schools.

The NCAA's reasoning is clear. Stung by increasing reports of college athletes who couldn't read or write, who skipped classes and who quit college altogether when their athletic careers were over, the organization decided strong support for academic standards was needed.

The question is: How could anyone — namely the protesting black educators — be upset with that position?

The black educators, along with a smattering of white university presidents and professors, claim that the new standards are racially discriminatory. They say that Proposition 48 will deny many young black athletes a chance to attend college and improve their lives — perhaps as many as 2,000 of them next year.

These educators argue, with some justification, that the SAT and ACT tests favor white, middle-class students. Many blacks score considerably lower on SAT and ACT tests than whites, on the average, but the scores go up when the same questions are rephrased in the idioms of black English.

But this doesn't mean the new academic rule is racist.

Proposition 48 is an attempt to force black and white athletes alike to get something out of college that will benefit them long after their playing days are over — an education. To that end, it will improve the lives of the young athletes who meet its standards. It will also re-establish the integrity of the universities which uphold those standards.

What's more, the rule doesn' prevent any athlete who has a low GPA or standardized test score from attending college or playing sports. He or she is free to go to a Division II or III school, or to attend a junior college in order to get a little academic seasoning before transferring to a larger school.

Proposition 48 may need some modifying touches. For instance, what does the NCAA plan to do about high schools that pump an athlete's high school grades in order to overcome an expected low SAT score? But it is not a step toward "athletic apartheid."

And it should not be scrapped.

THE BLADE
Toledo, OH, January 20, 1986

WHATEVER one might think of the latest effort by the National Collegiate Athletic Association to bring some order into the chaos of intercollegiate sports, it is a step in the right direction.

The new rules approved by college presidents at a meeting in New Orleans establish minimum academic standards for incoming college athletes. This addressed one facet of a two-pronged problem, the other being enforcement of existing NCAA rules governing recruiting and treatment of athletes after they have been awarded scholarships.

The new criteria for incoming athletes — 660 out of a possible 1,600 on the Scholastic Aptitude Test or 15 out of 36 on the American College Test in addition to a 1.8 overall grade average — are somewhat tougher than previous standards but not unrealistically nigh. These minimums will rise, but only slightly, over the next two years.

Opponents of the action are worried that the new standards will create an "apartheid" situation in American higher education by barring many black students from attending college on sports scholarships.

While that position may be understandable from one standpoint, it begs the real question, which is, what are colleges essentially for — to develop football and basketball players or graduate educated students?

One answer to that question is revealed in statistics which indicate that at some schools only a third of black male athletes who entered college have gone on to graduate. Data from other universities show that the graduation figure for such student-athletes is as high as 90 per cent. Much apparently depends on how standards are applied.

What about the gifted athlete who cannot meet the minimum standards but who might do so if given the opportunity? This issue was addressed by the NCAA presidents. Under the rule, these students can be admitted on scholarships but will not be allowed to play or practice in the first year. If they attain suitable grades during that period, they can then compete athletically, starting in their sophomore year.

That is fair enough, particularly in view of the fact that most schools provide academic help for athletes on scholarship, if needed, throughout their four years in college.

The important thing is that the new standards be applied fairly and equitably across the board. The time should be past when the top sports universities are the ones who can buy the best players.

The Chattanooga Times
Chattanooga, TN, January 23, 1986

When delegates to a meeting of the National Collegiate Athletic Association voted 206-94 last week to tighten the academic standards for athletes who enroll at Division I colleges, officials of predominantly black colleges, and some white schools, suggested that the decision amounted to "athletic apartheid," a reference to South Africa's policy of racial separation. The protests are unwarranted.

Under the rule, known as Proposition 48, the NCAA will require athletes to have a minimum high school grade point average of C. Also, they will have to score at least 700 points on the Scholastic Aptitude Test (or 15 on the American College Testing program). The standards will be phased in over three years, beginning this fall, and will include a provision under which higher GPAs could offset lower SAT or ACT scores. That is incentive enough to encourage athletes to study harder if they want to play college sports.

Even so, some critics argue that athletic programs provide universities with many benefits — national prestige, increased endowments by loyal fans and considerable revenue from televised games. Others contend it is unfair to use standardized tests because, they say, the tests are biased against blacks. As a result, so the argument goes, black athletes will be adversely affected in disproportionate numbers. Joseph Johnson, president of predominantly black Grambling College, charged that "there was a hidden agenda at this convention and that was to eliminate the number of black athletes on college campuses."

The problem is that such arguments against Proposition 48 gloss over the primary reason for attending college in the first place: to obtain a degree and certain skills that will allow graduates to compete in the marketplace. For many athletes, college is four years worth of practice and jetting around the country for games with other schools — and, incidentally, some academic courses geared to ensuring their continued eligibility.

Moreover, too many athletes are seduced by the dream that a career in professional sports awaits them after graduation; some have even left college early to sign lucrative professional contracts. Not until it's too late do most learn that relatively few athletes win such contracts. By then, their usefulness to the college has been used up and they are mostly left with memories. It's a cynical business, abetted by alumni associations and booster clubs whose chief concern is their team's win-loss record.

Proposition 48 is a racial issue only in the sense that educators agree that black students generally score lower on standardized tests than whites. Nevertheless, the NCAA hopes that the three year phase-in will cause higher standards to "trickle down" to high schools, thereby enabling athletes to meet the admission criteria. The rule also does not preclude Division I schools from giving athletic scholarships. But athletes will not be able to play or practice unless they establish satisfactory academic progress as freshmen, thus leaving them three years of eligibility.

Most important, Proposition 48 could ensure that athletes obtain marketable skills that will be more profitable in the long run than an ability to run off center or execute a hook shot. It's a long overdue reform.

Ueberroth Sets Drug Penalties; Options to Suspensions Offered

Baseball Commissioner Peter Ueberroth February 28, 1986 announced penalties for 21 players—including suspensions of 11 major league players—for their past involvement with illegal drugs. Among the 11 were such prominent players as Keith Hernandez of the New York Mets, Dave Parker of the Cincinnati Reds and Joaquin Andujar of the Oakland A's. The commissioner offered the 11 players an alternative to suspensions that included fines, random drug testing for the duration of their careers and community service work. Ten other players faced no suspensions but were required to undergo random drug testing for the rest of their careers. Within a week of the commissioner's announcement, all the players had accepted Ueberroth's demands.

Most of the players disciplined by Ueberroth had been involved in the 1985 federal trials of drug dealers in Pittsburgh. At the most publicized, that of Curtis Strong, seven current and former players had testified under immunity from prosecution about their drug use. Other players had been mentioned at the trial or had testified before the federal grand jury that returned indictments in the case. The widespread publicity generated by the Pittsburgh case caused a major upset and shocked baseball fans.

Before announcing his long-awaited action on those involved in the trial, Ueberroth had interviewed each of the 21 men eventually disciplined and several others. In announcing the disciplinary actions, Ueberroth divided the drug offenders into three categories. The most severe penalty—a one-year suspension from baseball unless the alternative penalties were chosen—was imposed on seven players whom Ueberroth said had been "involved in a prolonged pattern of drug abuse and...in some fashion facilitated the distribution of drugs in baseball."

SYRACUSE HERALD-JOURNAL
Syracuse, NY, March 4, 1986

Major league baseball Commissioner Peter Ueberroth's offer to allow a bunch of former (we're to believe) hopped-up foul balls to continue playing the National Pastime was more than fair to the players and teams involved.

Ueberroth gave seven players who were allegedly involved in distribution of cocaine the option of being suspended for a year or donating 10 percent of their annual salaries to organizations that combat drug abuse, submit to random drug testing for the remainder of their careers and do 100 hours of community work.

Four other players who used cocaine, but weren't involved in supplying the drug to others, were given the option of being suspended without pay for 60 days or forfeiting 5 percent of their salaries, contribute 50 hours of community service service and submit to random drug testing.

Another 10 players who were nominally involved with drugs must submit to mandatory drug testing as long as they are in baseball.

▽   ▽

A couple of those in the most serious grouping have indicated they may balk at Ueberroth's program. Keith Hernandez of the New York Mets said he will file a grievance to overturn the ruling, while Dave Parker of the Cincinnati Reds has compiled his own list of options, which include "complying, not complying, playing in Japan."

We're told Hernandez' objection is that he's a "private person" who would have difficulty in performing the community service. Tough luck, Mr. Sensitivity. As far as Parker's options, we doubt the Yokohama Giants would welcome a buzzhead with open arms, but if he's reluctant to adopt the commissioner's point of view, we'd much rather have him there than here. We're sure baseball will survive without any or all of these guys with the powdered noses.

It would be better if all big-league baseball players and the players' union got behind Ueberroth in trying to stamp out drug use in the big leagues. Ueberroth is saying drug use is not all right in the little corner of the world that he controls and penalties will be assessed those who do not abide by his rules.

▽   ▽

The effect is much wider, however, because what happens to the stars on our national sports scene is followed feverishly by fans, young and old. The ballplayers, whether they admit it or not, are aware of their impact on the fans. That's why so many are sought after for commercial endorsements, selling everything from razor blades to hot dogs to beer to chewing tobacco.

Whether we — or the athletes — like it, what a player does on and off the field is of public interest and can have wide and lasting impact. Athletes can't have it both ways; they can't accept the million-dollar salaries and national spotlight, without the responsibility of squeeky cleanness that goes along with superstardom.

It would be far and away better if the ballplayers decide to go along with Ueberroth. If the athletes can't agree to the commissioner's conditions, it would be better if they were just far away.

The Cincinnati Post
Cincinnati, OH, March 4, 1986

Even combative Bob Trumpy, host of WLW-AM's "Sportstalk" show, was having trouble Friday finding anyone who objected to Peter Ueberroth's discipline for 21 current and former baseball players—including the Reds' Dave Parker—who have been linked to drug use.

The decision was so fair that one wonders whether baseball commissioner Ueberroth is better suited for a judgeship than for political office, the future career with which his name has been most often associated.

Essentially, Ueberroth told the players: You've repented your sin of drug use, but you must do penance. You can play, but you must pay.

In Parker's case, the penance is distinctly painful. He will lose 10 percent of a year's salary, must volunteer for 100 hours of community service and must submit to random drug testing. But Parker's $100,000 loss will go to drug and alcohol abuse programs in the Cincinnati area, not to some petty-cash fund in the commissioner's office. And because it's a donation, Ueberroth says, it's tax deductible.

The drug testing is a more important aspect, though, because it will be a vital step toward ensuring that transgressions are not repeated. Ueberroth has sought drug testing for all players since Parker and others were implicated in a Pittsburgh cocaine trial last summer. The players' union has resisted, but the commissioner is finding ways to get his wish, slowly but surely.

Many of the contracts negotiated this spring have clauses requiring players to submit to drug tests. If the club owners refuse to erase such clauses in years to come, testing will, in effect, become mandatory—and no player can say that someone is changing the rules in the middle of the game.

We probably haven't seen the last of the cocaine clouds. New York's Keith Hernandez says he'll appeal Ueberroth's decision. And just a week ago, San Diego pitcher LaMarr Hoyt (he's the one who delayed Pete Rose's Ty-breaking hit by one day) checked into a drug treatment program.

Baseball fans know that hope springs eternal, though. Perhaps the worst of the cocaine storm is over and we can get down to the serious business of oiling the glove and rubbing pine tar—but not too much!—on the bat.

The Times-Picayune
The States-Item

New Orleans, LA, March 5,1986

Baseball Commissioner Peter Ueberroth has taken firm and promising action against drug abuse by big league baseball players. Last Friday, the commissioner conditionally suspended for one year seven well known players linked to drug use. He suspended four others for 60 days, but gave them an opportunity to avoid the penalty, and he said that 10 other players, who were not suspended, would have to agree to drug testing for the remainder of their careers.

The Ueberroth plan appears to have been carefully weighed. It contains elements of toughness, compassion and pragmatism. Rather than outright suspending or banning the offenders from baseball, he has offered them an opportunity to be a good influence on other players and to make amends to the national pastime and baseball fans. He has given them a chance to work against the drug menace that threatens to undermine public confidence in all professional sports.

One-year suspensions were imposed on Joaquin Andujar, Keith Hernandez, Dave Parker, Lonnie Smith, Jeff Leonard, Dale Berra and Enos Cabell. But they can continue to play if they donate 10 percent of their salaries to drug-prevention programs, agree to random drug testing for the rest of their careers and give 100 hours of community service in each of the next two years.

Players Al Holland, Lary Sorensen, Lee Lacy and Claudell Washington were suspended for 60 days. But Commissioner Ueberroth said they could avoid the penalty by donating 5 percent of their salaries, doing 50 hours of community service and agreeing to drug testing for the rest of their playing days.

The third group of players simply had to agree to drug testing for the rest of their careers.

Mr. Ueberroth's approach on a case-by-case basis, as he put it, is necessarily experimental. It could fail if the penalized players do not live up to the terms imposed. It is not a drug policy for all of baseball. It does not set specific penalties in advance so that other players will understand precisely what they face if they violate the policy. By contrast, the National Basketball Association's drug-abuse policy resulted in the "permanent" dismissal last Tuesday of Micheal Ray Richardson, pending a possible appeal in two years.

The 21 players cited by the baseball commissioner have an opportunity to demonstrate that something short of unforgiving suspensions or outright banishment from baseball will work to stop the baseball drug epidemic. To that extent, the penalty rightly places the tremendous burden and responsibility on the individual players involved to help right what has gone so terribly wrong with their career sport.

The Pittsburgh
PRESS

Pittsburgh, PA, March 2, 1986

Baseball Commissioner Peter Ueberroth has instituted the suspended suspension.

A baseball suspension now can be defined as a fine, because it can be assumed that none of the 12 players handed penalties for drug abuse would sit out any part of their careers.

The fines, 10 percent of their 1986 salaries for seven players and 5 percent for five others, amount to big bucks when compared with the salaries of most of the people who paid to see them perform while they were using drugs.

For instance, Dave Parker will have to give $87,500 to a Cincinnati drug-prevention center, but he will be left with an estimated base income of $787,500 for this baseball season. Dale Berra, even with his propensity to bobble everything he gets his hands on, still will be able to clutch more than $460,000 worth of paychecks this year after he gives about $51,000 to a New York drug center.

Unfortunately, Mr. Ueberroth, as commissioner, is the team owners' representative in major league baseball and the suspended suspensions reflect that alliance. These are valuable gate attractions he is dealing with, and outright suspension could affect both the win-loss and profit-loss ledgers.

He has, therefore, sent a poor message to young fans. If you are important enough, you can get away with drug abuse, or, even worse, buy your way out if you do get caught.

The players, of course, think even this action is too drastic and will file a grievance in an attempt to overthrow the ruling.

Meanwhile, Mr. Ueberroth made two more mistakes. He should have made certain that the players' donations to the drug centers be made non-tax-deductible. We fear the taxpayer will be subsidizing the fines if players, after turning the money over to non-profit drug centers, call the fines charitable donations.

And Mr. Ueberroth should have made them pay the fines to centers in the city where they were playing at the time of their addiction. Pittsburghers paid to see Dave Parker and Dale Berra play while they were abusing drugs. Pittsburgh, not Cincinnati and New York, should have the benefit of their fines.

The least we can say for Mr. Ueberroth's action is it was certainly charitable.

BUFFALO EVENING NEWS

Buffalo, NY, March 5, 1986

Baseball Commissioner Peter Ueberroth has meted out fair punishment for nearly two dozen major league ballplayers linked to the illegal use of drugs. In his first such action since becoming commissioner in 1984, Ueberroth balanced penalties with opportunities to earn a second chance. He needs to make it clear, however, that future drug abusers will not get off quite so lightly.

By allowing the seven players hit with the toughest penalties to avoid a one-year suspension, the commissioner, permitted them to continue to play ball and receive their lucrative salaries.

To earn that second chance, however, they must contribute 10 percent of their pay to drug rehabilitation facilities and perform drug-related community service for two years. And they must submit to random drug testing for the rest of their careers.

The monetary penalties are stiff, but not so stiff as missing an entire season would be. The community-service requirement can help turn the players' prominence into constructive efforts to deter youngsters tempted to make the same mistakes.

While noting that all the players he interviewed denied any current use of drugs, Ueberroth said the seven penalized most seriously had a "prolonged pattern of drug use" and also "in some fashion facilitated the distribution of drugs in baseball."

Drug abuse poses profound dangers, in sports and in society generally. Professional athletes who use illegal drugs harm themselves and the game that pays their salaries. And they can also mislead millions of youngsters who look up to them as heroes into thinking that drug use really isn't so bad.

The drug problem in professional sports doesn't affect only baseball, of course.

Just the other day the National Basketball Association expelled the second player this season for repeated use of drugs. And recent news reports say that 16 percent of the top 350 college seniors attending National Football League tryouts in January tested positive for drugs.

When you see results like that, said one respected coach, "you wonder what they are thinking about. How dumb can they be?" Pretty dumb, especially in not taking the risks of drug use seriously.

While the Ueberroth ruling is a step in the right direction, major league baseball must not stop there. In the future, players should be put on notice that if they use drugs, they will face mandatory suspensions from the game — with no opportunity to choose lesser alternatives as in the present cases.

In essence, professional baseball should require its athletes to make a choice — either play ball or continue to use drugs and lose that chance.

The Boston Herald

Boston, MA,
March 4, 1986

BASEBALL Commissioner Peter Ueberroth has shown once again he's a guy with all the right moves. Now if only the players' union leaders realize that in their opposition to drug testing they're way out in left field.

Ueberroth announced penalties for 21 players who had testified or were interviewed during last fall's cocaine trials in Pittsburgh. The penalties included donations of a portion of the player's salary (5 percent for some, 10 percent for others) to anti-drug efforts, time to be spent in community service, and submitting to routine drug testing in the future. Thus far at least 12 players have agreed to to the action.

The commissioner's proposal was fair, relevant to the offenses committed and put the entire sport on the right track.

But most important of all in announcing action in these particular cases Ueberroth also let it be known that he was taking the entire issue of drug testing out of the hands of the individual teams and making his office responsible.

"Rehabilitation must be independent of the team because what does a team do?" he asked. "It finds the first doctor that will say the player is cured so they can get him back in the lineup. I'm not in the business of winning; individual teams are."

Makes sense, right?

The move toward mandatory drug testing is gaining momentum. Some 350 players already have drug testing clauses in their contracts. An agent who represents some 90 players, including five disciplined by the commissioner, said he will urge the sport to adopt a uniform testing program.

Even some individual player representatives have come on board. Only the Major League Baseball Players Association leadership thus far remains opposed to drug testing.

It's time they too came on board for the good of their own members and of the sport.

ST. LOUIS POST-DISPATCH

St. Louis, MO, March 3, 1986

Baseball Commissioner Peter Ueberroth was firm but not unduly harsh in disciplining players who have been known to have drug problems. Some of the 11 who received the stiffest penalties almost instantly announced they would appeal through their union. But the players ignore the seriousness of the drug problem at their peril; and Mr. Ueberroth has sent clear signs on how they can hit their way out of the hole.

Seven players (three former Cardinals) who not only used drugs but "in some fashion facilitated the distribution of drugs in baseball" were given one-year, unpaid suspensions. The suspensions will not go into effect so long as the players agree to donate 10 percent of their salaries to drug programs, to submit to random drug testing throughout their careers and to contribute 100 hours of community service a year for two years. Lesser penalties were doled out to those with more limited drug involvement. Six of the seven testified in last summer's celebrated drug trial in Pittsburgh and were given immunity from prosecution. Mr. Ueberroth was right to see that the matter did not end there. Baseball cannot tolerate drug abuse and distribution by its highly paid stars.

An important facet of the drug testing is that it will be done through the commissioner's office, rather than by each team. Close to half of the 700 players in major-league baseball, according to Mr. Ueberroth, already agree to voluntary drug testing. The commissioner's office and players' union need to work out a program that would bring in the rest, for drugs are detrimental to the game and to every individual who becomes their victim.

FORT WORTH STAR-TELEGRAM

Fort Worth, TX, March 7, 1986

Baseball Commissioner Peter Ueberroth took an important, and long overdue, step when he conditionally suspended several major league baseball players for using cocaine. The punishment he meted out could have been sterner and probably should have been. But at least, major league baseball is now officially on record as opposing the use of "recreational" drugs.

Ueberroth suspended the players for a year but offered to lift the suspensions if the players agreed to certain conditions, including contributing 10 percent of their salaries to drug prevention programs and submitting to future drug tests.

Despite complaints from several of the players and the threat of legal action by the players union, Ueberroth's action appears quite fair. Too fair to suit the tastes of many observers.

Nationally syndicated columnist Carl Rowan this week described the punishment as far too lenient. Respondents to the Star Poll in this newspaper expressed overwhelming dismay (76 percent to 24 percent) that sterner measures weren't taken against the offending players.

Such sentiment is easy to understand, and we would share it if it weren't for a belief that Ueberroth knows what he is doing and that anytime a carrot-and-stick approach is used, the threat posed by the stick can be quite effective.

Other players have been put on notice: Ueberroth is not going to sit idly by and see the game destroyed by dopeheads. But he also is willing to give offenders a chance to straighten up and, through forfeiting parts of their salaries, help others fight drug dependency.

Players should realize something else, too. Fans are growing weary of seeing baseball's dirty linen flapping in the breeze, and the fans ultimately have far more power than Ueberroth. If they become disgusted enough to stop buying tickets to the games, baseball's cocaine-snorting oafs will be out on the street permanently.

When that happens, Ueberroth's carrot will look mighty sweet indeed.

The Chattanooga Times

Chattanooga, TN, March 11, 1986

Baseball Commissioner Peter Ueberroth tempered firmness with compassion in disciplining 11 players found to have used drugs, including some who helped distribute them. But he also sent the message that future infractions will be dealt with severely. A few of the players who received the harshest punishment have said they will appeal the penalties through their union. That is their right, of course, but it also indicates they have failed to perceive the seriousness of the problem.

Mr. Ueberroth gave each of the seven players who used and helped distribute drugs unpaid suspensions of a year. But he said he would suspend the sentence, so to speak, if the players would agree to donate 10 percent of their salaries to drug treatment programs, to submit to periodic drug testing for the rest of their professional careers, and to contribute 100 hours of community service a year for two years. The rest of the players whose involvement was more limited received lighter penalties.

Six of the seven players punished most severely testified last summer in that famous drug trial in Pittsburg — but in return for immunity from prosecution. It is to Mr. Ueberroth's credit that he made sure that was not the last word in the case. His actions last week affirm that baseball cannot and will not tolerate drug abuse within the sport, much less distribution by its well-paid players.

According to the commissioner, the drug testing will be done through his office and not by each team. It's also important that more than half of the 700 major league players have agreed to voluntary tests. The hope is that the commissioner's office and the players' union can agree on a program to persuade the rest of the players to volunteer. It's not just that drug use is bad for the players. It's also bad for the sport in the eyes of million of fans, young and old alike.

The San Diego Union

San Diego, CA, March 6, 1986

Baseball Commissioner Peter Ueberroth should be applauded for his efforts to crack down on major-league players who use illegal drugs. Last week's decision to punish 21 players for their well-documented drug use has sent a clear message to players and fans that the commissioner is serious about solving baseball's drug problem.

Commissioner Ueberroth ordered seven players to contribute 10 percent of their salaries and 200 hours of community service to anti-drug efforts or face one-year suspensions from baseball. Four other players were offered the choice of contributing 5 percent of their salaries and 50 hours of community service or receiving 60-day suspensions. These 11 players, and 10 others with known drug problems, also must submit to random drug testing for the remainder of their major-league careers.

One of the guilty players, Keith Hernandez of the New York Mets, has vowed to fight the commissioner's ruling by filing a grievance under baseball's collective-bargaining agreement.

Some columnists and commentators argue the Ueberroth order is too lenient. Some players, the Major League Players Association, and some sportswriters argue that the commissioner is being too tough.

These critics forget a significant fact. Several of these players could be in federal prison instead of spring training camp had they not been granted immunity for their testimony in a Pittsburgh drug trial last year. Confronted by hard evidence, and safe from prosecution, many admitted violating state and federal drug laws.

Although Commissioner Ueberroth has correctly identified drug abuse by players as one of baseball's most serious problems, major-league baseball still has no uniform anti-drug policy. Even so, some gains are being made. As many as one-half of the 650 major-league players now have drug-testing clauses in their contracts.

Nevertheless, drug-testing remains particularly troublesome to carry out. The Major League Players Association asserts that drug-testing clauses are invalid, that they violate baseball's collective-bargaining agreement.

Questions abound. Neither the commissioner nor most teams have decided or disclosed what would happen should a player fail a drug test. Would the player be sent to a rehabilitation center, fined, suspended, or booted from the team? And, how many tests can a player fail before he is punished? No one seems to know.

Contrast the uncertain drug policy in the baseball world with that of the National Basketball Association, which recently banned Michael Ray Richardson for life after his third violation of the league's anti-drug policy. Perhaps three chances is one too many, but at least the NBA has a policy. Three strikes and you're out; baseball players should understand that easily enough.

San Diego baseball fans are reassured that, among the 26 major-league teams, the Padres have one of the best anti-drug programs. Much credit for this goes to owner Joan Kroc, whose Operation Cork is a major contributor to the nationwide fight against drug and alcohol abuse. The Padres were the first of the major-league teams to implement drug testing for minor-league players. And team officials demonstrated patience and compassion in helping former second baseman Alan Wiggins overcome his cocaine addiction.

Significantly, the Padres have left no doubt that a second drug incident would not be tolerated. When Wiggins became a repeat offender, the Padres kept their word and cast him out, even though this cost them dearly. The message was clear: This team won't tolerate drug abuse.

Most Padre players apparently feel the same way. Twelve have signed contracts with drug-testing clauses. Several players whose contracts don't require drug testing, including such stars as outfielder Tony Gwynn and shortstop Garry Templeton, say they would willingly submit to the tests.

The Padres' policy is sufficiently meritorious to be a model for all professional sports teams. Random drug tests should be required of all players, first offenders should be provided the best treatment and counseling available, and second offenders should be sent packing.

St. Louis Review

St. Louis, MO, March 10, 1986

The recent actions of the Baseball Commissioner concerning drug use in the major leagues is a real breath of fresh air. Maybe it marks the end of the "ho-hum" attitude toward drug abuse among the idolized.

Major league players expect a lot from their fans: huge salaries, support, attendance, loyalty and glowing admiration. To date, this has been almost exclusively a one-way street. The Commissioner has decreed that we get more for our money than commercial spin-offs.

The old private life/professional life schizophrenia should be made a thing of the past. A person cannot live two different lives or have two sets of morals depending whether he is on the field or in the locker room.

One of the admirable parts of the Commissioner's decision is that it came from within the baseball industry itself. Hopefully the entire sport will rally behind the ruling and not try to justify the unjustifiable. When wrong has been done, those who are guilty should accept the consequences of their behavior. There may be some fine points to argue in this case, but the fact remains: something had to be done and what was done seems reasonable and fair.

Maybe the entertainment industry could learn a lesson from all this; government officials as well. How long can we see those who capture so many of the headlines be convicted of drug use and have it make no difference? Those who live off the public should pay damages to the public when they violate the public trust. How much good could be done in drug/alcohol treatment programs if rock stars convicted of drug use had to donate 10 percent of their earnings to drug prevention programs?

Of course, the real issue is not paying for mistakes, but learning from them. Baseball fans are willing to let bygones be bygones. Although it is wrong to conclude that "nobody got hurt," we would all be satisfied with improvement. This might be, it could be, it is, the best thing that could have come of this situation.

Len Bias, Top College Basketball Star, Dies After Cocaine Use

Len Bias, 22, University of Maryland basketball player who June 17 had been the second selection overall and the first by the champion Boston Celtics in the National Basketball Association's (NBA) annual draft of college players, collapsed in the early morning in a university dorm room in College Park, Md. June 19. He was pronounced dead of cardiac arrest at Leland Memorial Hospital in Riverside, Md. Early reports of Bias' death indicated that traces of cocaine had been found in the athlete's urine and that a bag containing white powder had been found in his leased car. State medical examiner John Smialek June 24 ruled that Bias had indeed died of cocaine intoxication. An overdose of cocaine can result in confusion, depression, headache and dizziness. During severe overdose there is circulatory collapse, respiratory failure and cardiac arrest. In cases of acute toxicity, death can occur in as little as two to three minutes or in as long as 30 minutes. Lethal doses vary according to the method of administration. Ingesting cocaine, which a later coroner's report determined Bias' administration to be, is more toxic than snorting it.

Bias, a Born-Again Christian, had recently passed drug tests administered to him by several NBA clubs. Bias had been named an All-America and Atlantic Coast Conference Player-of-the-Year during his senior season. Celtic star Larry Bird captured the feeling of much of the sports world when he called Bias' death "the cruelest thing I ever heard."

The sports world was shocked again June 27 when Don Rogers, 23, a defensive back for the Cleveland Browns, collapsed at his family's Sacramento, Calif. home and died within a few hours. The Sacramento County Coroner's Office June 30 officially announced that his death, which occurred a day before he was to be married, was "due to cocaine poisoning."

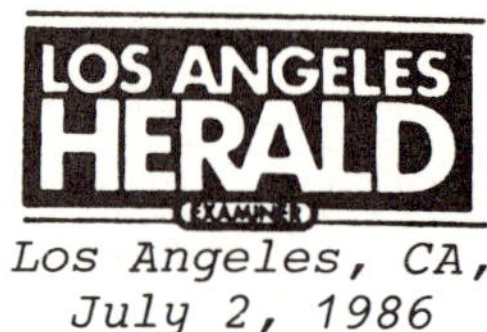

Los Angeles, CA,
July 2, 1986

It's unlikely that Len Bias and Don Rogers felt they were taking a gamble when they ingested what turned out to be fatal quantities of cocaine last month. But if any good can come out of the tragic deaths of these gifted athletes — both superbly conditioned and both, friends say, not regular drug users — it's to warn the rest of us that they were taking a far greater risk than was previously recognized.

It's long been understood that cocaine is psychologically addicting. But before the deaths of Bias, arguably the nation's best college basketball player, and Rogers, one of the NFL's finest defensive backs, few recognized how dangerous cocaine was physiologically.

Some medical researchers are becoming increasingly alarmed by cocaine's lethal nature: The drug can inhibit the heartbeat and interrupt brain functioning. The number of deaths attributed to cocaine has skyrocketed. There were 56 reported in L.A. County in 1985, compared to 5 in 1979. Moreover, the inadequate understanding of cocaine's deadliness probably has caused coroners to miss some of its victims. Researchers claim cocaine-induced heart attacks often are diagnosed as simple heart failure.

Only a handful of the 22 million Americans who have tried cocaine will pay the ultimate price. Still, some people are more sensitive to the drug, and they aren't necessarily protected if they use it in small amounts, or infrequently. Vulnerability to cocaine's fatal side effects is unpredictable. Worsening the risk is the fact that the new popularity of smoking the drug, rather than snorting it, makes it harder to control the amount consumed.

Neither Bias nor Rogers were felled by minute amounts of cocaine. Autopsies revealed that the quantities in both their bloodstreams were higher than normally considered fatal. But one mistake is all it takes, even for these two healthy young men who, their friends say, never used cocaine.

Bias and Rogers paid an awful price for their mistake. If it happened to them, it can happen to anyone.

THE SACRAMENTO BEE
Sacramento, CA, July 1, 1986

Don Rogers wasn't a drug addict. Neither was Len Bias. They were winners, stupendous athletes, both of them at the beginning of their prime, and good people, whose devastated families and teammates keep shaking their heads in disbelief: He wasn't like that, they keep saying. Each was as dedicated to his own good health as one would expect a star athlete to be. Except at one party, when each tried what far too many others also consider just a lark — safe as long as you keep it recreational. And each died.

Cocaine can do that. It's not like cigarettes that kill slowly over a lifetime of use or alcohol, which is dangerous only when abused. Cocaine can kill in one hit — besides what damage it does over the longer run to anyone who becomes addicted to it. Why hasn't the message gotten across?

There are answers. Cocaine is such an exhilarating high — it really does create that surge of prowess that it's advertised to — that all the downbeat public service messages about the toll it eventually takes are hard for anyone to believe who's tried it once or twice. And after years of drug education efforts that tried to scare kids with undiscriminating horror stories about every drug from marijuana to heroin, a sort of immunity to learning — the cry-wolf effect — has built up.

Too little of that "education" was honest; too little of it acknowledged what's unknown about why some people become addicted abusers and others can go on happily for a lifetime of moderate social drinking; too little was aimed at those who know what drugs do and think that they're smart enough to keep it under control.

A young person is easily left with the impression that if he isn't a raving maniac, if he's not forced into dealing in dark alleys with hoodlums, he's beat the downside; he's safe. It's not true. Cocaine is widely available — from the kind of with-it, successful people you would be pleased to call your friends. And you needn't have hit bottom yourself to be in danger from it. You can just be using it to play your best game. Or you can even know better than that, and just be using it for fun one night, celebrating your draft by the world-champion Boston Celtics or your upcoming wedding. And die.

It's not just the families and friends of Len Bias and Don Rogers who have to face that tragedy. The ignorance that killed those two most promising young men is widely shared. It is a sword hanging over all of us.

SYRACUSE
HERALD·JOURNAL
Syracuse, NY, June 23, 1986

You didn't have to be a basketball fan to be shocked by the tragic death of Len Bias. The former University of Maryland forward was the second player picked in last week's pro basketball draft. He was about to become a millionaire and a star for the world champion Boston Celtics. He was living, in his words, "a dream within a dream."

Two days later he was dead. For some reason the doctors couldn't immediately explain, his heart just stopped beating. Our first reaction when the bulletin came over the wire services was much the same as everyone's — a reluctance to believe it. Our second reaction, born of the times, was a suspicion that drugs were involved.

The next day, Bias' coach at Maryland, Lefty Driesell, told a national television audience: "From what I understood from the police there was a trace of cocaine in his urine.... If that's the case, it's completely out of character for Leonard Bias. I would be completely shocked."

Official confirmation awaits the completion of laboratory tests in several days. If they bear out the suspicions, Len Bias will have become another statistic. He will take his place with the other casualties of the cocaine epidemic. He may be better known than the school kids, professional people, laborers and skid-row bums that this "recreational" drug has claimed, but he's no less dead.

There is speculation that this may have been Bias' first experiment with cocaine. Friends say they never knew him to use drugs and he was only an occasional drinker. He knew his body was his future, and he took care of it. He may have made one mistake in an unguarded moment at a party. That's all it took.

Medical experts say it's quite possible for someone to die after a first experience with cocaine. even if it's only a small amount, and even if they have had no earlier evidence of heart disease. (Bias had recently been examined and found fit.) They don't really know why the drug affects some people in this way; they suspect it may have something to do with the sudden rise in blood pressure immedately after a toot.

There is an obvious lesson here for anyone contemplating trying cocaine, as well as habitual users. Sometimes, that first time — or the next time — leaves the user with no second chance.

Will people pay attention? Probably not. The consequences aren't given much thought when someone's offered that first hit — it's just a lark, after all — or when a junkie needs the stuff. Even a high-profile example of what can go wrong isn't likely to inspire much caution.

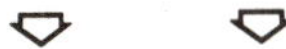

Cocaine is a plague that defies every attempt to control it. Every so often, some politician will declare "war on drugs," vowing to round up the pushers, bad-mouthing the countries that don't do more to halt the flow of what has become a major cash crop. It's a losing battle; the problem just gets bigger.

We are poorer for not have Len Bias around to entertain us on the basketball court for the next several years. We'd love to think he will become a martyr in the cause of ridding drug-abuse from society, that kids and adults everywhere will wise up after witnessing the kind of damage it can do.

It won't happen. If all it took was a tragedy to keep people from being stupid, no one would smoke cigarettes, or drink too much, or drive too fast.

There will continue to be drug victims wheeled into morgues with appalling frequency because they thought they were indestructible, that the worst only happened to "other people." It's a sad, frightening thing to contemplate.

The News and Courier
Charleston, SC, June 26, 1986

The sudden death last week of University of Maryland basketball star Len Bias was a shock. How could such a near-perfect athlete with no known physical problems — the top pick of the world champion Boston Celtics — die so young of cardiac arrest?

It was a mystery at first, but now the reason is clear. Len Bias died because he ingested an almost pure form of cocaine. He had been celebrating his selection as the No. 2 pick in the National Basketball Association draft. He was on the verge of becoming a multimillionaire. A dream of a lifetime was coming true for the 22-year-old Bias, but he would not live to see it through.

Cocaine — possibly "crack," the highly addictive and extremely dangerous form of the drug — was found in urine samples taken shortly after his death. Almost 12 grams of cocaine were in the car he had been using, according to preliminary reports. He suffered brain seizures, his heart began beating irregularly and stopped shortly after taking the drug, according to the medical examiner who conducted the autopsy. The final statistic to be recorded on Maryland's prized All-American is that he was the 16th person known to have died from cocaine use in the state in the last three years.

Len Bias' fate is refocusing the nation's attention on the dangers of cocaine, a drug that, once the euphoria wears off, can lead to depression, paranoia, psychological addiction, convulsions, brain seizures, heart attacks and death. Hopefully, the word will spread not only through the adult world but to the schools, the community gyms, the inner-city playgrounds and rural dirt courts where the game in which Len Bias excelled means so much to young people who are so susceptible to the temptations of drugs. Perhaps it will help some of them understand that no one, not even the fittest of the fit, is immune to the ravages of cocaine. Perhaps they will realize that the authorities are not crying "wolf" about this drug. Perhaps the glamor so wrongly associated with cocaine will be stripped away and the bitter truth will be shown.

Cocaine destroys lives. Playing around with it is a foolish and deadly game.

THE DENVER POST
Denver, CO, June 25, 1986

THE SADDEST sports story of the year — maybe of the decade — is now official: Maryland basketball star Len Bias was killed by cocaine.

Dr. John Smialek, Maryland state medical examiner, announced the results of the autopsy of Bias' body Tuesday. He ruled that the star athlete died of "cocaine intoxication which interrupted the normal electrical control of his heartbeat, resulting in the sudden onset of seizures and cardiac arrest."

No decent person can look at what happened to Bias and not feel sympathy for his family — and a twinge of fear at how viciously drugs can strike at even the strongest in our society. Smialek said there was no evidence of previous drug use by Bias or of an allergic reaction. He was killed outright by a normal snort of cocaine, pure and simple.

The story of one of the healthiest men in America taking a dangerous drug for what might have been his first time, and then suddenly dying, is a sad one. But maybe it takes a tragedy of this scale to expose the naked hypocrisy of those who have pleaded to "let the mystery of his death be buried with him" so as not to tarnish his memory.

There is no mystery in Len Bias' death — only a lesson. He used cocaine, and it killed him.

All the flowery tributes to the powerful body that moved so gracefully across basketball courts can't match the blunt force of Arthur Marshall, Prince George's County state's attorney, in summing up the meaning of the storybook life — and squalid death — of Len Bias:

"There's no surprises there at all. Anybody that takes a damn straw to their nose ought to think, 'It can happen to me if it can happen to Len Bias.' "

AKRON BEACON JOURNAL
Akron, OH, July 1, 1986

LEN BIAS is dead, Don Rogers is dead, and drug abuse is the reason. It doesn't matter if it was the first time or the 500th time these two young men used dangerous drugs; the result has the same tragic finality.

These two gifted athletes are not the only recent victims of drug abuse, only the most visible. Illegal drugs extract a huge toll each year in this country, in lost lives and careers. Most of those affected are anonymous except to their families and friends. They are merely statistics until the fate of a Don Rogers or Len Bias focuses national attention on this growing problem.

The temptation is to simply mourn the loss: So much promise and so little time to use it. And we look for scapegoats — the greedy world of pro sports that provides temptation after temptation; an educational system, indeed a whole society, that pampers and protects star athletes and isolates them from reality.

The blame can certainly be shared, but the prime culprit is the victim himself, who takes a chance and discovers too late that the odds are against him. And if the eulogies are true and these really are the fine, young men they are portrayed to be, then the problem is so out of control that we have to rethink the methods for dealing with it.

The Cleveland Browns, for which Don Rogers played defensive back, recognized the drug abuse in pro sports and organized a farsighted counseling program to deal with its victims. It's not enough.

Last summer, a parade of baseball players testified about how cocaine abuse affects the game. League officials wrung their hands, slapped some wrists, and declared the problem solved. It's not enough.

Neither will the abuse be taken care of solely through committees of the National Collegiate Athletic Association, drug awareness programs in public schools, or public appearances by Nancy Reagan, who has done much to raise consciousness on this problem. It might have to be admitted that the problem in sports is uncontrollable, too deeply ingrained in the way we make gods of celebrities and allow them to conform only to their own, special standards.

But it is clearly time for the government to launch a major campaign against drugs, similar to those against smoking and drunken driving. The government should certainly provide more funding for drug enforcement agencies, but the nation is unlikely to ever completely stop the flow of dangerous drugs.

Drug use simply has to be made socially unacceptable, and the users seen as pathetic. As long as they are portrayed as daring, if misguided, risk-takers, the appeal — and the tragedy — will continue.

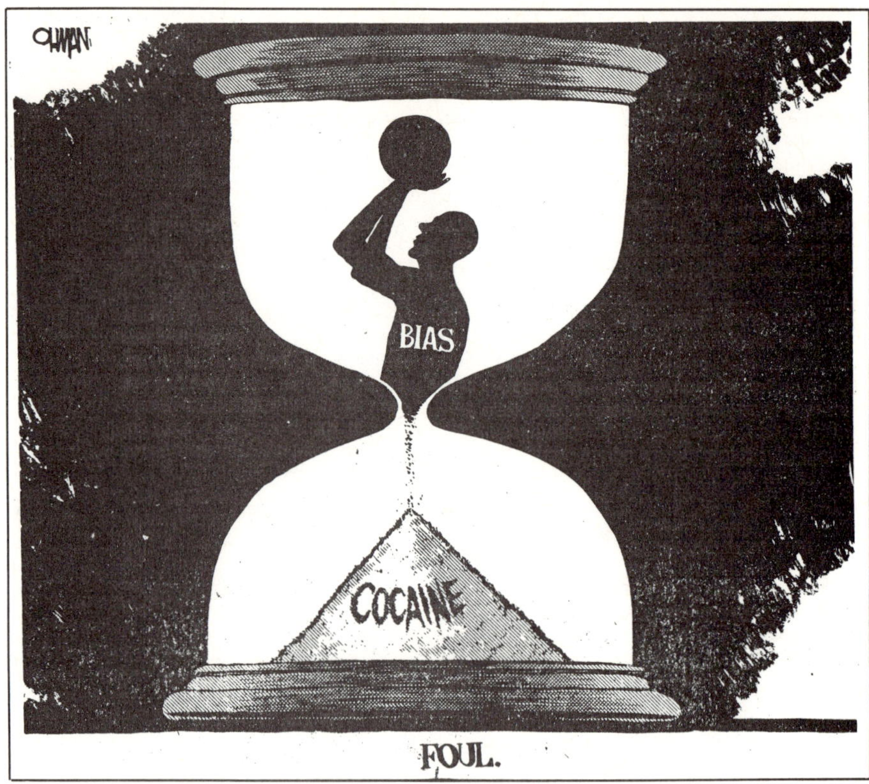

The Evening Gazette
Worcester, MA, June 30, 1986

Cocaine contributed to the death of Len Bias on the eve of a professional basketball career, but a secondary tragedy for some of his surviving teammates and others involves the continuing triumph of athletics over academics.

Many of the larger universities in National Collegiate Athletic Association 1-A programs are playing games with their athletes. They have adopted the philosophy that student-athletes aren't to be confused with students. They aren't held to the same standard; they aren't expected to graduate with the rest of their class. It is typical of the ways in which some young men, particularly those talented in football and basketball, are shortchanged on campuses where they are supposed to be preparing for productive lives, not just professional sports careers.

At the University of Maryland, where Bias played, most athletes are in a General Studies program. It's "a flexible educational structure for students who choose not to select a specific major." It means that students can take whatever courses and whatever subjects they choose. Bias had expressed an interest in majoring in art or interior design, but took General Studies because it was more compatible with basketball demands. Despite his own feeling that a degree would mean a great deal, Bias took recreation courses, reportedly chosen by his coaches. And he did not pass many of them.

The academic counselor for the Maryland athletics department, who resigned because she could not bring about a change in attitude among coaches, said Bias and another teammate stopped attending classes after the fall semester. They didn't make a pretense of being students.

Under NCAA rules, athletes must earn 24 credits a year towards a degree. That's four three-credit courses a semester. At Maryland, a 1.9 grade-point-average is good enough to stay in school. Wendy Whittemore, the counselor, said that all of the basketball players started the last academic year at 2.0, but many dropped to 1.5 averages after the fall semester and remained there through the November-to-March season. That's D-plus, C-minus range and technically they weren't qualified to continue as students.

She said there was depression and anger among team players because they were traveling a great deal and didn't have enough time to study. "All of them were feeling like a mountain had been shoveled on them and there was no way they were going to get out from under that."

Coaches certainly must take some of the responsibility for academic failure of their players just as they take credit to some degree for individual talents and team wins. Maryland basketball coach Lefty Driesell was quick to insist that drugs were not a problem with his team. That may be so, but he has been reticent about discussing the academic needs of his players.

In Driesell's words, "Len Bias was not failing. Someone wrote that he flunked all of his courses last spring, which is true, he did." Perhaps the basic problem is that the University of Maryland doesn't use the word "flunk" or "fail" but says a student is "academically dismissed." That gives students, particularly athletes, the opportunity to take courses over at night or in summer school without a blemish on their records.

The previous counselor at Maryland, who quit last year, said the coaches' attitudes toward academics were detrimental, although they probably would deny it. He said Driesell and others frequently asked about class attendance, but only to be sure that players were going to be eligible.

Len Bias was not alone in his academic swamp. Eleven of 18 college seniors drafted by National Basketball Association teams a few weeks ago did not graduate in four academic years. They attended various colleges and universities. Some were many credits short of attaining a degree. That's a sad, tragic commentary on what and where some university and college priorities are for athletes these days.

The Times-Picayune
The States-Item
New Orleans, LA, June 21, 1986

There is no mystery why the sudden death of 22-year-old Len Bias shocked the sports world and all others familiar with his exploits as a University of Maryland basketball player. It is simple: He was a young man of extraordinary athletic abilities, an apparently superb physical specimen on the threshold of an outstanding and very lucrative professional career. He was on top of his world.

One day he was seen on national television celebrating his drafting by the National Basketball Association champion Boston Celtics. Two days later, the television cameras showed his shrouded body being wheeled to an ambulance.

The news would have been no less shocking or sad had death come suddenly to an equally promising and celebrated young opera star, politician, musician or novelist.

We are saddened because a young man died unexpectedly at the very threshold of a career universally expected to be one for the record books. The sense of sadness and shock is compounded because of a national preoccupation with youth that often exaggerates its strengths and virtues. As anyone who has survived it knows, youth can be more vulnerable than age. Deaths like that of Len Bias remind us that we are all mortal regardless of age.

Yet there is a mystery associated with, or at least suggested by, the death of this splendid young athlete. While there are indications that the condition that killed Len Bias may have been founded on a congenital heart disorder, there are also suggestions that it might have been triggered by the use of cocaine.

Traces of the drug reportedly were found in his urine. A police spokesman says the death is being treated as "suspicious" and a homicide investigation is under way.

The wider mystery, then, is why so many youths, including many of uncommon promise, cannot seem to resist the dangerous lure of illegal drugs. Indications that Len Bias might even have experimented with drugs evoked almost as much disbelief as his death among his university and professional associates. "Drugs weren't part of the lifestyle of the Lenny Bias that I knew," said Richard M. Dull, the Maryland athletic director.

Similar expressions of disbelief came from Boston Celtics officials, who had placed great value on the player's strength of character in making him the second player they chose in the NBA draft.

No one is suggesting that Len Bias was anything close to being a regular drug user. Further tests might indicate that drugs had nothing to do with his death. But the suspicion of drug use in connection with this tragedy nevertheless calls attention to the pervasiveness of the drug problem.

The mystery remains why so many athletes, including many with their fortunes already assured, as well as other youths cannot seem to avoid the flame of drugs. Anyone can die at any time. But no one has to risk everything on drugs any more than he or she has to jump off the nearest bridge. The mystery is why so many people can't seem to get that through their heads.

Richmond Times-Dispatch
Richmond, VA, June 25, 1986

"One of the cruelest things I've ever heard" was the reaction of Boston Celtics superstar Larry Bird to the shocking news last week that 22-year-old Len Bias of the University of Maryland had died of cardiac arrest just two days after the champion Celts had made him their top choice in the National Basketball Association draft. Yesterday's report by the Maryland medical examiner confirmed that a cruel substance called cocaine killed Len Bias. "Cocaine intoxication," the culmination of an all-night celebratory binge in a dormitory room, made an athlete's strong heart stop beating.

One of the cruelest things about this death is that Mr. Bias, from all indications, was not a hardened drug user. He was a superbly conditioned athlete who had been tested recently by the Celtics and three other NBA teams and found to be drug-free. According to friends and relatives, he was a born-again Christian who led an exemplary life and who had warned young people away from drugs. Evidently he succumbed to temptation and made his one fatal mistake in a moment of weakness when he was exhilarated by realization of his dream but also thoroughly fatigued by all the hullabaloo.

Cruel though it may be, remembrances of Len Bias the brilliant athlete must take second place to this stark warning to all who might be tempted to experiment with cocaine: Your first sniff can very well be your last. Dr. Paul D. Thompson, a Brown University cardiologist who has studied sudden death in athletes, told Newsweek that cardiac arrest is a real possibility when a person's system isn't used to the potent stimulant. Furthermore, even before the Bias autopsy, an official of the National Institute of Drug Abuse reported steady increases nationally in cocaine-related deaths and observed that "perfectly healthy young people, with no other risk factors like being overweight, have died of heart attack after snorting cocaine."

Or, as Maryland state's attorney Arthur Marshall, who is leading a criminal investigation in Prince George's County of the Bias death, put it: "Anybody that takes a damn straw to their nose ought to think it can happen to me if it can happen to Len Bias."

As for that investigation, Mr. Marshall has convened a grand jury that will seek testimony from players and acquaintances who may know something about how Len Bias died but who have not been forthcoming with police. He's indicated that he would consider granting immunity from prosecution for someone who used drugs but not for someone who supplied them. The person or persons who gave Mr. Bias the fatal cocaine could be charged with manslaughter. Good. There's nothing cruel about that.

The Louisville Times
Louisville, KY, June 26, 1986

There is a special poignancy in the death of University of Maryland basketball star Len Bias. Here was a young man destined to taste fame and fortune as a professional athlete who has become the most prominent recent victim of the deadly taste of cocaine.

Mr. Bias was an exceptionally talented 22-year-old whom the Boston Celtics would have made a millionaire within a few months. Instead, according to Maryland's chief medical examiner, Mr. Bias died as a result of what was said to be his first encounter with cocaine. The tragedy emphasizes that the drug is a scourge, as emergency room doctors in many communities will confirm, that no longer recognizes social and economic boundaries.

The highly publicized details of Mr. Bias's collapse have revealed cocaine — once regarded as a pricy, but relatively harmless, recreational drug favored by jet setters, baseball players and other well-to-do folk — to be a capricious and indiscriminate killer.

Mr. Bias's vulnerability to the drug should be all the more alarming to others tempted to experiment with it, or with the currently popular and more potent form known as "crack," because he was as healthy and physically fit as a young man can be. The numerous medical exams that preceded the National Basketball Association draft showed no sign of trouble.

But cocaine, which Mr. Bias's friends believe he used that night for the first time to celebrate his recent good fortune, caused his heart to stop beating. And, according to the medical report, he did not die of an overdose. Indeed, the level of the substance in his blood was considered about average.

That is what makes cocaine so insidious. Its effects on the brain and cardiovascular system can without warning kill or hurt people who show every sign of being in excellent health. Users can die from heart attacks, strokes and severe allergic reactions. Anyone with a heart problem is especially vulnerable and should shun cocaine and seek thrills elsewhere.

Cocaine-related deaths and "episodes" requiring medical treatment are increasing in many cities and in the country as a whole because the price of the drug has declined to the point where it is within reach of even low income citizens.

Despite federal attempts to control drug trafficking and the best efforts of local police, moreover, cocaine and "crack" can be easily obtained. Mr. Bias and his companions are said to have bought it on a street in Washington that is literally a drug bazaar. University of Maryland students have told reporters that its use on campus is widespread.

Mr. Bias was a role model for young men and women who admired his skills and his drive for success. His death should serve as a bitter reminder that what at the moment seems to be a harmless "high" can instantly put an end to the brightest hopes.

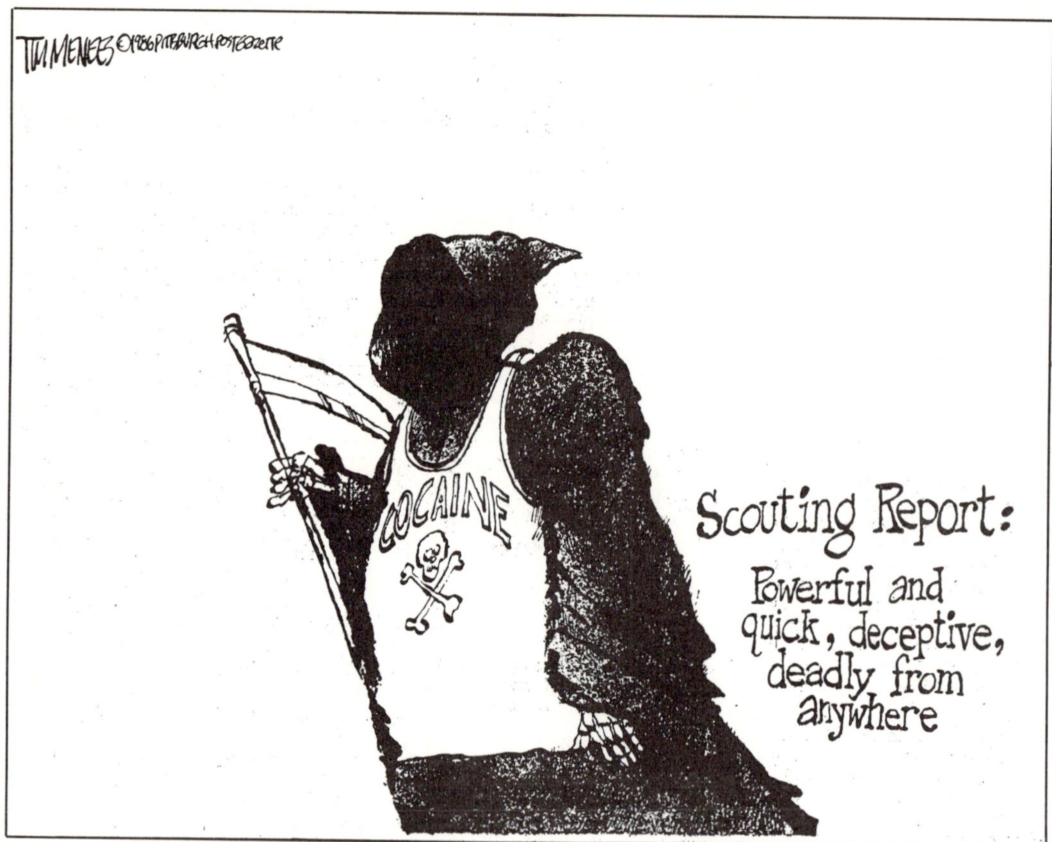

THE LINCOLN STAR

Lincoln, NE, July 1, 1986

Many varied experiences are provided by the world of sports, and sometimes they are so large as to affect life in general. Such is surely true in the case of the two young athletes who recently celebrated a high point in their lives and reaped sudden death.

On June 19, Len Bias died of complications from ingesting cocaine, shortly after celebrating being drafted by the champion Boston Celtics. Bias was a No. 2 draft and one of the handful of top players coming out of the collegiate ranks.

On June 27, Don Rogers died, ending a brilliant professional football career that was just getting started. Coroner's toxicologist James Beede said, "Yes, there was cocaine found in the body. Obviously, it was a lethal dose."

The night before he died, Rogers had been out late, attending a premarital bachelor's party.

In the past four years of record, three men have died of cocaine-related complications in Nebraska. Officials agree that cocaine also may have caused deaths that officially have been attributed to other things.

THE SIGNIFICANCE of Bias' and Rogers' deaths is in the circumstances, as well as the sheer dreadfulness of the events. Both were young, vibrant and at the pinnacle of success.

Both died within hours after celebrating joyous developments in their lives. The pattern, say experts in such matters, is not uncommon.

Very often, people will give drugs a try when they are especially up or down, seeking still higher euphoria or escape from despair or desperation. Once a mind-altering drug such as cocaine is tried, the tendency is to try it again and, perhaps, repeatedly.

With sufficient repetition, cocaine can produce deadly bodily reactions such as heart stoppage or ruptured blood vessels. Cocaine is far more than a moment of artificial exaltation.

AS ROGERS and Bias might have been, one may be lulled into a false idea of cocaine's safety by seeing others use the drug. Cocaine has been glorified as the essence of the drug culture, including the alarming growth in the use of "crack," a cocaine product of especially deadly potential.

Being prominent individuals and in the peak of physical condition, Bias and Rogers are very unfortunate examples of the pitfalls of drug use — even a single experiment with it. No one had any knowledge of any previous drug use by either of those two young men.

Once again, the message is clear — drugs and alcohol can be and often are deadly if abused or when taken beyond proper medical supervision. One experience with an illegal drug and you put your life on the line.

Alcohol still claims more lives in one way or another, but the illegal drugs are devastating to their users. Perhaps the untimely deaths of these two sports figures will serve through their high notoriety as a life-saving caution to others who might think about trying a drug just once to see what it's like.

That one careless experiment could be the end of your life.

THE INDIANAPOLIS STAR

Indianapolis, IN, June 29, 1986

The cocaine death of all-American basketball player Len Bias may save some lives.

It aroused much nonsensical philosophizing and blame-laying, as drug deaths of celebrities do. The silliest response of all blamed warnings against drug abuse for luring people into abusing drugs.

Drug abuse has been killing people for ages. So has alcohol abuse. It's no secret. Why get nasty with people who tell green kids about it?

People abuse drugs and alcohol for fun. They do lots of foolish things for fun. We live in a fun-loving age. People hungry for fun ignore what happened to John Belushi, Jimmi Hendrix, Janis Joplin, Elvis Presley and David Kennedy.

Fun can be risky. Alcohol abuse kills nearly 100,000 Americans a year. Drug abuse kills fewer, but it is moving up on the chart.

There is no sure way to make a big dent in drug and alcohol abuse. Drug suppliers can be caught and supplies seized. But new connections soon replace them. Alcohol is legal.

Finally, there are warnings. Fun-seekers laugh at warnings. But people who don't want more Len Bias types to die young will keep up the warnings.

One consequence is a move for surprise drug tests for athletes. A rugged practice of that might have saved Len Bias.

There is no moral to this story of the untimely death of a promising young athlete. What happened is the moral.

WORCESTER TELEGRAM.
Worcester, MA, July 5, 1986

The tragedy that befell Len Bias in a university dormitory room speaks to his life in the classroom. His failure to grasp the message of cocaine destruction is stacked up alongside the college's failure to educate him. He failed in a moment of indiscretion; his university failed when it put athletics above academics.

This basketball star is not the exception, rather the rule in the world of big-time college sports where gate receipts prevail over all other considerations.

At the close of his senior year at the University of Maryland, Len Bias was 21 credits short of earning a degree. That's not unusual for athletes competing in many NCAA 1-A programs. Of 12 players on the same basketball team with Bias, five had flunked out of school. Only one of three seniors on the Georgia Tech basketball team graduated this spring. None of the three seniors on Clemson's team or the two seniors playing for North Carolina State graduated. Of the 18 seniors drafted in the first round by National Basketball Association teams this year, only seven were graduates. That is appalling.

It denotes massive irresponsibility and cynical exploitation of young athletes. Superstars win games, and winning games means money to colleges and universities. Big-name athletes, all-stars and all-America players are heroes to alumni. They make fund-raising successful.

A player of Bias' caliber could bring up to $15 million to a large institution with national exposure and television rights. It is easy to understand why college administrators and trustees find such a bonanza irresistable. They find ways to ease star athletes through three years of college, only to run into dead ends in the senior year. The norm for athletes in such situations is to spend another year in school or to drop out without a degree.

Some college heroes go on to fame and fortune in professional sports; Bias would have earned an estimated $2 million a year in salary and endorsements playing for the Boston Celtics. But what of the less fortunate yet talented who face life unprepared because they spent their college years playing games? Who is responsible for their future? Who is responsible for the cynical process that compromises education — the sole purpose of a college or university — for a fast buck? How long before these sports factories, hypocritically disguised as institutions of higher education, come to their senses?

Is the "mania of college sports a form of mental illness that infects coaches, college presidents, boards of trustees, state legislators and the press," as one observer suggests? The institutions that resist the disease, including those in Central Massachusetts, deserve much credit. Those that succumb to the temptation and sacrifice the integrity of the academic process invite the sort of just criticism they now receive.

LEXINGTON HERALD-LEADER
Lexington, KY, July 2, 1986

The use of cocaine hasn't come to a screeching halt as the result of the two recent, sudden deaths of athletes who took the drug. Nor is it likely to do so. The influence of cocaine on American culture is too profound, its image too glamorous and swank, for drug dealers to simply fold their tents and slink away.

Nevertheless, the deaths of basketball star Len Bias and football player Don Rogers, both of which have been linked with cocaine, are the kind of tragic examples that drug-education programs can't buy. These were young men in fighting trim, both dead within hours after taking the drug.

There are those who maintain that the impact of such highly publicized deaths will be minimal, rather like seeing a car wreck and then again driving recklessly only moments later. That's a poorly reasoned example. Driving is almost mandatory in the United States. Cocaine use is not. The drug is expensive, addictive, often dangerously difficult to obtain and occasionally packed with impurities. In no way is driving a Ford Escort with the seat belt unfastened like walking the high wire of cocaine purchase and use.

Ingesting cocaine is not a physical need, at least not initially. It is dangerously chic, though. Two big-time deaths may serve to increase the thrill for some, to heighten their feeling of beating the odds. But what about a third celebrity death due to cocaine consumption? Or a fourth?

True, making a really major dent in U.S. cocaine consumption will take more than the deaths of Bias and Rogers, prominent though they have been. But the deaths of celebrities, although not earth-shattering occurrences in themselves, help to publicly focus the dangers of various national perils. When actor Rock Hudson died of AIDS, that disease was brought home to millions of Americans who previously felt it to be an exotic, distant affliction, like the plague. When the luminaries fall, it's far easier to see how the kid next door is at risk, too.

The Star-Ledger
Newark, NJ, June 26, 1986

At 22, Lenny Bias had it made. A superbly gifted athlete, he had just been drafted by the renowned Boston Celtics, this year's winner of the National Basketball Association championship. And he was about to be made an instant millionaire, the assured economic result of being the second player taken in the college draft.

But Lenny Bias never made it. He died from a snort of cocaine that caused his heart to beat erratically, brought on violent seizures and finally a cardiac arrest that killed him. Ironically, he had taken the fatal drug at a college party to celebrate the promising future he was about to embark on as a professional basketball player.

The premature death of Lenny Bias is a lamentable commentary on a society deeply and cruelly enmeshed in a depressing drug culture. There is strong evidence of widespread drug use that is taking place not only on college campuses but in high schools as well.

Drug use is perhaps even more highly visible in American professional sports, where efforts to establish some monitoring mechanisms have been generally thwarted by powerful, resistant player unions. But, then again, it is highly unlikely that drug use among athletes is more extensive than in other social areas; it attracts greater attention because of sports celebrities.

The exalted status of sports in American life should have some redeeming meaning in the aftermath of the drug death of Lenny Bias. The notoriety should serve in a meaningful manner to focus public attention on the deadly implications of drug abuse, the addictive dependence on cocaine and heroin that has become a way of life for far too many Americans of all ages.

Even the most rigorous law enforcement will not be enough to effectively stanch the flood tide of drugs pouring across the borders into the United States. And as long as there are users, there will be drug pushers to supply their demands.

Drug education and rehabilitation programs could be key initiatives in any concerted public effort in trying to finally abate a life-threatening, endemic drug culture that made Lenny Bias the latest of its tragic victims.

Rozelle Urges Drug Testing Plan; Concern Mounts After Bias' Death

The dispute over drug testing mounted in July 1986 when National Football League (NFL) Commissioner Pete Rozelle announced his intention to immediately implement a $1 million per year program that called for each player to submit to two random regular-season urinalysis tests for cocaine, marijuana, opiate, amphetamine and alcohol use. Under the program, a first positive test for substances other than amphetamines would require a player to undergo 30 days of counseling and additional testing at half pay. A second positive test would lead to a 30-day unpaid suspension, and a third would get the player banned from the NFL. Reinstallment of a three-time loser would be at Rozelle's discretion.

Suggesting that Rozelle was using the recent cocaine-related deaths of former Maryland basketball star Len Bias and Cleveland Browns safety Don Rogers to push his plan, the National Football League Players Association objected to the commissioner's unilateral action, saying that it violated the existing agreement between players and management. Although a number of players expressed public support for drug testing, the union didn't buckle under, agreeing to "expedited arbitration" on Rozelle's action. But before arbitrator Richard Kasher of Philadelphia could hold his hearings, Rozelle withdrew his bid. In the meantime, players reporting to summer training camps would be subjected to urinalysis drug testing, which was allowed during the preseason under the league's then current labor agreement signed in 1982.

ARGUS-LEADER

*Sioux Falls, SD,
July 10, 1986*

Professional football players are in tough field position.

The players' union is in the no-win situation of resisting Commissioner Pete Rozelle's plan to start randomly testing players for drug use.

That unfairly taints the National Football League Players Association as favoring

Editorial

drug use, which isn't the case. The union considers the program an unauthorized change in its collective bargaining agreement. The association might have a point, but that's for a judge to decide.

There is no doubt about one thing: the need for drug-testing programs in professional sports.

Among private employers, professional sports have a heavier-than-normal responsibility of keeping ranks clean from drugs because professional athletes serve as role models for youth.

There are too many bad examples for girls and boys. Too many sports heroes have been arrested and convicted in drug and alcohol-related incidents. Too many stars' lives have been shattered. Len Bias, Don Rogers and too many people outside of sports have died.

Rozelle has the right idea. He's trying to impose the strongest anti-drug program in sports.

Under his plan, urine specimens would be taken from players in preseason physicals and in spot-checks during the season. Any player whose drug problem required hospitalization would be suspended for 30 days at half pay. A second hospitalization would mean removal from the roster for 30 days without pay. A player would be banned from the league if he tested positive again.

Gene Upshaw, president of the players association, says the union is not opposed to all anti-drug plans but wants to negotiate a program through collective bargaining. The union has filed a grievance to block Rozelle's plan, which is scheduled to be implemented this month when players go to training camp.

How all this will come out is uncertain, but the need for an anti-drug program like Rozelle's is clear.

THE PLAIN DEALER

Cleveland, OH, July 10, 1986

According to The Washington Post, these are boom times for companies making drug testing equipment. That's in large part because of announcements such as the one this week from National Football League Commissioner Pete Rozelle. The NFL, he said, immediately will begin an enhanced screening program involving all of the league's more than 1,100 players.

Already, there are cries that Rozelle unfairly is making athletes pay for what is a broader problem of society at large. It is argued that the tests are a degrading invasion of the privacy of the players who don't do drugs. The players' union says it will file a grievance because the testing program alters playing conditions as outlined by the 1982 union contract, and that any such changes should be subject to negotiations.

Rozelle counters by saying players, in negotiations, would not accept a testing program that went far enough to deal with the league's drug problem. He claims authority to act under the league's constitution, which gives him power to deal with conduct he finds detrimental to the league's integrity.

There's no question that widespread drug use is a public relations problem for football. In the wake of drug stories that hounded the New England Patriots following last year's Super Bowl—the team admitted that 12 of its players had used illegal drugs during the season—it was only a matter of time before Rozelle acted, as have officials of other sports such as professional tennis, swimming and track and field.

Few people are so naive as to think Rozelle's move will eliminate drugs from professional football. Fewer people are so naive as to think the NFL program will have any impact at all on society at large. But that's not the point. Football players represent huge capital investments, and Rozelle has clear evidence that too many of those investments are going sour because of drug use. He is acting to protect the interest of owners and the sport. Clearly, he should be able to do so.

The program proposed this week seeks to identify the scope of the problem and to establish treatment programs for individuals involved. Those with serious problems identified in the initial tests will be removed from the team roster for 30 days and admitted to hospitals. Those with less serious problems will be counseled for 30 days. If they test positive after that, they also will be removed from the roster for 30 days. If future tests continue to show problems, a player could be banned for at least a year.

An invasion of privacy for a group of employees? Perhaps. But these aren't ordinary employees. They earn high salaries and have a lot of free time on their hands. They play before huge crowds and television audiences.

Rozelle makes a convincing case for strong action. There is a need for the league to provide medical help for those who need it, to keep small drug problems from becoming bigger drug problems, and to improve football's image.

DAILY NEWS
New York, NY, July 9, 1986

Is there anyone left in America who doesn't know that drugs—*especially* cocaine—have ripped through professional sports like a blitzing linebacker? Most athletes have money to burn. The coke is available—it's flooding the nation. And peer pressure to abstain has just about vanished--a new survey reports that by their mid-20s "some 75% to 80% of today's young adults have tried an illicit drug." Terrifying!

Yet incredibly, the Players Association of the NFL fails to get the message. NFL Commissioner Pete Rozelle announced Monday a mandatory drug testing program for all players, including two unscheduled urinalyses each season, with lifetime suspensions for three-time losers.

But the players union is fighting the plan. Dumb! That's not helping players—just the opposite. The addicts need treatment, which the plan includes. Nonusers need protection from drugged-up opponents who play out of control.

Pro athletes hold a special place in society, especially among kids. Many members of the players union say they understand the drug threat—and support Rozelle's plan. If the leaders don't, they're very stupid. Or something worse.

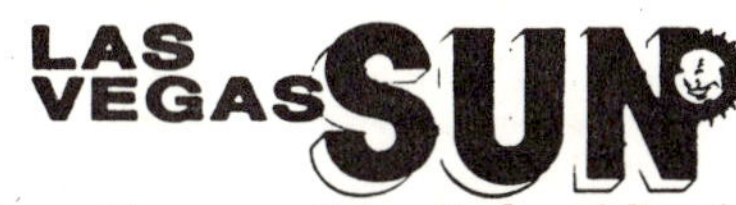

Las Vegas, NV, July 13, 1986

Has it come to this? Mandatory drug testing in the National Football League?

Any time something is "mandatory," there is immediate controversy. If we are *forced* to do something, we often object to it, whether or not it's beneficial to us.

Many players are opposed to the new drug testing plan because they claim it was shoved down their throats. They say, however, they're willing to talk about the issue.

Indeed, the issue must be carefully looked at by both sides. While individuals' rights must be protected, one fact remains: The NFL has not been able to make a serious dent in what is said to be widespread drug usage among its players. Hence, the reason for the proposed *mandatory* testing.

Two tragic deaths

The tragic deaths of basketball star Len Bias and Cleveland Browns' safety Don Rogers have made a serious issue even more serious. The deaths triggered a flood of calls to hotlines across the country from users and parents seeking assurances and more information about cocaine's deadly properties.

Before, players known to be using drugs were fined and/or jailed. Now, they are finding out they may have to pay a higher price for drug usage: their lives. If nothing else, these latest tragedies should tell us that drug use is indeed deadly.

For example, cocaine, which seems to be "the drug of the '80s," is rapidly absorbed into the brain and triggers a rise in the heart rate. Muscle contractions can lead to seizures, causing the user to stop breathing or producing irregular heartbeats leading to heart failure.

Perhaps the NFL would be wise to tackle the problem's very roots. Why do some athletes have a burning need to use drugs? Is the pressure too great? Do they have trouble coping with the instant "status" that comes with six-figured contracts and the trappings that go along with being a "superhero?"

Some say the problem is just symptomatic of drug use in society. It's in the classrooms, boardrooms and playgrounds of America. Why single out athletes?

Whether they like it or not, American athletes are heroes and role models for today's youths. Youngsters want to be like them. They want to feel the roar of the crowd as they run 90 yards for a game-breaking touchdown or hit a grand slam. For many youths, these sports figures represent the American dream.

Tests mandatory at UNLV

What about the right of an individual to do what he wants on his own time? Well, continued drug use carries with it long-lasting effects. And if it begins to alter an athlete's ability to perform his job or tarnishes the image of sports, it becomes the business of the NFL, college or high school.

For two years, UNLV has had mandatory drug testing of its athletes. Now the university plans to broaden its program to include not only testing, but recommendations on counseling and treatment. Such followup is a must if a college is truly interested in helping its athletes develop to their full potential — both on and off the football field or basketball court.

Just because a university has such a program doesn't mean its athletes have a drug problem. But it may be a good way to keep one from developing.

The key is prevention. Start young. Emphasize the *real* effects of drugs on the mind and body, and maybe young athletes will think twice before reaching for them. Hopefully, those feelings will spill over into the general youth population not involved in sports.

The increased concern triggered by Bias' and Rogers' drug-related deaths may be short-lived — until someone else dies.

Whatever their differences, the NFL and players should come to an agreement quickly on the need for a program to curtail drug use — before it's too late for the athlete the testing was designed to help.

The Boston Herald
Boston, MA, July 9, 1986

THREE cheers for NFL Commissioner Pete Rozelle. Enough talk, enough negotiating, enough playing Mr. Nice Guy in the wake of a problem that just won't go away — a problem that grows worse with every passing season.

Rozelle announced a seven-step, league-wide drug testing plan to deal with this problem that we have all come to realize is costing too many lives. It was the bold stroke the sport needed.

Under the plan all NFL players will be subject to random drug tests beginning with the start of training camp this month. All confirmed users would be placed under medical care. Those requiring hospitalization would be removed from team rosters for 30 days, losing half salary the first time it happens, full salary the second time and after one more positive test would be banned from the league.

All draft-eligible college players would also be tested, thus setting the standard early in the game. And the system set up by Rozelle would have the effect of distancing individual teams from the testing and treatment segments. That is both practical and courageous. After all, the self-interest of clubs in having players return to the line-up is an undeniable fact of life.

As usual the player's union — which is apparently more concerned with preserving its prerogatives than with the health of its members and the reputation of the sport they play — is insisting that Rozelle's plan goes well beyond what was negotiated in their contract. It's a sadly narrow vision that will not see what has become all too apparent to most fans.

Rozelle, in announcing his plan, said that NFL players "fit the target group" for drug use by virtue of age, money and time — the off-season, after all is six months long and their high salaries make even cocaine readily available.

Surely the player's union can understand that. Surely even they must concede that those who are abusing drugs need help, and that Rozelle's no-nonsense plan will provide it.

The Courier-Journal
Louisville, KY, July 9, 1986

AFTER THE SUDDEN, shocking deaths of basketball star Len Bias and Cleveland Browns defensive back Don Rogers, many professional football players and other athletes should welcome a program of mandatory drug testing. The fans, especially those with sons and daughters who seek to emulate the immensely talented players in the professional leagues, surely will.

No one should be deluded into thinking that mandatory testing is in itself a cure for the drug plague that seems to have millions of Americans in its grip. Many questions remain about the legality and propriety of an investigative technique that can intrude on individual privacy in a particularly unpleasant way and regularly produces inaccurate results.

Still, the struggle to control and discourage the use of illegal and lethal drugs must be escalated, and the world of professional sports is an obvious target. Although the National Football League Players Association is initially resisting the idea, the random testing program announced this week by NFL Commissioner Pete Rozelle appears to safeguard the rights and well-being of the athletes. It places considerable emphasis on helping players overcome drug habits while establishing the principle that the league won't tolerate serious and continuing abuse.

Although Mr. Rozelle's first priority is to prop up the sagging reputation of the sports business, his plan is basically humanitarian. To the extent that fear of getting caught deters nose guards and running backs from smoking crack or injecting crank, the tests will save lives and preserve careers. Above all, it will help to sever the link between drugs and success — the fatal connection that induces young athletes to celebrate their proudest achievements with a snort of cocaine.

Indeed, testing, drug education and counseling need to begin long before players reach the professional ranks and assume that drug use is one of the prerogatives of their exalted status. It's entirely appropriate, then, for the University of Kentucky to build on its already established drug program and for the University of Louisville to plan a greatly expanded effort. Other institutions should follow their lead.

Privacy issues remain and could become more troubling if other businesses try drug testing in a big way. But the fact remains that athletes, because of their often privileged position in our society and the adulation they receive, have an obligation to observe high standards of behavior and can reasonably be expected to forfeit some of their privacy. Mr. Rozelle is not asking much of citizens who have been given a great deal and whose lives may be saved by the measures he proposes.

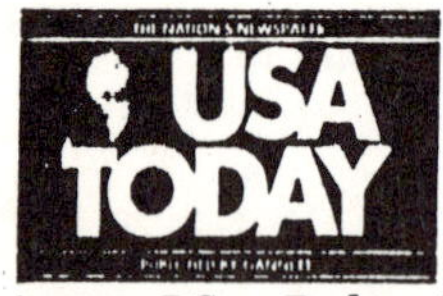

Washington, DC, July 15, 1986

Sometime tonight in Houston, Tim Raines will step on to the field to play for the National League in baseball's annual classic, the All-Star Game.

The Montreal Expos star is one of baseball's best players. He's hitting .331, he's scored 51 runs, he's stealing bases. But a few years ago, Tim Raines was a far different player. When he should have run, he stood still. When he should have thrown, he held the ball. In short, he was out of it.

The culprit? You guessed it — cocaine.

Raines was lucky. He got help; he kicked his habit. But as we all know now, other gifted athletes were not so lucky. Maryland basketball star Len Bias is dead; a grand jury is trying to figure out where he got his cocaine. Don Rogers of the Cleveland Browns planned to be on his honeymoon this week. Killer cocaine turned that wedding into a wake.

Left unchecked, drugs could destroy sports.

Recognizing that, National Football League Commissioner Pete Rozelle last week announced a plan to require random drug testing of players.

The NFL's plan is well thought out and has safeguards. An independent expert, a physician, oversees testing. Confirmed users get medical care. And penalties escalate: After three serious drug episodes, players are banned.

Although the NFL plan is a good start, it's not without flaws. It doesn't include an adequate test for steroids, the dangerous strength-builders players use. And it lacks a deterrent for amphetamine use.

But it's still a step forward. The NFL has recognized the danger and acted. Among pro leagues, only basketball has a thorough testing plan. Every league needs one.

Some people reject drug testing under any circumstances. They say it is an unwarranted invasion of privacy.

Yes, drug testing means some innocent athletes will give up part of their privacy. But if testing deters drug use — and surely it does — the gain will be worth it. Instead of blindly fighting tests, professional athletes should work with their leagues to devise fair tests that prevent abuses.

Athletes, as Rozelle said, are very vulnerable to drugs. They are young, rich, and have a lot of free time. And pushers aren't dumb. That's why they try to hook a kid like Len Bias: It makes it easier to hook other kids. Having a star use drugs helps sales — just like a shoe endorsement.

It's obvious pro sports has a serious drug problem. The roster of stars who have been damaged or destroyed grows ever longer. In basketball, Micheal Ray Richardson, John Lucas, and Quintin Dailey are suffering. In football, Mercury Morris and Tony Peters were victims. In baseball, Tim Raines was once in such sad shape he would only slide headfirst, to protect the cocaine in his back pocket.

It's time to get tough. Sports czars must send drug abusers this simple message: "You will be tested. If you're hooked, you will be treated. If you can't beat it, you're through."

Let's get the druggies out of sports. Let's kick the habit. Let's learn to say no to drugs — once and for all.

AKRON BEACON JOURNAL
Akron, OH, July 13, 1986

WHAT'S happening with professional athletes and drugs is part of a growing dilemma for American society.

Some facts are clear: Drugs kill. And cocaine, one of the most seductive, kills and destroys lives and families faster than many other drugs.

In the glittering world of professional sports, the graves of Don Rogers and Len Bias are mute testimony to the destruction of such drugs.

A story published today, on the front page of this section of the newspaper, sounds a chilling warning for anyone using or tempted to use cocaine. We hope it will be read in every household. In addition, the National Institute of Drug Abuse has just warned of an alarming increase in the number of cocaine-related deaths and injuries across the country.

How should society deal with this growing problem? How should the heads of pro sports or businesses or colleges deal with it?

Pete Rozelle, the commissioner of the National Football League, has now taken one approach, forced on him by frustration and the glamour of athletic stardom. Much to the dismay of the players' union, he proposed random drug tests of all players during the season. If a player tests positive three times, he will be banned permanently from the game — although he could apply for reinstatement after one year.

The plan is quite simple, and in the wake of recent events, many will readily agree with its approach. However, beneath the surface of Mr. Rozelle's plan lurk several difficult and complex issues for a free society. And although the focus is currently on athletes, the issue of drug testing is important to all of us. There are already estimates that 25 percent of American businesses now require some type of drug testing for employees or prospective employees. Other companies are having considerable success, not with testing, but with voluntary programs for employees who are drug abusers.

An important issue in all this is individual privacy. Some argue that it is raised as a shield for drug users. But that misses the point. Most Americans do not abuse drugs, and the tradition of presuming that someone is innocent should not be easily eroded. The concern is that random drug tests would violate the fundamental notions of due process, that a person should not be searched without reasonable cause.

Mr. Rozelle acknowledged that his plan would sacrifice a player's privacy. His justification was that professional athletes are role models in society and thus are required to meet a higher standard of behavior. It's true pro players are role models. But is that necessarily a good thing? Some believe society's adoration of young athletes is part of the problem and that it may be time to take them down from their pedestal.

Dealing with drug abuse is as complex as explaining why promising young people turn to cocaine. Where do drug tests fit in? It's not an easy question. Beyond concern about the precedent that would be set, many are skeptical about their reliability and wonder whether the tests are truly a deterrent against drug use.

Others have shown how cocaine disappears from the body more quickly than marijuana. That in turn suggests that mandatory testing of athletes or others in the workplace may identify those who use drugs less dangerous than cocaine while missing some high-risk people who have been using cocaine. Is that either sensible or fair?

Pro football is but one arena of human endeavor. The real dilemma for society as a whole is how best to handle the dangers of drug use and whether most Americans, including the majority who do not use or abuse drugs, are willing to give up individual privacy as a means of combatting this evil.

WORCESTER TELEGRAM.

Worcester, MA, July 12, 1986

There will be a lot of yelling and screaming about rights and player contracts, but Pete Rozelle's drug program for the National Football League should be adopted. Despite the obligatory protests about drug testing, most professional football players know in their hearts that the actions must be taken.

The National Basketball Association has already headed down the road of drug testing with penalties for major infractions. The post-Super Bowl flap about drug users among the New England Patriots made it inevitable that football had to clean house.

Rozelle's program is tough but fair. He has appointed Dr. Forest Tennant, a nationally recognized expert in the field of chemical dependency, as NFL drug adviser with authority to create and run a league-wide program. The program will begin with urine tests required of all draft-eligible college players, all players at the pre-season training camps and any player if there is presumed drug use. There will be two unannounced tests of each player during the season. To avoid any charges of bad or inaccurate tests, Rozelle has hired the top nationwide network of laboratories to collect and analyze specimens, each coded to conceal identities. The league office and the teams' administrative personnel will be left out of the drug testings as much as possible.

If and when a player is identified as using drugs — prohibited substances, as the program says — the first concern will be to put the user under medical care, confidentially when treatment can be on an out-patient basis. If a player has been treated and is again found using drugs, he may be removed from the playing field. In extreme cases, players may be banished permanently from the league.

Professional sports, from players to team owners, have to get a handle on drug use. Rozelle seems willing to be a lightning rod. He states frankly that he is taking these actions without negotiating with players or owners. But most people affiliated with professional sports agree that something has to be done and there is no diplomatic way to get agreement for testing procedures.

The presence of professional football players spaced out on drugs is a physical danger to everybody on the field — the player himself, his teammates and the opponents. The image of a drugged player does irreparable harm to the youth who idolize and imitate him. The highly paid athlete who spends grandly on illicit drugs corrupts the public good. Players on drugs cause a loss of faith that could put professional sports out of the picture in the future.

Pete Rozelle has taken the only route he could in launching a complex drug testing program for the National Football League. Let's hope it works.

Rockford Register Star

Rockford, IL, July 15, 1986

The National Football League will delay its random but mandatory rule that players must submit to drug tests twice a season, which is about as near as the NFL and its union are to agreeing on this critical move.

That's an opportunity lost, an opportunity in which both sides might have said, "Drugs are bad for business, bad for players, bad for sports, bad for anybody who uses them."

Maybe Commissioner Pete Rozelle did jump the gun in announcing his new drug policy. Maybe an arbitrator, whom both sides agreed should examine Rozelle's authority and whether it includes ordering drug tests, will find a contractual base for ruling "yes" or "no" on the new policy.

But surely, neither side wants to countenance drug abuse, which is a point that can be lost in the current standoff. Neither side can ignore the deaths of Len Bias or Don Rogers, a point that also could get lost.

The argument which tends to obscure professional football's genuine concern about heroin and cocaine and "pot" is the old one of territorial imperative — who controls the turf?

Considering that lives are at risk as well as athletic prowess, not to mention professional football's image, players and bosses might have sought a more collegial way to determine how drug tests fit into their mutual concerns.

But that didn't happen. And the arbitrator's ruling isn't expected until mid-September when the season already has commenced. Too bad. The intervening time lost is momentum lost in the fight against drugs in a critical sport.

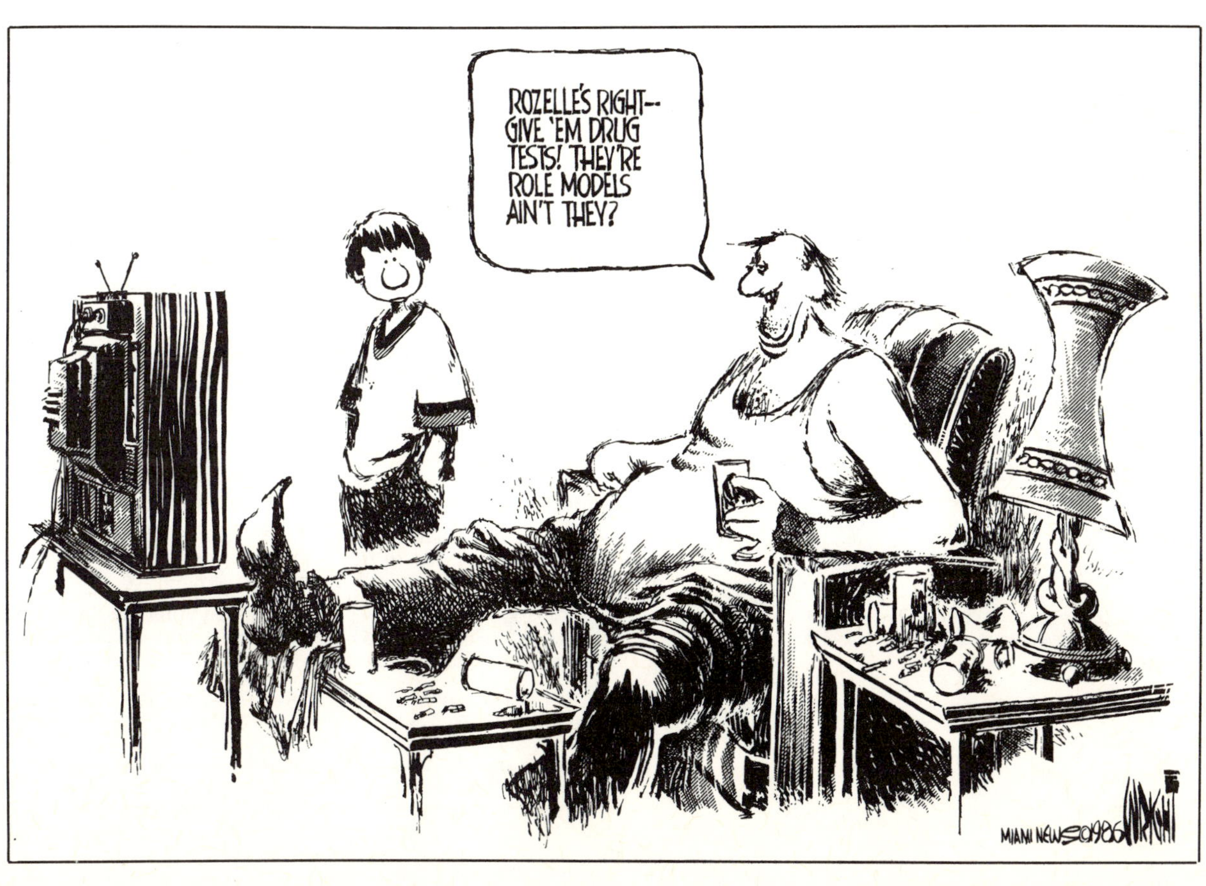

the Charleston Gazette

Charleston, WV, July 15, 1986

THE commissioner of the National Football League has announced a more rigorous program of drug-testing. Players are to be tested once at pre-season training camps and twice, unannounced, during the regular season.

Players who test positive three times will be barred from competition for a year, after which they may ask to play again. If a player's test shows a positive result, he will be subject to additional unannounced testing at any time.

Pete Rozelle's announcement hasn't been graciously received by Gene Upshaw, the players' elected union representative. Rozelle, says Upshaw, has defied the 1982 agreement that allows only the single testing of players at training camps. Terms of the agreement are binding and can't be changed during its life except by mutual consent.

An arbiter will settle the dispute within the next 60 days.

Players won't win friends among the American public fighting Rozelle. Technically they may be correct. If players are wise, however, they will yield and go along with Rozelle.

This society is sick, sick, sick, sick from drugs.

Upshaw asks on behalf of players: Why should athletes be singled out among a whole society to stop the sickness?

The answer is because athletes are privileged members of this society, role models if you please, upon whom millions of youngsters look reverently and talk of becoming.

Football heroes, if they don't have an obligation to compatriots who make possible their fine salaries, assuredly do have an obligation to the millions of youths who worship them. It's known as noblesse oblige. If players have never heard of the term — high time they did.

Nobody has to be a football player. It is a privileged position. As such it carries with it certain responsibilities. Drug taking in the United States has reached staggering heights. (Never mind that the federal government is handling the problem in the one way guaranteed to make it worse: boosting the profit motive instead of trying to decrease it or eliminate it. Still, other segments of society must combat the evil and hope Congress ultimately comes to its senses.)

Rozelle, for the game's sake, as he says, has the obligation — especially after last year's Super Bowl performance by a team with an unknown number of players regularly taking drugs — to try to oust them in professional football.

Don't football owners have a right to expect from an athlete a weekly effort uninfluenced and unimpaired by drugs? Of course, they do. So do fans.

Upshaw, if he wishes to serve the players, will quickly find a way to cooperate with Rozelle rather than buck him.

Seattle Post-Intelligencer

Seattle, WA, July 9, 1986

National Football League Commissioner Pete Rozelle has raised a new and persuasive reason for requiring mandatory drug tests of NFL players, in saying "Our concern is the health and welfare of the players — those taking drugs and those injured by those taking drugs."

It marked the first time Rozelle has made the argument that players risk potential injuries from fellow players who are under the influence of drugs, but it is a perfectly rational one. A football player whose judgment is impaired or who is immune to pain as a result of drugs can be lethal on the playing field.

Although the announced drug-testing program — which includes two random urinalysis tests each season and counseling and treatment for those in need of it — is in the best interests of the vast majority of NFL players as well as the future of the sport itself, the players' association will resist it. The association argues that the mandatory testing program violates a 1982 collective bargaining agreement, which expires next January and which presently is being renegotiated.

The NFL owners should stand fast in insisting that the Rozelle program be incorporated in a new agreement, if not adopted this season. Drug testing is a reasonable condition of employment in professional sports for a number of reasons, not the least of which is Rozelle's concern for athletes who must share the field with drugged-up or "wired" competitors.

The Birmingham News

Birmingham, AL, July 14, 1986

It is a shame that highly paid professional football players must be tested for drug abuse to protect the sport's reputation and credibility. But apparently a sufficient number of players are using illegal drugs to threaten the National Football League.

So Commissioner Pete Rozelle's announcement of an anti-drug program is welcome. Equally unwelcome is the players' union's response that it will fight such a program, because it is not defined in the union's player contract and, in fact, violates the contract.

The union, as well as individual members, should be as interested as Rozelle in the health of the league. The union should also be the first to recognize that drug abusers are highly vulnerable to other abuses. Given the high cost of cocaine and other drugs, it is not inconceivable that some drug abuser could engage in point-shaving to fix a game for the benefit of crooked gamblers. Such an incident could so damage the credibility of professional football that years would be required for its recovery.

Rozelle believes he's on solid ground in ordering random drug testing for each of the 28 teams in the league. He points to two provisions — one in the by-laws and another in the union contract — which give him "the obligation and the authority to protect the health and welfare of the players and to preserve the public confidence in the NFL."

In brief, Rozelle's plan mandates random testing during the 1986 season and will begin with training camp physicals this month. Any player requiring hospitalization for substance abuse will be removed from the team's roster for 30 days and will receive 50 percent of his pay for that period.

A second hospitalization would mean removal from the roster for another 30 days with no pay. If the player relapses and tests positive again, he will be permanently banned from playing in the NFL.

The commissioner has set aside $1 million to finance the program, which will be directed by a medical expert on drugs and drug abuse, so its implementation will cost the players nothing.

We suspect that only a small minority of NFL players are regular drug abusers and that many of the fine men on the rosters will applaud the commissioner's plan privately if not publicly. Drugs are a health problem among athletes as much as pulled muscles, fractured bones or flu. That being the case, why is it inappropriate to test for drugs but not inappropriate to test for diabetes, heart disease, hearing loss, etc.?

The Dallas Morning News
Dallas, TX, July 8, 1986

It is time for professional sports to declare war on drugs. And that is exactly what National Football League Commissioner Pete Rozelle has done in a sweeping package of proposals aimed at getting illicit narcotics out of pro football.

The league hopes to curtail widespread drug usage among players by conducting at least two random tests during the year. Players who test positive for drugs would be sent to rehabilitation centers and be fined two game checks — or about $25,000. A second offense would carry a fine of as much as $50,000. And those players found to be using drugs a third time would face a potential lifetime suspension from the NFL.

These are tough rules.

They are sure to be protested by the NFL Players Association. But tough measures are needed to deal with a problem that is said to be reaching epidemic proportions in professional athletics.

The deaths of basketball star Len Bias and Cleveland Browns Don Rogers due to cocaine intoxication serve as tragic testimony that athletic organizations on the collegiate and professional levels must get serious about drug abuse.

Rozelle has said that drug prevention and saving lives are not collective-bargaining issues with him. Officials of the National Basketball Association and Major League Baseball should be ready to take the same hard-line approach.

DESERET NEWS
Salt Lake City, UT, July 9-10, 1986

With its opposition to Commissioner Pete Rozelle's new drug testing program, the NFL players' union is in a no-win situation.

If the new plan had gone unchallenged, the union could have permitted a precedent for Rozelle's taking broader unilateral action affecting other terms of employment for the National Football League players.

But by resisting the program, the NFL Players Association is giving itself a black eye by making it look like the union doesn't take the drug abuse problem in professional football seriously enough.

It would be a big mistake, however, to shrug off that problem even though only a minority of all the players are involved.

The Rozelle program comes amid an NFL offseason that has been rocked by the acknowledgement following the Super Bowl that several New England Patriots had taken drugs, and by the recent death of Cleveland Browns defensive back Don Rogers from a cocaine-induced cardiac arrest.

Does anyone seriously believe that only those teams and players are involved in drug abuse? Of course not. That's why NFL coaches, executives, and even some players are hailing Rozelle's plan to make the NFL the first professional sports league to require random drug testing.

Under the new program, which takes effect immediately, there will be two random drug tests during the regular season. A test during training camp given under a 1982 program will continue. Players testing positively for drugs three times will be banned from the NFL for a minimum of one year.

By contrast, the National Basketball Association has a 1984 program under which players are tested only if there is "reasonable suspicion" of drug use. Then, an independent expert hired by the NBA can order tests. A player treated for drug abuse three times is banned from the league for a minimum of two years.

The National Hockey League has no drug testing program, though one is being worked on. In professional baseball, there is no drug testing program for major league players, though there is one for players in the minor leagues.

The cocaine-related deaths of Don Rogers and of Maryland college basketball star Len Bias, the top draft pick of the Boston Celtics, ought to prompt tougher and more widespread drug programs.

Decades of experience have shown that athletes are often drawn to drugs for relaxation, to improve their performance, or both. The drugs include steroids, alcohol, and amphetamines as well as narcotics.

Big league athletes often serve as role models for young Americans. Some of those youngsters seem bound to learn the folly of drug abuse from the deaths of Rogers and Bias. But the message won't be complete as long as some superstars get away with playing with drugs without suffering more than a comparatively small nick in their oversized salaries.

THE SACRAMENTO BEE
Sacramento, CA, July 14, 1986

After years of drug rumors, drug arrests and drug exposes, National Football League Commissioner Pete Rozelle has finally discovered that football has a problem. But is he, or anybody else in football, truly serious about it?

The drug problem in football is not just a matter of image, of coked-out football stars setting a bad example for the young, though that cannot be far from the mind of the NFL's master publicist. It's a question, first and foremost, Rozelle now says, of the health and safety of players. A 250-pound linebacker bulked up on anabolic steroids, wired on "speed" and oblivious to pain is a danger, not only to himself, but to every other player on the field. The lore of football is replete with stories of injuries inflicted by players full of chemical courage.

Unfortunately, Rozelle's plan falls short of coming to grips with the problem. Amphetamines aren't on the list of drugs that can lead to player punishments, and the tests won't even screen for steroids. Rozelle's program would punish a casual pot smoker, but not a ferocious safety who gets his playing macho and muscle from pills.

Equally disappointing has been the response of the NFL players' union. In filing a grievance against the program Rozelle wants to impose, the union is treating drug testing as a bargaining chip to be traded in exchange for something the players want from the owners.

An end to drug use in football is something the union itself should be demanding. It is the players who weekly risk being injured by opponents high on speed; it is the players who've been victimized by subtle, and sometimes direct, pressure from their teams to use dangerous steroids, stimulants and painkillers to gain a competitive edge. At least one players' agent has threatened to sue league owners on behalf of his clients if action isn't taken to stop drug use for competitive advantage. Why isn't the union as aggressive in protecting its members?

The best answer to football's drug problem is not random testing imposed by the commissioner from on high, but a joint commitment by players and owners to put player health and safety ahead of winning. The union could end the current impasse by volunteering to participate in a mandatory program of post-game testing, as in track and field, designed to screen for use of steroids, cocaine, amphetamines and other substances that make football more dangerous. In return, owners should agree to drug penalties, not just on athletes, but on teams that condone or encourage drug use. If drugs are a threat to the integrity of football, as they surely are, it's time for everybody to get serious.

Index